50% OFF
Online Medical-Surgical Nurse Prep Course!

By Mometrix

Dear Customer,

We consider it an honor and a privilege that you chose our Medical-Surgical Nurse Practice Questions. As a way of showing our appreciation and to help us better serve you, we are offering **50% off our online Med-Surg Prep Course**. Many online prep courses are needlessly expensive and don't deliver enough value. With our course, you get access to the best Medical-Surgical Nurse prep material, and **you only pay half price**.

We have structured our online course to perfectly complement your printed practice questions. The Med-Surg Prep Course contains **in-depth lessons** that cover all the most important topics, **90+ video reviews** that explain difficult concepts, over **900+ online practice questions** to ensure you feel prepared, and more than **350+ digital flashcards**, so you can study while you're on the go.

Online Medical-Surgical Nurse Prep Course

Topics Covered:

- Assessment and Diagnosis
  - o Physical Assessment
  - o Laboratory Testing
- Planning, Implementation, and Evaluation
  - o Patient Education
  - o Dialysis
- Professional Role
  - o Therapeutic Communication
  - o Nursing Ethics
- And More!

Course Features:

- Medical-Surgical Nurse Study Guide
  - o Get content that complements our best-selling study guide.
- Full-Length Practice Tests and Flashcards
  - o With over 900 online practice questions and 350+ digital flashcards, you can test yourself again and again.
- Mobile Friendly
  - o If you need to study on the go, the course is easily accessible from your mobile device.

To receive this discount, visit us at mometrix.com/university/medsurg or simply scan this QR code with your smartphone. At the checkout page, enter the discount code: **msn50off**

If you have any questions or concerns, please contact us at support@mometrix.com.

Sincerely,

TEST PREPARATION

FREE Study Skills Videos/DVD Offer

Dear Customer,

Thank you for your purchase from Mometrix! We consider it an honor and a privilege that you have purchased our product and we want to ensure your satisfaction.

As part of our ongoing effort to meet the needs of test takers, we have developed a set of Study Skills Videos that we would like to give you for <u>FREE</u>. These videos cover our *best practices* for getting ready for your exam, from how to use our study materials to how to best prepare for the day of the test.

All that we ask is that you email us with feedback that would describe your experience so far with our product. Good, bad, or indifferent, we want to know what you think!

To get your FREE Study Skills Videos, you can use the **QR code** below, or send us an **email** at studyvideos@mometrix.com with *FREE VIDEOS* in the subject line and the following information in the body of the email:

- The name of the product you purchased.
- Your product rating on a scale of 1-5, with 5 being the highest rating.
- Your feedback. It can be long, short, or anything in between. We just want to know your impressions and experience so far with our product. (Good feedback might include how our study material met your needs and ways we might be able to make it even better. You could highlight features that you found helpful or features that you think we should add.)

If you have any questions or concerns, please don't hesitate to contact me directly.

Thanks again!

Sincerely,

Jay Willis
Vice President
jay.willis@mometrix.com
1-800-673-8175

Medical-Surgical Nurse Exam

SECRETS

Study Guide
Your Key to Exam Success

Written and edited by the Mometrix Nursing Certification Test Team

Printed in the United States of America

This paper meets the requirements of ANSI/NISO Z39.48-1992 (Permanence of Paper).

Mometrix offers volume discount pricing to institutions. For more information or a price quote, please contact our sales department at sales@mometrix.com or 888-248-1219.

Mometrix Media LLC is not affiliated with or endorsed by any official testing organization. All organizational and test names are trademarks of their respective owners.

Paperback
ISBN 13: 978-1-61072-013-7
ISBN 10: 1-61072-013-X

Ebook
ISBN 13: 978-1-62120-312-4
ISBN 10: 1-62120-312-3

DEAR FUTURE EXAM SUCCESS STORY

First of all, **THANK YOU** for purchasing Mometrix study materials!

Second, congratulations! You are one of the few determined test-takers who are committed to doing whatever it takes to excel on your exam. **You have come to the right place.** We developed these study materials with one goal in mind: to deliver you the information you need in a format that's concise and easy to use.

In addition to optimizing your guide for the content of the test, we've outlined our recommended steps for breaking down the preparation process into small, attainable goals so you can make sure you stay on track.

We've also analyzed the entire test-taking process, identifying the most common pitfalls and showing how you can overcome them and be ready for any curveball the test throws you.

Standardized testing is one of the biggest obstacles on your road to success, which only increases the importance of doing well in the high-pressure, high-stakes environment of test day. Your results on this test could have a significant impact on your future, and this guide provides the information and practical advice to help you achieve your full potential on test day.

Your success is our success

We would love to hear from you! If you would like to share the story of your exam success or if you have any questions or comments in regard to our products, please contact us at **800-673-8175** or **support@mometrix.com**.

Thanks again for your business and we wish you continued success!

Sincerely,
The Mometrix Test Preparation Team

> **Need more help? Check out our flashcards at:**
> **http://mometrixflashcards.com/MedicalSurgical**

TABLE OF CONTENTS

Introduction

Thank you for purchasing this resource! You have made the choice to prepare yourself for a test that could have a huge impact on your future, and this guide is designed to help you be fully ready for test day. Obviously, it's important to have a solid understanding of the test material, but you also need to be prepared for the unique environment and stressors of the test, so that you can perform to the best of your abilities.

For this purpose, the first section that appears in this guide is the **Secret Keys**. We've devoted countless hours to meticulously researching what works and what doesn't, and we've boiled down our findings to the five most impactful steps you can take to improve your performance on the test. We start at the beginning with study planning and move through the preparation process, all the way to the testing strategies that will help you get the most out of what you know when you're finally sitting in front of the test.

We recommend that you start preparing for your test as far in advance as possible. However, if you've bought this guide as a last-minute study resource and only have a few days before your test, we recommend that you skip over the first two Secret Keys since they address a long-term study plan.

If you struggle with **test anxiety**, we strongly encourage you to check out our recommendations for how you can overcome it. Test anxiety is a formidable foe, but it can be beaten, and we want to make sure you have the tools you need to defeat it.

1

Secret Key #1 – Plan Big, Study Small

There's a lot riding on your performance. If you want to ace this test, you're going to need to keep your skills sharp and the material fresh in your mind. You need a plan that lets you review everything you need to know while still fitting in your schedule. We'll break this strategy down into three categories.

Information Organization

Start with the information you already have: the official test outline. From this, you can make a complete list of all the concepts you need to cover before the test. Organize these concepts into groups that can be studied together, and create a list of any related vocabulary you need to learn so you can brush up on any difficult terms. You'll want to keep this vocabulary list handy once you actually start studying since you may need to add to it along the way.

Time Management

Once you have your set of study concepts, decide how to spread them out over the time you have left before the test. Break your study plan into small, clear goals so you have a manageable task for each day and know exactly what you're doing. Then just focus on one small step at a time. When you manage your time this way, you don't need to spend hours at a time studying. Studying a small block of content for a short period each day helps you retain information better and avoid stressing over how much you have left to do. You can relax knowing that you have a plan to cover everything in time. In order for this strategy to be effective though, you have to start studying early and stick to your schedule. Avoid the exhaustion and futility that comes from last-minute cramming!

Study Environment

The environment you study in has a big impact on your learning. Studying in a coffee shop, while probably more enjoyable, is not likely to be as fruitful as studying in a quiet room. It's important to keep distractions to a minimum. You're only planning to study for a short block of time, so make the most of it. Don't pause to check your phone or get up to find a snack. It's also important to **avoid multitasking**. Research has consistently shown that multitasking will make your studying dramatically less effective. Your study area should also be comfortable and well-lit so you don't have the distraction of straining your eyes or sitting on an uncomfortable chair.

The time of day you study is also important. You want to be rested and alert. Don't wait until just before bedtime. Study when you'll be most likely to comprehend and remember. Even better, if you know what time of day your test will be, set that time aside for study. That way your brain will be used to working on that subject at that specific time and you'll have a better chance of recalling information.

Finally, it can be helpful to team up with others who are studying for the same test. Your actual studying should be done in as isolated an environment as possible, but the work of organizing the information and setting up the study plan can be divided up. In between study sessions, you can discuss with your teammates the concepts that you're all studying and quiz each other on the details. Just be sure that your teammates are as serious about the test as you are. If you find that your study time is being replaced with social time, you might need to find a new team.

Secret Key #2 – Make Your Studying Count

You're devoting a lot of time and effort to preparing for this test, so you want to be absolutely certain it will pay off. This means doing more than just reading the content and hoping you can remember it on test day. It's important to make every minute of study count. There are two main areas you can focus on to make your studying count.

Retention

It doesn't matter how much time you study if you can't remember the material. You need to make sure you are retaining the concepts. To check your retention of the information you're learning, try recalling it at later times with minimal prompting. Try carrying around flashcards and glance at one or two from time to time or ask a friend who's also studying for the test to quiz you.

To enhance your retention, look for ways to put the information into practice so that you can apply it rather than simply recalling it. If you're using the information in practical ways, it will be much easier to remember. Similarly, it helps to solidify a concept in your mind if you're not only reading it to yourself but also explaining it to someone else. Ask a friend to let you teach them about a concept you're a little shaky on (or speak aloud to an imaginary audience if necessary). As you try to summarize, define, give examples, and answer your friend's questions, you'll understand the concepts better and they will stay with you longer. Finally, step back for a big picture view and ask yourself how each piece of information fits with the whole subject. When you link the different concepts together and see them working together as a whole, it's easier to remember the individual components.

Finally, practice showing your work on any multi-step problems, even if you're just studying. Writing out each step you take to solve a problem will help solidify the process in your mind, and you'll be more likely to remember it during the test.

Modality

Modality simply refers to the means or method by which you study. Choosing a study modality that fits your own individual learning style is crucial. No two people learn best in exactly the same way, so it's important to know your strengths and use them to your advantage.

For example, if you learn best by visualization, focus on visualizing a concept in your mind and draw an image or a diagram. Try color-coding your notes, illustrating them, or creating symbols that will trigger your mind to recall a learned concept. If you learn best by hearing or discussing information, find a study partner who learns the same way or read aloud to yourself. Think about how to put the information in your own words. Imagine that you are giving a lecture on the topic and record yourself so you can listen to it later.

For any learning style, flashcards can be helpful. Organize the information so you can take advantage of spare moments to review. Underline key words or phrases. Use different colors for different categories. Mnemonic devices (such as creating a short list in which every item starts with the same letter) can also help with retention. Find what works best for you and use it to store the information in your mind most effectively and easily.

Secret Key #3 – Practice the Right Way

Your success on test day depends not only on how many hours you put into preparing, but also on whether you prepared the right way. It's good to check along the way to see if your studying is paying off. One of the most effective ways to do this is by taking practice tests to evaluate your progress. Practice tests are useful because they show exactly where you need to improve. Every time you take a practice test, pay special attention to these three groups of questions:

- The questions you got wrong
- The questions you had to guess on, even if you guessed right
- The questions you found difficult or slow to work through

This will show you exactly what your weak areas are, and where you need to devote more study time. Ask yourself why each of these questions gave you trouble. Was it because you didn't understand the material? Was it because you didn't remember the vocabulary? Do you need more repetitions on this type of question to build speed and confidence? Dig into those questions and figure out how you can strengthen your weak areas as you go back to review the material.

 Additionally, many practice tests have a section explaining the answer choices. It can be tempting to read the explanation and think that you now have a good understanding of the concept. However, an explanation likely only covers part of the question's broader context. Even if the explanation makes perfect sense, **go back and investigate** every concept related to the question until you're positive you have a thorough understanding.

As you go along, keep in mind that the practice test is just that: practice. Memorizing these questions and answers will not be very helpful on the actual test because it is unlikely to have any of the same exact questions. If you only know the right answers to the sample questions, you won't be prepared for the real thing. **Study the concepts** until you understand them fully, and then you'll be able to answer any question that shows up on the test.

It's important to wait on the practice tests until you're ready. If you take a test on your first day of study, you may be overwhelmed by the amount of material covered and how much you need to learn. Work up to it gradually.

On test day, you'll need to be prepared for answering questions, managing your time, and using the test-taking strategies you've learned. It's a lot to balance, like a mental marathon that will have a big impact on your future. Like training for a marathon, you'll need to start slowly and work your way up. When test day arrives, you'll be ready.

Start with the strategies you've read in the first two Secret Keys—plan your course and study in the way that works best for you. If you have time, consider using multiple study resources to get different approaches to the same concepts. It can be helpful to see difficult concepts from more than one angle. Then find a good source for practice tests. Many times, the test website will suggest potential study resources or provide sample tests.

Practice Test Strategy

If you're able to find at least three practice tests, we recommend this strategy:

UNTIMED AND OPEN-BOOK PRACTICE

Take the first test with no time constraints and with your notes and study guide handy. Take your time and focus on applying the strategies you've learned.

TIMED AND OPEN-BOOK PRACTICE

Take the second practice test open-book as well, but set a timer and practice pacing yourself to finish in time.

TIMED AND CLOSED-BOOK PRACTICE

Take any other practice tests as if it were test day. Set a timer and put away your study materials. Sit at a table or desk in a quiet room, imagine yourself at the testing center, and answer questions as quickly and accurately as possible.

Keep repeating timed and closed-book tests on a regular basis until you run out of practice tests or it's time for the actual test. Your mind will be ready for the schedule and stress of test day, and you'll be able to focus on recalling the material you've learned.

Secret Key #4 – Pace Yourself

Once you're fully prepared for the material on the test, your biggest challenge on test day will be managing your time. Just knowing that the clock is ticking can make you panic even if you have plenty of time left. Work on pacing yourself so you can build confidence against the time constraints of the exam. Pacing is a difficult skill to master, especially in a high-pressure environment, so **practice is vital**.

Set time expectations for your pace based on how much time is available. For example, if a section has 60 questions and the time limit is 30 minutes, you know you have to average 30 seconds or less per question in order to answer them all. Although 30 seconds is the hard limit, set 25 seconds per question as your goal, so you reserve extra time to spend on harder questions. When you budget extra time for the harder questions, you no longer have any reason to stress when those questions take longer to answer.

Don't let this time expectation distract you from working through the test at a calm, steady pace, but keep it in mind so you don't spend too much time on any one question. Recognize that taking extra time on one question you don't understand may keep you from answering two that you do understand later in the test. If your time limit for a question is up and you're still not sure of the answer, mark it and move on, and come back to it later if the time and the test format allow. If the testing format doesn't allow you to return to earlier questions, just make an educated guess; then put it out of your mind and move on.

On the easier questions, be careful not to rush. It may seem wise to hurry through them so you have more time for the challenging ones, but it's not worth missing one if you know the concept and just didn't take the time to read the question fully. Work efficiently but make sure you understand the question and have looked at all of the answer choices, since more than one may seem right at first.

Even if you're paying attention to the time, you may find yourself a little behind at some point. You should speed up to get back on track, but do so wisely. Don't panic; just take a few seconds less on each question until you're caught up. Don't guess without thinking, but do look through the answer choices and eliminate any you know are wrong. If you can get down to two choices, it is often worthwhile to guess from those. Once you've chosen an answer, move on and don't dwell on any that you skipped or had to hurry through. If a question was taking too long, chances are it was one of the harder ones, so you weren't as likely to get it right anyway.

On the other hand, if you find yourself getting ahead of schedule, it may be beneficial to slow down a little. The more quickly you work, the more likely you are to make a careless mistake that will affect your score. You've budgeted time for each question, so don't be afraid to spend that time. Practice an efficient but careful pace to get the most out of the time you have.

Secret Key #5 – Have a Plan for Guessing

When you're taking the test, you may find yourself stuck on a question. Some of the answer choices seem better than others, but you don't see the one answer choice that is obviously correct. What do you do?

The scenario described above is very common, yet most test takers have not effectively prepared for it. Developing and practicing a plan for guessing may be one of the single most effective uses of your time as you get ready for the exam.

In developing your plan for guessing, there are three questions to address:

- When should you start the guessing process?
- How should you narrow down the choices?
- Which answer should you choose?

When to Start the Guessing Process

Unless your plan for guessing is to select C every time (which, despite its merits, is not what we recommend), you need to leave yourself enough time to apply your answer elimination strategies. Since you have a limited amount of time for each question, that means that if you're going to give yourself the best shot at guessing correctly, you have to decide quickly whether or not you will guess.

Of course, the best-case scenario is that you don't have to guess at all, so first, see if you can answer the question based on your knowledge of the subject and basic reasoning skills. Focus on the key words in the question and try to jog your memory of related topics. Give yourself a chance to bring the knowledge to mind, but once you realize that you don't have (or you can't access) the knowledge you need to answer the question, it's time to start the guessing process.

It's almost always better to start the guessing process too early than too late. It only takes a few seconds to remember something and answer the question from knowledge. Carefully eliminating wrong answer choices takes longer. Plus, going through the process of eliminating answer choices can actually help jog your memory.

Summary: Start the guessing process as soon as you decide that you can't answer the question based on your knowledge.

How to Narrow Down the Choices

The next chapter in this book (**Test-Taking Strategies**) includes a wide range of strategies for how to approach questions and how to look for answer choices to eliminate. You will definitely want to read those carefully, practice them, and figure out which ones work best for you. Here though, we're going to address a mindset rather than a particular strategy.

Your odds of guessing an answer correctly depend on how many options you are choosing from.

Number of options left	5	4	3	2	1
Odds of guessing correctly	20%	25%	33%	50%	100%

You can see from this chart just how valuable it is to be able to eliminate incorrect answers and make an educated guess, but there are two things that many test takers do that cause them to miss out on the benefits of guessing:

- Accidentally eliminating the correct answer
- Selecting an answer based on an impression

We'll look at the first one here, and the second one in the next section.

To avoid accidentally eliminating the correct answer, we recommend a thought exercise called **the $5 challenge**. In this challenge, you only eliminate an answer choice from contention if you are willing to bet $5 on it being wrong. Why $5? Five dollars is a small but not insignificant amount of money. It's an amount you could afford to lose but wouldn't want to throw away. And while losing $5 once might not hurt too much, doing

it twenty times will set you back $100. In the same way, each small decision you make—eliminating a choice here, guessing on a question there—won't by itself impact your score very much, but when you put them all together, they can make a big difference. By holding each answer choice elimination decision to a higher standard, you can reduce the risk of accidentally eliminating the correct answer.

The $5 challenge can also be applied in a positive sense: If you are willing to bet $5 that an answer choice *is* correct, go ahead and mark it as correct.

Summary: Only eliminate an answer choice if you are willing to bet $5 that it is wrong.

Which Answer to Choose

You're taking the test. You've run into a hard question and decided you'll have to guess. You've eliminated all the answer choices you're willing to bet $5 on. Now you have to pick an answer. Why do we even need to talk about this? Why can't you just pick whichever one you feel like when the time comes?

The answer to these questions is that if you don't come into the test with a plan, you'll rely on your impression to select an answer choice, and if you do that, you risk falling into a trap. The test writers know that everyone who takes their test will be guessing on some of the questions, so they intentionally write wrong answer choices to seem plausible. You still have to pick an answer though, and if the wrong answer choices are designed to look right, how can you ever be sure that you're not falling for their trap? The best solution we've found to this dilemma is to take the decision out of your hands entirely. Here is the process we recommend:

Once you've eliminated any choices that you are confident (willing to bet $5) are wrong, select the first remaining choice as your answer.

Whether you choose to select the first remaining choice, the second, or the last, the important thing is that you use some preselected standard. Using this approach guarantees that you will not be enticed into selecting an answer choice that looks right, because you are not basing your decision on how the answer choices look.

This is not meant to make you question your knowledge. Instead, it is to help you recognize the difference between your knowledge and your impressions. There's a huge difference between thinking an answer is right because of what you know, and thinking an answer is right because it looks or sounds like it should be right.

Summary: To ensure that your selection is appropriately random, make a predetermined selection from among all answer choices you have not eliminated.

Test-Taking Strategies

This section contains a list of test-taking strategies that you may find helpful as you work through the test. By taking what you know and applying logical thought, you can maximize your chances of answering any question correctly!

It is very important to realize that every question is different and every person is different: no single strategy will work on every question, and no single strategy will work for every person. That's why we've included all of them here, so you can try them out and determine which ones work best for different types of questions and which ones work best for you.

Question Strategies

☑ READ CAREFULLY

Read the question and the answer choices carefully. Don't miss the question because you misread the terms. You have plenty of time to read each question thoroughly and make sure you understand what is being asked. Yet a happy medium must be attained, so don't waste too much time. You must read carefully and efficiently.

☑ CONTEXTUAL CLUES

Look for contextual clues. If the question includes a word you are not familiar with, look at the immediate context for some indication of what the word might mean. Contextual clues can often give you all the information you need to decipher the meaning of an unfamiliar word. Even if you can't determine the meaning, you may be able to narrow down the possibilities enough to make a solid guess at the answer to the question.

☑ PREFIXES

If you're having trouble with a word in the question or answer choices, try dissecting it. Take advantage of every clue that the word might include. Prefixes can be a huge help. Usually, they allow you to determine a basic meaning. *Pre-* means before, *post-* means after, *pro-* is positive, *de-* is negative. From prefixes, you can get an idea of the general meaning of the word and try to put it into context.

☑ HEDGE WORDS

Watch out for critical hedge words, such as *likely, may, can, sometimes, often, almost, mostly, usually, generally, rarely,* and *sometimes.* Question writers insert these hedge phrases to cover every possibility. Often an answer choice will be wrong simply because it leaves no room for exception. Be on guard for answer choices that have definitive words such as *exactly* and *always.*

☑ SWITCHBACK WORDS

Stay alert for *switchbacks.* These are the words and phrases frequently used to alert you to shifts in thought. The most common switchback words are *but, although,* and *however.* Others include *nevertheless, on the other hand, even though, while, in spite of, despite,* and *regardless of.* Switchback words are important to catch because they can change the direction of the question or an answer choice.

☑ FACE VALUE

When in doubt, use common sense. Accept the situation in the problem at face value. Don't read too much into it. These problems will not require you to make wild assumptions. If you have to go beyond creativity and warp time or space in order to have an answer choice fit the question, then you should move on and consider the other answer choices. These are normal problems rooted in reality. The applicable relationship or explanation may not be readily apparent, but it is there for you to figure out. Use your common sense to interpret anything that isn't clear.

Answer Choice Strategies

⊘ ANSWER SELECTION

The most thorough way to pick an answer choice is to identify and eliminate wrong answers until only one is left, then confirm it is the correct answer. Sometimes an answer choice may immediately seem right, but be careful. The test writers will usually put more than one reasonable answer choice on each question, so take a second to read all of them and make sure that the other choices are not equally obvious. As long as you have time left, it is better to read every answer choice than to pick the first one that looks right without checking the others.

⊘ ANSWER CHOICE FAMILIES

An answer choice family consists of two (in rare cases, three) answer choices that are very similar in construction and cannot all be true at the same time. If you see two answer choices that are direct opposites or parallels, one of them is usually the correct answer. For instance, if one answer choice says that quantity x increases and another either says that quantity x decreases (opposite) or says that quantity y increases (parallel), then those answer choices would fall into the same family. An answer choice that doesn't match the construction of the answer choice family is more likely to be incorrect. Most questions will not have answer choice families, but when they do appear, you should be prepared to recognize them.

⊘ ELIMINATE ANSWERS

Eliminate answer choices as soon as you realize they are wrong, but make sure you consider all possibilities. If you are eliminating answer choices and realize that the last one you are left with is also wrong, don't panic. Start over and consider each choice again. There may be something you missed the first time that you will realize on the second pass.

⊘ AVOID FACT TRAPS

Don't be distracted by an answer choice that is factually true but doesn't answer the question. You are looking for the choice that answers the question. Stay focused on what the question is asking for so you don't accidentally pick an answer that is true but incorrect. Always go back to the question and make sure the answer choice you've selected actually answers the question and is not merely a true statement.

⊘ EXTREME STATEMENTS

In general, you should avoid answers that put forth extreme actions as standard practice or proclaim controversial ideas as established fact. An answer choice that states the "process should be used in certain situations, if..." is much more likely to be correct than one that states the "process should be discontinued completely." The first is a calm rational statement and doesn't even make a definitive, uncompromising stance, using a hedge word *if* to provide wiggle room, whereas the second choice is far more extreme.

⊘ BENCHMARK

As you read through the answer choices and you come across one that seems to answer the question well, mentally select that answer choice. This is not your final answer, but it's the one that will help you evaluate the other answer choices. The one that you selected is your benchmark or standard for judging each of the other answer choices. Every other answer choice must be compared to your benchmark. That choice is correct until proven otherwise by another answer choice beating it. If you find a better answer, then that one becomes your new benchmark. Once you've decided that no other choice answers the question as well as your benchmark, you have your final answer.

⊘ Predict the Answer

Before you even start looking at the answer choices, it is often best to try to predict the answer. When you come up with the answer on your own, it is easier to avoid distractions and traps because you will know exactly what to look for. The right answer choice is unlikely to be word-for-word what you came up with, but it should be a close match. Even if you are confident that you have the right answer, you should still take the time to read each option before moving on.

General Strategies

⊘ Tough Questions

If you are stumped on a problem or it appears too hard or too difficult, don't waste time. Move on! Remember though, if you can quickly check for obviously incorrect answer choices, your chances of guessing correctly are greatly improved. Before you completely give up, at least try to knock out a couple of possible answers. Eliminate what you can and then guess at the remaining answer choices before moving on.

⊘ Check Your Work

Since you will probably not know every term listed and the answer to every question, it is important that you get credit for the ones that you do know. Don't miss any questions through careless mistakes. If at all possible, try to take a second to look back over your answer selection and make sure you've selected the correct answer choice and haven't made a costly careless mistake (such as marking an answer choice that you didn't mean to mark). This quick double check should more than pay for itself in caught mistakes for the time it costs.

⊘ Pace Yourself

It's easy to be overwhelmed when you're looking at a page full of questions; your mind is confused and full of random thoughts, and the clock is ticking down faster than you would like. Calm down and maintain the pace that you have set for yourself. Especially as you get down to the last few minutes of the test, don't let the small numbers on the clock make you panic. As long as you are on track by monitoring your pace, you are guaranteed to have time for each question.

⊘ Don't Rush

It is very easy to make errors when you are in a hurry. Maintaining a fast pace in answering questions is pointless if it makes you miss questions that you would have gotten right otherwise. Test writers like to include distracting information and wrong answers that seem right. Taking a little extra time to avoid careless mistakes can make all the difference in your test score. Find a pace that allows you to be confident in the answers that you select.

⊘ Keep Moving

Panicking will not help you pass the test, so do your best to stay calm and keep moving. Taking deep breaths and going through the answer elimination steps you practiced can help to break through a stress barrier and keep your pace.

Final Notes

The combination of a solid foundation of content knowledge and the confidence that comes from practicing your plan for applying that knowledge is the key to maximizing your performance on test day. As your foundation of content knowledge is built up and strengthened, you'll find that the strategies included in this chapter become more and more effective in helping you quickly sift through the distractions and traps of the test to isolate the correct answer.

Now that you're preparing to move forward into the test content chapters of this book, be sure to keep your goal in mind. As you read, think about how you will be able to apply this information on the test. If you've already seen sample questions for the test and you have an idea of the question format and style, try to come up with questions of your own that you can answer based on what you're reading. This will give you valuable practice applying your knowledge in the same ways you can expect to on test day.

Good luck and good studying!

Assessment and Diagnosis

Nursing Process

PURPOSE OF NURSING ASSESSMENT

Nursing assessment evaluates patient data to help in diagnosis and treatment. The nurse assesses baseline health and medical history to be sure the patient will be safe. The nurse also determines what limitations the patient may have in terms of understanding or cooperation. Nursing assessment is an ongoing process, which includes baseline information, information on the patient's response and recovery to the intervention, and continued efforts to maintain the patient's health. The nurse can collaborate with other team members to help in this assessment.

PURPOSE OF NURSING DIAGNOSIS AND PLANNING

Nursing diagnosis is directed at patient comfort and outcome. With a diagnosis, nurses establish nursing interventions that are needed for the patient to be safe and comfortable. The nurse uses the diagnosis to direct therapies and to anticipate potentially needed interventions.

Planning allows the nurse to outline the methods needed to achieve patient goals. This accounts for alternative therapies that may be needed, setting priorities, satisfactory outcomes to be achieved, and expectations for discharge. The nurse needs to document the plan. The plan outlines nursing responsibilities, possible interventions, and expected outcomes.

IMPLEMENTATION OF NURSING PLAN

Implementing the nursing plan requires a measure of fluidity. The original plan is based on initial data. As new data is accumulated, however, the original plan may be modified. There is a need to incorporate individual needs of the patient as the plan proceeds. Different interventions may be called for depending on individual responses or limitations. The nurse needs to continually monitor the patient's response and status to be able to offer appropriate nursing interventions. Documentation is essential at every step of the way. The information can be useful in further treatment of the individual. It can also be used to assess the process so that improvements or adjustments can be made. The documentation may also be used for research purposes to further the knowledge of nursing practice. The record may become necessary for legal purposes as well.

EVALUATION PROCESS

In order to provide the best care for the patient, the nurse must **evaluate** the process in effect. This entails reviewing procedures and interventions in relation to standards of care, quality of care, and patient outcomes. Critical evaluation of the nursing process can lead to changes that may improve the quality of care for patients and/or identify personnel issues that need to be addressed. Modifying care plans is important to maintaining effective patient care. Deficiencies may be noted and can, therefore, be addressed. This underscores the importance of adequate documentation. In order to evaluate the process, the nurse must have access to the documentation to assess the present process. This evaluation may lead to changes that improve the quality of care in the nursing unit.

15

Health History Collection

COMPONENTS OF HEALTH HISTORY

There are several different components that must be included in a nursing **health history**:

- The **biographic element** of the nursing health history includes the patient's name, age, physical address, sex, marital status, occupational status, religious preference, healthcare financing, and regular physician.
- The **chief complaint** is the next aspect of the history and involves the reason the patient is seeking care.
- Following this, the **history of the present illness** details the current health problem, including date of onset, description of symptoms, and any aggravating factors.
- **Past medical history** entails asking about the patient's usual health status, past medical or surgical problems, immunization status, current medications, allergies (including medication allergies), and family history.
- A detailed **family history** is important as it may reveal risk factors for certain medical conditions such as heart disease, diabetes, arthritis, hypertension, or mental disorders.
- The **review of systems** is used to obtain a full, systematic report by the patient on subjective symptoms. For example, in inquiring about the cardiovascular system, the nurse notes positive or negative answers regarding chest pain and other symptoms or problems that are pertinent to heart function and circulation.
- The patient's **lifestyle** is another important component of the nursing health history and includes habits, diet, sleep, hobbies, and the patient's ability to perform the activities of daily living.
- A **social history** is the component of the nursing health history that details family relationships, ethnicity, educational level, economic status, and the condition of the patient's home and environment.
- The nursing health history also includes the patient's **psychological status** and the patient's **usual means of obtaining healthcare.**

OBTAINING A HEALTH HISTORY

The health history assessment and review of systems help to identify nursing care needs:

- First, check the patient's chart for information gathered by other health professionals and note any areas that need clarification prior to the patient interview.
- Use the written tool provided by the facility to record the history, customizing it to the patient.
- Record any changes in this information during the patient's hospital stay.
- Plan the time of the interview with the patient when there are not critical care needs that must be met first.
- Take time to alleviate patient's anxiety and establish rapport and trust.
- Approach the patient with an attitude of respect and sincere caring.
- Listen to the patient and use effective therapeutic communication skills during the interview.
- Review all areas of the health history with the patient and then ask for any other information that may be important. The family may be able to fill in missing information if the patient is unable to do so.

Physical Assessment

NORMAL STRUCTURE AND FUNCTION ACROSS THE LIFESPAN

It is vital to understand the normal structure and function of anatomy and physiology across the lifespan, from infants to geriatric patients, when performing a nursing assessment. For example, normal pulse rates and blood pressure ranges for a newborn are vastly different from those for an adult. A healthy newborn will have a resting heartbeat of 70-190 beats per minute, but this standard changes to 60-100 beats per minute in adults. It is important to recognize the normal differences in skin color and hue, and the development of dentition and muscle function across the lifespan. There are standard developmental stages from infancy to adolescence, as well as documented normal changes in geriatric physiology.

ORGANS THAT MAINTAIN HOMEOSTASIS IN THE BODY

The organs of homeostatic function include the following:

- **Lungs**: The lungs help maintain acid-base balance by releasing CO_2. They also remove water via expired air.
- **Kidneys**: The kidneys maintain fluid balance in the body by filtering the blood and releasing fluid as needed. Electrolyte levels are maintained in the same way. Wastes and toxins are removed from the blood and body in the urine. The pH of the blood is maintained via the retention of hydrogen ions.
- **Heart**: The heart must pump blood with sufficient force to properly perfuse all organs and to push enough blood through the kidneys for filtering.
- **Adrenal glands**: Aldosterone and cortisol are produced by the adrenals to cause the kidneys to retain sodium and fluids.
- **Pituitary**: The pituitary stores and releases antidiuretic hormone (ADH) from the hypothalamus to direct the kidneys to retain fluids to maintain cellular osmotic pressure.
- **Parathyroid**: Parathyroid hormone maintains calcium and phosphate levels by causing calcium absorption by the intestines and renal tubules and from the bones as needed.

DAILY GAIN AND LOSS OF FLUIDS

The body's fluid gains and losses should be about equal on a daily basis to maintain fluid and electrolyte balance. This can be monitored by measuring **intake** and **output** (I&O), but a number of other factors must be considered as well:

Fluid gains are as follows:

- Food people eat each day contains about 1000 mL of fluid.
- Fluids they drink average 1300 mL per day.
- Metabolic processes produce about 300 mL per day.

Fluid losses are as follows:

- Fluid is lost via the kidneys by production of 1-2 L of urine daily.
- The skin sweats and this evaporates an average of 600 mL daily, but this can increase up to 1000 mL/hr in hot and dry climates, during fever, or as a result of burns. Fluid loss can decrease in hot humid conditions.
- Exhaled air accounts for 300-400 mL of fluid loss daily.
- Fluids lost in stools total about 100-200 mL daily.

PHYSICAL EXAMINATION TECHNIQUES

The **physical exam** is an important element of nursing assessment. The physical assessment needs to be organized and systematic and should be age- and developmentally-appropriate. The physical exam may be a complete physical exam, a system-specific exam, or an exam of a specific body part. The basic **techniques** of a physical exam are inspection, palpation, auscultation, and percussion. The nurse makes a visual, aural, and olfactory assessment of the patient. This includes paying attention to the patient's skin tone, breathing sounds, and breath odor. Palpation includes techniques for touching the patient's body in order to get physical information such as temperature, skin tone and condition, or swelling in the glands. Auscultation is the examination of sounds within the body, such as heart tones, wheezing or crackling in the lungs, or bowel sounds. Auscultation is usually performed with a stethoscope. Percussion involves making quick taps to parts of the body with the fingers to ascertain the shape and condition of organs, identify areas of tenderness, or assess reflexes.

PALPATION

Use of palpation can provide valuable details during physical assessment of the patient:

- Be sure to wash and warm the hands prior to touching the patient.
- Do not use gloves unless you anticipate contact with bodily fluids.
- Explain the process and how it will feel and instruct the patient to relax the muscles if appropriate. Provide warmth and privacy during palpation.
- Use light palpation to feel the cervical lymph nodes and thyroid glands and to feel the superficial blood vessels for thrills.
- Place your hands on the chest to detect heart vibrations and to feel tactile fremitus during speech.
- Palpate the relaxed abdomen to identify structures and their borders and any masses or nodules on otherwise smooth organ surfaces.
- Utilize both hands to palpate the female reproductive organs by pushing organs into the reach of the other hand.

Palpation to identify organs and structures takes practice. Each patient is different but after you palpate many patients, the similarities in organ borders and consistency can be determined.

PALPATING FOR TACTILE FREMITUS

The act of speaking causes the chest wall to vibrate. This vibration can be felt by placing your hands lightly on the chest wall over a section of the lungs bilaterally while the patient repeats the letter "e" or the numbers "99." The amount of vibration felt depends on the weight of the patient, the muscle mass of the chest and back, gender, deepness of the voice, and condition of the lungs. **Tactile fremitus** is greater over major airways and normal lung tissue. It is less over lungs full of air or with emphysema or a pneumothorax. Lung consolidation will produce increased fremitus. The nurse should not feel for fremitus over the sternum or scapula. The areas above and below the breasts and above, medial to, and below the scapulae should be tested.

PERCUSSION

Percussion is striking part of the body to set the chest or abdominal wall into motion, producing sound that helps to locate underlying organs and reveal whether they are dense or filled with air or fluid. The sounds produced include:

- **Tympany**: Hollow drum sound produced when the organ contains air (stomach, intestines)
- **Resonance**: Hollow, low-pitched sound of normal lungs
- **Hyperresonance**: Low-pitched sound of lungs with emphysema or pneumothorax (louder than resonance)
- **Dullness**: "thud" heard over dense structures such as the liver
- **Flatness**: sound heard over muscles or bones such as in the thigh

Percussion is performed by placing the middle finger of one hand over the area and striking it with the middle finger of the opposite hand. It can be used to find the margins of an organ or area of pathology by repeatedly striking areas near to each other and listening for changes in sound representing the edge of the organ. The extent of lung consolidation can be determined in this manner.

AUSCULTATION

Auscultation is listening to sounds within the body through either the bell or the diaphragm of the stethoscope. These sounds differ in the following ways:

- **Intensity**: The level of sound in terms of loudness
- **Frequency**: Low or high pitch of the sound
- **Quality**: Helps to distinguish between rumbling and musical-type sounds

The **bell** of the stethoscope is best when listening for the lower frequency sounds of heart murmurs or bruit, with the bell placed lightly on the skin. The **diaphragm** is best for high-pitched sounds, such as heart or lung sounds or bowel sounds, with the diaphragm placed firmly on the skin. The nurse should not touch the tubing or place the end of the stethoscope in contact with cloth or hair, or extra sounds will be heard that may obscure the sounds transmitted.

Cardiovascular Assessment

ASSESSMENT OF THE CARDIOVASCULAR SYSTEM

Cardiovascular assessment includes questioning the patient for any family history of death at a young age or other cardiovascular diseases. Elderly African-American males are at highest risk for cardiovascular problems. One must question the patient about edema, chest pain, dyspnea, fatigue, vertigo, syncope or other changes in consciousness, weight gain, and leg cramps or pain. If chest pain is a symptom, one must ask about the intensity, timing, location, any radiation, quality, meaning to the patient, factors that aggravate or alleviate the pain, nausea, dyspnea, diaphoresis, or any other accompanying symptoms. Physical assessment includes assessment of vital signs, heart and lung sounds, skin assessment, radial, popliteal, and pedal pulses, circulation and sensation of extremities, and auscultation of the aorta, renal, iliac, and femoral arteries for bruits. Blood should be taken for a lipid profile and electrolytes. The patient must be helped to modify risk factors such as hypertension, smoking, diabetes, obesity, hyperlipidemia, inactivity, and stress.

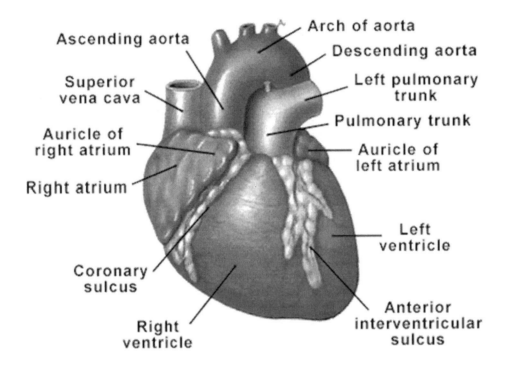

Review Video: <u>Cardiovascular Assessment</u>
Visit mometrix.com/academy and enter code: 323076

Review Video: <u>Circulatory System</u>
Visit mometrix.com/academy and enter code: 376581

Review Video: <u>Heart Blood Flow</u>
Visit mometrix.com/academy and enter code: 783139

ASSESSMENT OF HEART SOUNDS

Auscultation of heart sounds can help to diagnose different cardiac disorders. Areas to auscultate include the aortic area, pulmonary area, Erb's point, tricuspid area, and the apical area. The **normal heart sounds** represent closing of the valves.

- The **first heart sound** (S1) "lub" is closure of the mitral and tricuspid valves (heard at apex/left ventricular area of the heart).
- The **second heart sound** (S2) "dub" is closure of the aortic and pulmonic valves (heard at the base of the heart). There may be a slight splitting of the S2.

The time between S1 and S2 is systole and the time between S2 and the next S1 is diastole. Systole and diastole should be silent although ventricular disease can cause gallops, snaps, or clicks and stenosis of the valves or failure of the valves to close can cause murmurs. Pericarditis may cause a friction rub.

Additional heart sounds:

- **Gallop rhythms**: S3 commonly occurs after S2 in children and young adults but may indicate heart failure or left ventricular failure in older adults (when heard with patient lying on left side). S4 occurs before S1, during the contracting of the atria when there is ventricular hypertrophy, found in coronary artery disease, hypertension, or aortic valve stenosis.
- **Opening snap**: Unusual high-pitched sound occurring after S2 with stenosis of mitral valve from rheumatic heart disease
- **Ejection click**: Brief high-pitched sound after S1; aortic stenosis
- **Friction rub**: Harsh, grating holosystolic sound; pericarditis
- **Murmur**: Sound caused by turbulent blood flow from stenotic or malfunctioning valves, congenital defects, or increased blood flow. Murmurs are characterized by location, timing in the cardiac cycle, intensity (rated from Grade I to Grade VI), pitch (low to high-pitched), quality (rumbling, whistling, blowing) and radiation (to the carotids, axilla, neck, shoulder, or back).

CARDIAC MONITORING

Cardiac monitoring includes the evaluation of different intervals and segments on the electrocardiogram:

- **QT interval**: This is the complete time of ventricular depolarization and repolarization, which begins with the QRS segment and ends when the Y wave is completed. Typically, duration usually ranges from 0.36 to 0.44 seconds, but this may vary depending on the heart rate. If the heat rate is rapid, the duration is shorter and vice versa. Certain medications can prolong the QT interval, in such cases monitoring this is critical. A prolonged QT interval puts the patient at risk for R-on-T phenomenon, which can result in dangerous arrhythmias.
- **ST segment**: This is an isoelectric period when the ventricles are in a plateau phase, completely depolarized and beginning recovery and repolarization. Deflection is usually isoelectric, but may range from -0.5 to +1mm. If the ST segment is ≥0.5 mm below the baseline, it is considered depressed and may be an indication of myocardial ischemia. Depression may also indicate digitalis toxicity. If the ST segment is elevated ≥1 mm above baseline, this is an indication of myocardial injury.

MAP

The MAP **(mean arterial pressure)** is most commonly used to evaluate perfusion as it shows pressure throughout the cardiac cycle. Systole is one-third and diastole two-thirds of the normal cardiac cycle. The MAP for a blood pressure of 120/60 is calculated as follows:

$$\text{MAP} = \frac{\text{Diastole} \times 2 + \text{Systole}}{3}$$

$$\text{MAP} = \frac{60 \times 2 + 120}{3} = \frac{240}{3} = 80$$

Normal range for mean arterial pressure is 70-100 mmHg. A MAP of greater than 60 mmHg is required to perfuse vital organs, including the heart, brain, and kidneys.

Oxygen Saturation as it Relates to Hemodynamic Status

Hemodynamic monitoring includes monitoring **oxygen saturation** levels, which must be maintained for proper cardiac function. The central venous catheter often has an oxygen sensor at the tip to monitor oxygen saturation in the right atrium. If the catheter tip is located near the renal veins, this can cause an increase in right atrial oxygen saturation; and near the coronary sinus, a decrease.

- Increased oxygen saturation may result from left atrial to right atrial shunt, abnormal pulmonary venous return, increased delivery of oxygen or decrease in extraction of oxygen.
- Decreased oxygen saturation may be related to low cardiac output with an increase in oxygen extraction or decrease in arterial oxygen saturation with normal differences in the atrial and ventricular oxygen saturation.

Electrocardiogram

The electrocardiogram records and shows a graphic display of the electrical activity of the heart through a number of different waveforms, complexes, and intervals:

- **P wave**: Start of electrical impulse in the sinus node and spreading through the atria, muscle depolarization
- **QRS complex**: Ventricular muscle depolarization and atrial repolarization
- **T wave**: Ventricular muscle repolarization (resting state) as cells regain negative charge
- **U wave**: Repolarization of the Purkinje fibers

A modified lead II ECG is often used to monitor basic heart rhythms and dysrhythmias:

- Typical placement of leads for 2-lead ECG is 3-5 cm inferior to the right clavicle and left lower ribcage. Typical placement for a 3-lead ECG is (RA) right arm near shoulder, (LA) V₅ position over 5th intercostal space, and (LL) left upper leg near groin.

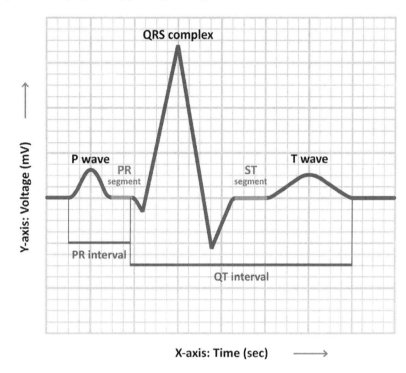

ADMINISTRATION OF 12-LEAD ECG

The electrocardiogram provides a graphic representation of the electrical activity of the heart. It is indicated for chest pain, dyspnea, syncope, acute coronary syndrome, pulmonary embolism, and possible MI. The standard **12 lead ECG** gives a picture of electrical activity from 12 perspectives through placement of 10 body leads:

- 4 limb leads are placed distally on the wrists and ankles (but may be placed more proximally if necessary).
- Precordial leads:
  - V1: Right sternal border at 4th intercostal space
  - V2: Left sternal border at 4th intercostal space
  - V3: Midway between V2 and V4
  - V4: Left midclavicular line at 5th intercostal space
  - V5: Horizontal to V4 at left anterior axillary line
  - V6: Horizontal to V5 at left midaxillary line

In some cases, additional leads may be used:

- Right-sided leads are placed on the right in a mirror image of the left leads, usually to diagnose right ventricular infarction through ST elevation.

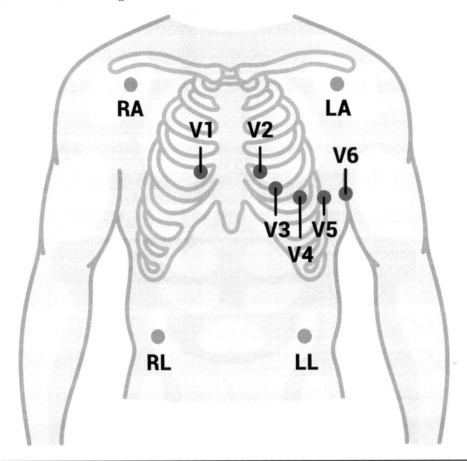

Review Video: 12 Lead ECG
Visit mometrix.com/academy and enter code: 962539

CARDIAC OUTPUT

Cardiac output (CO) is the amount of blood pumped through the ventricles during a specified period. Normal cardiac output is about 5 liters per minutes at rest for an adult. Under exercise or stress, this volume may multiply 3 or 4 times with concomitant changes in the heart rate (HR) and stroke volume (SV). The basic formulation for calculating cardiac output is the heart rate (HR) per minute multiplied by the stroke volume (SR), which is the amount of blood pumped through the ventricles with each contraction. The stroke volume is controlled by preload, afterload, and contractibility.

$$CO\left(\frac{\text{mL}}{\text{min}}\right) = HR\left(\frac{\text{beats}}{\text{min}}\right) \times SV\ (\text{mL})$$

The heart rate is controlled by the autonomic nervous system. Normally, if the heart rate decreases, stroke volume increases to compensate. The exception to this would be cardiomyopathies, so bradycardia results in a sharp decline in cardiac output.

CARDIAC INDEX

Cardiac index (CI) is the cardiac output (CO) divided by the body surface area (BSA). This is essentially a measure of cardiac output tailored to the individual, based on height and weight, measured in liters/min per square meter of BSA.

- Normal value: 2.2–4.0 L/min/m²

STROKE VOLUME

Stroke volume (SV) is the amount of blood pumped through the left ventricle with each contraction, minus any blood remaining inside the ventricle at the end of systole.

- Normal values: 60–70 mL
- Formula:

$$SV \text{ (mL)} = CO\left(\frac{mL}{min}\right) \div HR\left(\frac{beats}{min}\right)$$

PULMONARY VASCULAR RESISTANCE AND EJECTION FRACTION

Pulmonary vascular resistance (PVR) is the resistance in the pulmonary arteries and arterioles against which the right ventricle has to pump during contraction. It is the mean pressure in the pulmonary vascular bed divided by blood flow. If PVR increases, SV decreases.

- Normal value: 1.2–3.0 units or 100–250 dynes/sec/cm⁵

Ejection Fraction (EF) is the percentage of the total blood volume of the heart that is pumped out with each beat. Dramatically decreased values indicate heart failure.

- Normal value: 60–70%

PRELOAD AND AFTERLOAD

Preload refers to the amount of elasticity in the myocardium at the end of diastole when the ventricles are filled to their maximum volume and the stretch on the muscle fibers is the greatest. The preload value is based on the volume in the ventricles. The amount of preload (stretch) affects stroke volume because as stretch increases, the resultant contraction also increases (Frank-Starling Law). Preload may decrease because of dehydration, diuresis, or vasodilation. Preload may increase because of increased venous return, controlling fluid loss, transfusion, or intravenous fluids.

Afterload refers to the amount of systemic vascular resistance to left ventricular ejection of blood and pulmonary vascular resistance to right ventricular ejection of blood. Determinants of afterload include the size and elasticity of the great vessels and the functioning of the pulmonic and aortic valves. Afterload increases with hypertension, stenotic valves, and vasoconstriction.

MINIMALLY/NON-INVASIVE HEMODYNAMIC MONITORING

Hemodynamic monitoring and evaluation of cardiac function is an important component of the care of the critically ill patient. **Minimally or non-invasive** alternatives to traditional invasive means of hemodynamic monitoring (such as the use of a pulmonary artery catheter) include esophageal Doppler, arterial pressure based cardiac output monitoring, and impedance cardiography. **Esophageal Doppler** is a minimally invasive option used in surgical patients to monitor descending aortic blood flow and estimate cardiac output. A probe is inserted into the esophagus and then connected to a monitor, where waveform shapes produced by aortic blood flow are displayed.

Arterial pressure based cardiac output monitors (APCO's) use an algorithm to estimate cardiac output through the analysis of the arterial pressure waveform. The radial or femoral artery is accessed using a standard arterial catheter and no external calibration is needed.

Impedance cardiography is a non-invasive method of hemodynamic monitoring in which sensors placed on the body use electrical signals to measure the level of change in impedance in the thoracic fluid. A waveform is generated and is then used to calculate cardiac output and stroke volume, as well as ten additional hemodynamic parameters.

INTRAARTERIAL BLOOD PRESSURE MONITORING

Intraarterial blood pressure monitoring uses a catheter to measure systolic, diastolic, and mean arterial pressures (MAP) continuously. Before catheter insertion, collateral circulation must be assessed by Doppler or the Allen test (radial). Complications include arterial vasospasm, hematoma formation, hemorrhage (accidental disconnect), catheter occlusion, compartment syndrome, retroperitoneal bleed (femoral site), and thrombus/embolus.

Set up: The line should be connected to the monitor as well as a pressure bag set at 300 mmHg with no longer than 3 feet of stiff, noncompliant tubing to ensure accuracy. The transducer is leveled at the phlebostatic axis of the patient. The line should be kept free of any air or bubbles, and re-zeroed every four hours and with a change of patient position.

Pressure Bag

Pressure Transducer and Automatic Flushing System (set at the level of the midaxillary line)

Saline Filled Non-Compressible Tubing

Arterial Line

Waveform: A normal ABP waveform should be smooth and regular, with a dicrotic notch. To test, perform a "square-wave" or "Fast Flush" test; flush the line while watching the monitor. There should be a square shape, followed by two oscillations and a return to normal waves. A missing dicrotic notch indicates a blockage of some kind (thrombus, plaque, and vasospasm) or low pressure in the bag. Too many oscillations or an increased sharpness of the wave indicates under dampening and is caused by increased SVR or too long of tubing.

ASSESSMENT OF LOWER EXTREMITIES

Assessment of lower extremities includes a number of different elements:

- **Appearance** includes comparing limbs for obvious differences or changes in skin or nails as well as evaluating for edema, color changes in skin, such as pallor or rubor. Legs that are thin, pale, shiny, and hairless indicate peripheral arterial disease.
- **Perfusion** should be assessed by checking venous filling time and capillary refill, skin temperature (noting changes in one limb or between limbs), bruits (indicating arterial narrowing), pulses (comparing both sides in a proximal to distal progression), ankle-brachial index and toe-brachial index.
- **Sensory function** includes the ability to feel pain, temperature, and touch.
- **Range of motion** of the ankle must be assessed to determine if the joint flexes past 90° because this is necessary for unimpaired walking and aids venous return in the calf.
- **Pain** is an important diagnostic feature of peripheral arterial disease, so the location, intensity, duration, and characteristics of pain are important.

ASSESSMENT OF PULSE AND BRUIT

Evaluation of the pulses of the **lower extremities** is an important part of assessment for peripheral arterial disease/trauma. Pulses should be first evaluated with the patient in supine position and then again with the legs dependent, checking bilaterally and proximal to distal to determine if intensity of pulse decreases distally. Pedal pulses should be examined at both the posterior tibialis and the dorsalis pedis. The pulse should be evaluated as to the rate, rhythm, and intensity, which is usually graded on a 0 to 4 scale:

0 = pulse absent
1 = weak, difficult to palpate
2 = normal as expected
3 = full
4 = strong and bounding

Pulses may be **palpable** or **absent** with peripheral arterial disease. Absence of pulse on both palpation and Doppler probe does indicate peripheral arterial disease.

Bruits may be noted by auscultating over major arteries, such as femoral, popliteal, peroneal, and dorsalis pedis, indicating peripheral arterial disease.

ASSESSING PERFUSION OF LOWER EXTREMITIES

Assessment of perfusion can indicate venous or arterial abnormalities:

- **Venous refill time**: Begin with the patient lying supine for a few moments and then have the patient sit with the feet dependent. Observe the veins on the dorsum of the foot and count the seconds before normal filling. Venous occlusion is indicated with times greater than 20 seconds.
- **Capillary refill**: Grasp the toenail bed between the thumb and index finger and apply pressure for several seconds to cause blanching. Release the nail and count the seconds until the nail regains normal color. Arterial occlusion is indicated with times of more than 2 to 3 seconds. Check both feet and more than one nail bed.
- **Skin temperature**: Using the palm of the hand and fingers, gently palpate the skin, moving distally to proximally and comparing both legs. Arterial disease is indicated by decreased temperature (coolness) or a marked change from proximal to distal. Venous disease is indicated by increased temperature about the ankle.

ABI

PROCEDURE

The ankle-brachial index **(ABI) examination** is done to evaluate peripheral arterial disease of the lower extremities.

1. Apply BP cuff to one arm, palpate brachial pulse, and place conductivity gel over the artery.
2. Place the tip of a Doppler device at a 45-degree angle into the gel at the brachial artery and listen for the pulse sound.
3. Inflate the cuff until the pulse sound ceases and then inflate 20 mmHg above that point.
4. Release air and listen for the return of the pulse sound. This reading is the brachial systolic pressure.
5. Repeat the procedure on the other arm and use the higher reading for calculations.
6. Repeat the same procedure on each ankle with the cuff applied above the malleoli and the gel over the posterior tibial pulse to obtain the ankle systolic pressure.
7. Divide the ankle systolic pressure by the brachial systolic pressure to obtain the ABI.

Sometimes, readings are taken both before and after 5 minutes of walking on a treadmill.

INTERPRETING RESULTS

Once the ABI examination is completed, the ankle systolic pressure must be divided by the brachial systolic pressure. Ideally, the BP at the ankle should be equal to that of the arm or slightly higher. With peripheral arterial disease the ankle pressure falls, affecting the ABI. Additionally, some conditions that cause calcification of arteries, such as diabetes, can cause a false elevation.

Calculation is simple:

$$ABI = \frac{\text{Ankle systolic}}{\text{Brachial systolic}}$$

The degree of disease relates to the **score**:

- >1.4: Abnormally high, may indicate calcification of vessel wall
- 1.0–1.4: Normal reading, asymptomatic
- 0.9–1.0: Low reading, but acceptable unless there are other indications of PAD
- 0.8–0.9: Likely some arterial disease is present
- 0.5–0.8: Moderate arterial disease
- < 0.5: Severe arterial disease

Respiratory Assessment

ASSESSMENT OF THE RESPIRATORY SYSTEM

If significant respiratory distress is present, one must stabilize the patient before doing a **respiratory history** or ask family if available:

- Question the patient about risk factors, such as smoking, exposure to smoke or other inhaled toxins, past lung problems, and allergies.
- Ask the patient about symptoms of respiratory problems, such as dyspnea, cough, sputum production, fatigue, ability to do ADLs and IADLs, and chest pain.
- Determine how long symptoms have been present, the length of periods of dyspnea, aggravating and alleviating factors, and the severity of symptoms.

When performing a **physical assessment**, one should assess vital signs, posture, pulse oximetry, check nails for clubbing, do a skin assessment, listen to lung sounds via auscultation and percussion, and look for accessory muscle use, signs of anxiety, and edema. Depending on condition, blood may be drawn for arterial blood gases, electrolytes, and CBC. Sputum cultures may be obtained.

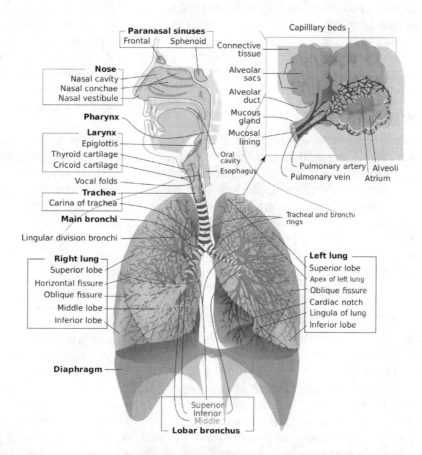

Review Video: <u>Respiratory System</u>
Visit mometrix.com/academy and enter code: 783075

29

PRIMARY AND SECONDARY MUSCLES USED FOR BREATHING

Muscles used for breathing are separated into primary and secondary muscle groups.

- The **primary muscle groups** are those that are used in normal, quiet breathing. When patients are in respiratory distress and breathing is more difficult, secondary muscle groups become activated. The muscles considered primary for breathing are the diaphragm and the external intercostal muscles. These muscles act by changing the pressure gradient, allowing the lungs to expand and air to flow in and out.
- The **secondary muscle groups** include the sternocleidomastoid, scaleni, internal intercostals, obliques, and abdominal muscles. These secondary muscle groups work when breathing is difficult, both in inspiration and expiration, in cases such as obstructions or bronchoconstriction. Use of these secondary muscle groups can often be seen on exam and may be described as see-saw or abdominal breathing (when the abdominal muscles are being used during exhalation) or retractions as the muscles activate and can be seen between rigid structures such as bone.

NORMAL PHYSIOLOGICAL AIRWAY CLEARANCE

Normal airway clearance is caused by various aspects of the respiratory system. A thin layer of mucus lines the airways as a protective mechanism against debris and helps trap foreign objects before they enter the lower airways. Proper hydration keeps the mucosa adequately moist so it can trap foreign debris. As this debris lands in the mucus, the cilia in the respiratory tract act as an "elevator" to push the debris up to the larynx, where it can either be coughed up or swallowed and digested. An intact cough reflex is necessary for the debris to stimulate the cough, and normal muscle strength and nerve innervation of the diaphragm is required to produce a sufficiently forceful cough.

VENTILATION/PERFUSION RATIO

In order to maintain homeostasis, the respiratory and cardiac systems need to maintain a careful balance. The **ventilation/perfusion ratio** indicates that ventilation of the lungs and perfusion to the lungs are within a normal balance. A normal ventilation/perfusion ratio is equal to 0.8. A ventilation/perfusion ratio higher than normal is indicative of ventilation that is too high, perfusion that is too low, or some combination of the two. This can occur because of hyperventilation (either physiological or caused by healthcare practitioners due to incorrect ventilator settings), pulmonary embolism, or hypotension. Essentially, a high ventilation/perfusion ratio means that there is more ventilation than perfusion. If the ventilation/perfusion ratio is lower than normal, then ventilation is too low, perfusion is too high, or some combination of the two. This can be caused by atelectasis, pneumonia, or lung disease. Whatever the cause, a low ventilation/perfusion ratio indicates that there is more perfusion than ventilation.

NORMAL AND ABNORMAL BREATH SOUND TERMS

Normal breath sounds can be divided into three types. Vesicular breath sounds are low, soft sounds that can normally be heard over the peripheral lung space. Bronchovesicular breath sounds are moderate pitch breath sounds that are normally heard in the upper lung fields. Tracheal breath sounds are higher in pitch and heard over the trachea. Abnormal breath sounds are also known as adventitious lung sounds. Wheezes are high-pitched, expiratory sounds caused by air flowing through an obstructed airway. Stridor is also high-pitched, but is usually heard on inspiration in the upper airways. Coarse crackles are caused by an excessive amount of secretions in the airway and can be heard on inspiration and expiration. Fine crackles occur late in the expiratory phase and usually occur when the peripheral airways are being "popped" back open.

> **Review Video: Lung Sounds**
> Visit mometrix.com/academy and enter code: 765616

DIAGNOSTIC PROCEDURES AND TOOLS USED DURING PULMONARY ASSESSMENT

The diagnostic procedures and tools used during assessment of **pulmonary and thoracic trauma/disease** will vary according to the type and degree of injury/disease, but may include:

- **Thorough physical examination** including cardiac and pulmonary status, assessing for any abnormalities.
- **Electrocardiogram** to assess for cardiac arrhythmias.
- **Chest x-ray** should be done for all those with injuries to check for fractures, pneumothorax, major injuries, and placement of intubation tubes. X-rays can be taken quickly and with portable equipment so they can be completed quickly during the initial assessment.
- **Computerized tomography** may be indicated after initial assessment, especially if there is a possibility of damage to the parenchyma of the lungs.
- **Oximetry and atrial blood gases** as indicated.
- **12-lead electrocardiogram** may be needed if there are arrhythmias for more careful observation.
- **Echocardiogram** should be done if there is apparent cardiac damage.

CAPNOGRAPHY WITH END-TIDAL CO_2 DETECTOR

Capnometry utilizes an **end-tidal CO_2 (ETCO) detector** that measures the concentration of CO_2 in expired air, usually through pH sensitive paper that changes color (commonly purple to yellow). Typically, the capnometer is attached to the ETT and a bag-valve-mask (BVM) ventilator attached. The capnogram provides data in the shape of a waveform that represents the partial pressure of exhaled gas. It is often used to confirm placement of endotracheal tubes as clinical assessment is not always sufficient, and it is a noninvasive mode of monitoring carbon dioxide in the respiratory cycle. Information provided by the capnogram includes:

- $PaCO_2$ level
- Type and degree of bronchial obstruction, such as COPD (waveform changes from rectangular to a fin-like)
- Air leaks in the ventilation system
- Rebreathing precipitated by need for new CO_2 absorber
- Cardiac arrest
- Hypothermia or reduced metabolism

The normal capnogram is a waveform that represents the varying CO_2 level throughout the breath cycle:

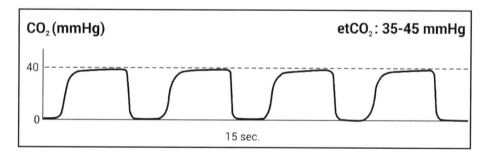

ARTERIAL BLOOD GASES

Arterial blood gases (ABGs) are monitored to assess effectiveness of oxygenation, ventilation, and acid-base status and to determine oxygen flow rates. Partial pressure of a gas is that exerted by each gas in a mixture of gases, proportional to its concentration, based on total atmospheric pressure of 760 mmHg at sea level. Normal values include:

- Acidity/alkalinity (pH): 7.35-7.45
- Partial pressure of carbon dioxide ($PaCO_2$): 35-45 mmHg

- Partial pressure of oxygen (PaO_2): ≥80 mmHg
- Bicarbonate concentration (HCO_3^-): 22-26 mEq/L
- Oxygen saturation (SaO_2): ≥95%

The relationship between these elements, particularly the $PaCO_2$ and the PaO_2 indicates respiratory status. For example, $PaCO_2$ >55 and the PaO_2 <60 in a patient previously in good health indicates respiratory failure. There are many issues to consider. Ventilator management may require a higher $PaCO_2$ to prevent barotrauma and a lower PaO_2 to reduce oxygen toxicity.

Endocrine Assessment

ASSESSING FOR ENDOCRINE DISORDERS

The **endocrine system** comprises organs that produce hormones that are critical to growth, sexual development, and metabolism, so changes in these areas are suggestive of endocrine disorders. While symptoms may vary widely, there are often generalized symptoms that can be associated with most endocrine disorders. One should question the patient about fatigue and ability to perform ADLs, heat or cold intolerance, changes in sexual libido, sexual functioning, and secondary sexual characteristics, weight fluctuation, sleep problems, decreased concentration and memory, and mood changes. During the physical exam, one should assess the patient for edema, "moon" face or "buffalo hump," exophthalmos, hair loss, female facial hair, enlarged trunk with thin extremities, and enlarged hands and feet. Vital signs should be assessed for hypo or hypertension, and one should assess for changes in skin appearance and vision.

THYROID IMAGING

Thyroid imaging plays a critical role in assessment of many thyroid diseases. This test may be used to determine the uptake characteristics of the thyroid gland in addition to the size and shape of the gland. In addition, **thyroid imaging** may determine how much iodine-131 is needed in order to safely ablate the gland when necessary. The radioactive iodine uptake scan (RAIU) is basically administration of iodine-123 with imaging performed 8 and 24 hours later:

Uptake of radioactive iodine is increased in disorders such as Graves' disease, "hot" nodules of various etiologies (including toxic multinodular goiter), TSH-secreting pituitary tumor, and iodine deficiency.

Uptake of radioactive iodine is decreased in the setting of thyroiditis and iodine excess.

Ultrasound imaging is used in thyroid disease to determine the size and structure of a thyroid nodule, such as to determine uniformity of shape, irregular contour, solid/cystic structure, and depth.

Neurological Assessment

ASSESSMENT OF THE NEUROLOGICAL SYSTEM

Assessment of the neurological system includes:

- Assess the **health history** for any trauma, falls, alcoholism, drug abuse, medications taken, and family history of neurological problems.
- Ask about any presenting **neurological symptoms**, the circumstances in which they occur, whether they fluctuate, and any associated factors, such as seizures, pain, vertigo, weakness, abnormal sensations, visual problems, loss of consciousness, changes in cognition, and motor problems.

Assessment includes determining the level of consciousness and cognition. Posture and movements are assessed for abnormalities. Facial expression and movement are noted. Cranial nerve assessment is done. The patient is assessed for strength, coordination, and balance and the ability to perform ADLs. One should assess for clonus and test all reflexes, including Babinski, gag, blink, swallow, upper and lower abdominal, cremasteric in males, plantar, perianal, biceps, triceps, brachioradialis, patellar and ankle. Peripheral sensation is tested by touching the patient with cotton balls and the sharp and dull ends of a broken tongue blade.

> **Review Video: Nervous System**
> Visit mometrix.com/academy and enter code: 708428

ASSESSING FUNCTIONAL STATUS

Functional abilities include the acts needed to meet basic needs and perform *activities of daily living* (ADLs), such as eating and elimination, as well as those *activities that are essential to independent living* (IADLs), such as shopping. A thorough assessment of the patient's functional abilities will identify areas that should be concentrated upon during rehabilitation. One should observe the patient as he/she performs these functions and record the following:

- Degree of independence shown
- Ability to complete activity without rest
- Nerve function
- Muscle function and strength
- Motion
- Coordination
- Cardiac status
- Respiratory status
- Assistance required to complete activity

The facility usually provides one of the tools available to record a functional assessment. The most common tool used is the Functional Independence Measure (FIM). Other tools available include the Barthel Index, the PULSES Profile, and the Patient Evaluation Conference System.

AMERICAN STROKE ASSOCIATION CLASSIFICATION SYSTEM FOR THE EXTENT OF BRAIN ATTACK INJURY

The American Stroke Association developed a **brain attack outcome classification system** to standardize descriptions of stroke injuries:

- **Number of impaired domains** (Potentially affected neurological domains: motor, sensory, vision, language, cognition, and affect): Level 0: no domains impaired; Level 1: one domain impaired; Level 2: two domains impaired; Level 3: greater than 2 domains impaired.
- **Severity of impairment**: A (minimal or no neurological deficit due to stroke); B (mild/moderate deficit); or C (severe deficit). Note: When more than one domain is affected, severity is measured by the domain with the most impairment.

Assessment of function determines the ability to **live independently**:

- **I**: Independent in basic activities of daily living (BADL), such as bathing, eating, toileting, and walking; and instrumental activities of daily living (IADL), such as telephoning, shopping, maintaining a household, socializing, and using transportation
- **II**: Independent in BADL but partially dependent in IADL
- **III**: Partially dependent in BADL (less than 3 areas) and IADL
- **IV**: Partially dependent in BADL (3 or more areas)
- **V**: Completely dependent in BADL (5 or more areas) and IADL

Level III requires much assistance and Levels IV and V cannot live independently.

ADMINISTRATION OF THE NIHSS

The **National Institutes of Health Stroke Scale (NIHSS)** is administered with careful attention to directions. The examiner should record the answers and avoid coaching or repeating requests, although demonstration may be used with aphasic patients. The scale comprises 11 sections, with scores for each section ranging from 0 (normal) to 2, 3, or 4:

- **Level of consciousness**: Response to noxious stimulation (0-3), request for month and his/her age (0-2), request to open and close eyes, grip and release unaffected hand (0-2)
- **Best gaze**: Horizontal eye movement (0-2)
- **Visual**: Visual fields (0-3)
- **Facial palsy**: Symmetry when patient shows teeth, raises eyebrows, and closes eyes (0-3)
- **Motor, arm**: Drift while arm extended with palms down (0-4)
- **Motor, leg**: Leg drift at 30 degrees while patient supine (0-4)
- **Limb ataxia**: Finger-nose and heel-shin (0-2)
- **Sensory**: Grimace or withdrawal from pinprick (0-2)
- **Best language**: Describes action of pictures (0-3)
- **Dysarthria**: Reads or describes words on list (0-2)
- **Distinction and inattention**: Visual spatial neglect (0-2)

GLASGOW COMA SCALE

The Glasgow coma scale (GCS) measures the depth and duration of coma or impaired level of consciousness and is used for post-operative assessment. The GCS measures three parameters: best eye response, best verbal response, and best motor response, with a total possible score that ranges from 3 to 15:

Eye opening	4: Spontaneous
	3: To verbal stimuli
	2: To pain (not of face)
	1: No response

35

Verbal	5: Oriented
	4: Conversation confused, but can answer questions
	3: Uses inappropriate words
	2: Speech incomprehensible
	1: No response
Motor	6: Moves on command
	5: Moves purposefully respond pain
	4: Withdraws in response to pain
	3: Decorticate posturing (flexion) in response to pain
	2: Decerebrate posturing (extension) in response to pain
	1: No response

Injuries/conditions are classified according to the total score: 3-8 Coma; ≤8 Severe head injury likely requiring intubation; 9-12 Moderate head injury; 13-15 Mild head injury.

Review Video: **Glasgow Coma Scale**
Visit mometrix.com/academy and enter code: 133399

CRANIAL NERVES

	Name	Function	PE Test
I	Olfactory	Smell	Test olfaction
II	Optic	Visual acuity	Snellen eye chart; Accommodation
III	Oculomotor	Eye movement/ pupil	Pupillary reflex; Eye/eyelid motion
IV	Trochlear	Eye movement	Eye moves down & out
V	Trigeminal	Facial motor/ sensory	Corneal reflex; Facial sensation; Mastication
VI	Abducens	Eye movement	Lateral eye motion
VII	Facial	Facial expression; Taste	Moves forehead, closes eyes, smile/frown, puffs cheeks; Taste
VIII	Vestibulo-cochlear (Acoustic)	Hearing; Balance	Hearing (Weber/Rinne tests); Nystagmus
IX	Glosso-pharyngeal	Pharynx motor/sensory	Gag reflex; Soft palate elevation
X	Vagus	Visceral sensory, motor	Gag, swallow, cough
XI	Accessory	Sternocleidomastoid and trapezius (motor)	Turns head & shrugs shoulders against resistance
XII	Hypoglossal	Tongue movement	Push out tongue; move tongue from side to side

ICP AND MONROE-KELLIE HYPOTHESIS

Increasing **intracranial pressure (ICP)** is a frequent complication of brain injuries, tumors, or other disorders affecting the brain, so monitoring the ICP is very important. Increased ICP can indicate cerebral edema, hemorrhage, and/or obstruction of cerebrospinal fluid. The **Monroe-Kellie hypothesis** states that in order to maintain a normal ICP, a change in volume in one compartment must be compensated by a reciprocal change in volume in another compartment. There are 3 compartments in the brain: the brain tissue, cerebrospinal fluid (CSF), and blood. The CSF and blood can change more easily to accommodate changes in pressure than tissue, so medical intervention focuses on cerebral blood flow and drainage. Normal ICP is 1-15 mmHg on transducer or 13.6–203.9 mmH$_2$O on manometer. As intracranial pressure increases, **symptoms** include:

- Headache
- Alterations in level of consciousness
- Restlessness

- Slowly reacting or nonreacting dilated or pinpoint pupils
- Seizures
- Motor weakness
- Cushing's triad (late sign):
  - Increased systolic pressure with widened pulse pressure
  - Bradycardia in response to increased pressure
  - Decreased respirations

ICP MONITORING DEVICES

The intracranial pressure (ICP) **monitoring device** may be placed during surgery or a ventriculostomy performed in which a burr hole is drilled into the frontal area of the scalp and an **intraventricular catheter** threaded into the lateral ventricle. The intraventricular catheter may be used to monitor ICP and to drain excess CSF. Other monitoring devices include:

- **Intracranial pressure monitor bolt** (subarachnoid bolt) is applied through a burr hole with the distal end of the monitor probe resting in the subarachnoid space.
- **Epidural monitors** are placed into the epidural space.
- **Fiberoptic monitors** may be placed inside the brain.

The intraventricular catheter is the most accurate. CSF may be drained continuously or intermittently and must be monitored hourly for amount, color, and character. For ICP measurement, the patient's head must be elevated to 30-45° and the transducer leveled to the tragus of the ear or outer canthus of the eye, depending on facility policy.

CEREBRAL BLOOD FLOW, MAP, AND CPP

Cerebral blood flow, or the blood supply to the brain at any given moment, is influenced directly by one's **mean arterial pressure** (MAP). A MAP of greater than 60 mmHg is required to perfuse vital organs, including the brain. A MAP that falls below 60 mmHg risks ischemia and infarction. An excessively high MAP (greater than 100 mmHg) can also cause damage. A high MAP can result in increased oxygen demands by the heart, vascular injury, end organ damage, and stroke.

Cerebral perfusion pressure (CPP) is the pressure required to maintain adequate blood flow to the brain. CPP is based on mean arterial pressure (MAP) and intracranial pressure (ICP). Elevated ICP can be associated with a reduction in CPP.

$$CPP = MAP - ICP$$

- Normal CPP: 60-100 mmHg.
- <60 mmHg: Hypoperfusion occurs, resulting in focal or global ischemia.
- <30 mmHg: Hypoperfusion is marked and incompatible with life.
- >100 mmHg: Leads to hypertensive encephalopathy and cerebral edema (particularly if CPP >120 mmHg); Patients with chronic hypertension tolerate a higher level of CPP.

Gastrointestinal Assessment

ASSESSMENT OF THE GASTROINTESTINAL SYSTEM

Assessment of the gastrointestinal system includes:

- Ask about personal and family history of gastrointestinal problems and risk factors, such as alcoholism, smoking, drug and medicine use, and poor dietary habits.
- Ask about symptoms, such as GI discomfort, flatus, nausea, vomiting, diarrhea, and abdominal pain.
- Determine the defecation pattern and ask about weight fluctuations.

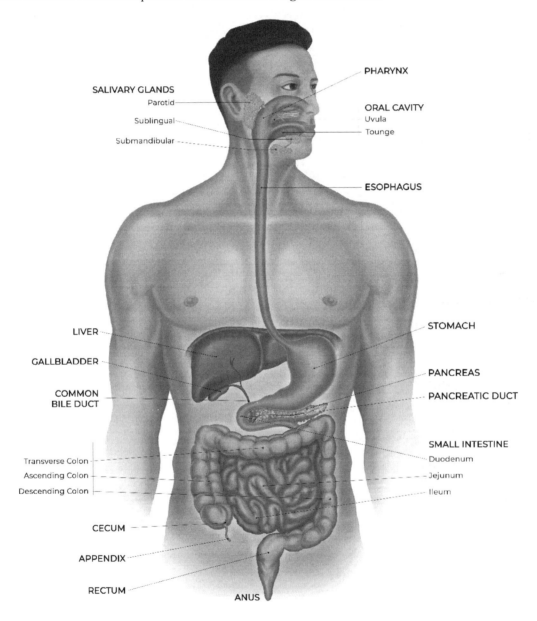

When performing a **physical assessment**, one must assess oral mucosa, tongue, teeth, pharynx, thyroid and parathyroid glands, skin color, moisture, turgor, nodules or lesions, bruises, scars, abdominal shape, and bowel sounds, assessing the abdomen in all 4 quadrants using the stethoscope diaphragm. The number of sounds heard determine if the intestines are functioning:

- **Absent**: no sounds in 3-5 minutes
- **Hypoactive**: only one sound in 2 minutes
- **Normal**: sounds heard every 5-20 seconds
- **Hyperactive**: 5-6 sounds in <30 seconds

One should examine the anal region for fissures, inflammation, tears, and dimples. Blood may be drawn for liver function studies, lipid profile, iron studies, CBC.

> **Review Video: Gastrointestinal System**
> Visit mometrix.com/academy and enter code: 378740

ASSESSMENT FOR GALLBLADDER AND PANCREATIC DISEASE

Gallbladder and pancreatic assessments are prompted by the appearance of symptoms. Symptoms of gallbladder disease include epigastric discomfort following fatty food intake, abdominal distension, right upper quadrant pain, which may be colicky, nausea, and vomiting. Pain may occur intermittently.

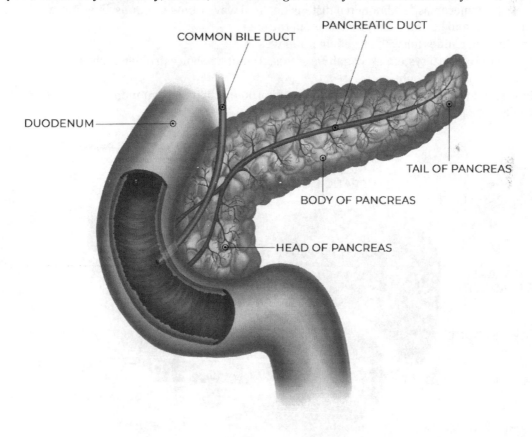

The patient with pancreatitis may have acute onset of severe abdominal pain, back pain, extensive vomiting, and dyspnea. Pancreatitis is most often related to gallstones or alcoholism, so history of alcohol use and examination for gallstones must be done:

- Assess for RUQ tenderness and mass, bowel sounds, and abdominal guarding.
- Assess the vital signs for hypotension, tachycardia, or fever and note any anxiety, agitation, or confusion.
- Note signs of hypoxia.
- Assess the skin for jaundice and bruising on the flanks and near the umbilicus.
- Blood is drawn to assess amylase and lipase, CBC, calcium, glucose, and bilirubin.

ASSESSMENT FOR LIVER DISEASE

The liver must be 70% damaged before lab tests show abnormalities. Assessment of risk factors and early symptoms are important to identify early disease. Risk factors for liver disease include alcoholism and drug abuse, risky sexual practices, exposure to infection or environmental toxins, and travel to countries with poor sanitation. One should question the patient about symptoms of liver disease, such as fatigue, itching, abdominal pain, anorexia, weight gain, fever, blood in stools or black stools, sleep problems, lack of menstruation, and lack of libido. Physical assessment includes checking vital signs and skin for scratches, pallor, jaundice, dryness, bruising, petechiae, abdominal veins and spider angiomas, and red palms:

- Assess for gynecomastia, abdominal distension, fluid waves, bowel sounds, liver margins, tenderness, consistency, and hardness and sharpness of the edge.
- Examine extremities for wasting, edema, and weakness.
- Assess neurological system for cognitive status, tremors, balance problems, slurred speech.
- Identify testicular atrophy.
- Blood should be drawn for serum enzymes and proteins, bilirubin, ammonia, clotting factors, and lipid profile.

ASSESSMENT OF NUTRITIONAL STATUS

Assessment of nutritional status begins with an assessment of the patient's intake. The patient is asked to report intake for the previous 24 hours. This may indicate the need for a **food diary** over a period of time:

- Compare the patient's nutritional intake with the requirements of the USDA's MyPlate.
- Measure height and weight and check against a BMI table to help determine nutritional status.
- Measure waist circumference.
- Assess the patient for physical signs of poor nutrition such as muscle wasting, obesity, hair breakage and loss, poor skin turgor, ulcers, bruising, and loss of subcutaneous tissue.
- Assess mucous membranes and condition of teeth, abdomen, extremities, and thyroid gland.

Nutritional status is connected to endocrine disease, infections, other acute and chronic diseases, digestion, absorption, excretion, and storage of nutrients, so these areas must also be assessed. Blood testing should include proteins, transferrin, electrolytes, vitamins A and C, carotene, and CBC. Test urine for creatinine, thiamine, riboflavin, niacin, albumin, and iodine.

ASSESSING NUTRITIONAL STATUS OF HOSPITALIZED PATIENTS

Assessing the nutritional status of the hospital inpatient is an important part of forming a care plan. The two screening tools that are most commonly used are the **Subjective Global Assessment (SGA)** and the **Prognostic Nutritional Index (PNI)**. The SGA provides a nutritional assessment based on both the patient history and current symptoms. The patient is asked about any changes in weight and is also asked questions about his or her diet. The presence of symptoms that may lead to weight loss and poor nutritional status, such as diarrhea, nausea, and vomiting, as well as water retention (edema) and muscle wasting (cachexia), is also included in the SGA. The PNI is also used as an indicator of malnutrition and is especially helpful in determining how well a patient will recover from surgery. The PNI assesses nutritional status through the measurement of serum proteins such as albumin and transferrin combined with a skinfold measurement and a cutaneous hypersensitivity test as an indicator of immune function.

Genitourinary Assessment

ASSESSMENT OF KIDNEYS AND URINARY TRACT

Assessment of kidneys and urinary tract includes:

- Assess the health history for family urinary system disease and risk factors, such as previous urinary disease, increased age, immobility, hypertension, diabetes, chemical exposure, chronic disease, radiation to the pelvis, STDs, alcohol or drug use, and complications of pregnancy and delivery.
- Determine daily fluid intake.
- Question symptoms such as flank or abdominal pain, hesitancy, urgency, difficulty or straining with voiding, difficulty emptying the bladder, urinary incontinence, fatigue, SOB, exercise intolerance from anemia, fever, chills, blood in the urine, and GI symptoms.

Physical assessment includes vital signs, kidney and bladder palpation, and percussion over the bladder after urination:

- Palpate for ascites and edema.
- Measure the DTRs and check gait and ability to walk heel-to-toe.
- Examine the genitalia and check the urethra and vagina for herniation, irritation, or tears.

Urine specimen is obtained via clean catch midstream technique for analysis and culture if indicated. Blood is taken for a CBC, and in males, prostate-specific antigen (PSA) levels will also be measured via blood specimen.

Review Video: Urinary System
Visit mometrix.com/academy and enter code: 601053

KIDNEY REGULATORY FUNCTIONS REGARDING FLUID BALANCE

Kidney regulatory functions include maintaining **fluid balance**. Fluid excretion balances intake with output, so increased intake results in a large output and vice versa:

- **Osmolality** (the number of electrolytes and other molecules per kg/urine) measures the concentration or dilution. With dehydration, osmolality increases; with fluid retention, osmolality decreases. With kidney disease, urine is dilute and the osmolality is fixed.
- **Specific gravity** compares the weight of urine (weight of particles) to distilled water (1.000). Normal urine is 1.010-1.025 with normal intake. High intake lowers the specific gravity, and low intake raises it. In kidney disease, it often does not vary.
- **Antidiuretic hormone** (ADH/vasopressin) regulates the excretion of water and urine concentration in the renal tubule by varying water reabsorption. When fluid intake decreases, blood osmolality rises, and this stimulates the release of ADH, which increases reabsorption of fluid to return osmolality to normal levels. ADH is suppressed with increased fluid intake, so less fluid is reabsorbed.

ASSESSING SEXUAL HEALTH AND PREFERENCES

Bringing up the topic of sex gives a patient permission to ask questions and openly discuss **sexual concerns**:

- Ask for permission to ask questions about sexual health and preferences during the gynecological/urological portion of the health history.
- If the patient refuses, go on with the rest of the health history, otherwise continue.
- Ask first if the person has sex with men, women, or both.
- Be nonjudgmental and do not assume that those who are elderly or disabled do not have sex. Use layman terms according to the patient's age and education level.
- Ask if the person is having any problems with relationships or sexual intercourse.
- Ask if the person has ever been forced to have sex or if is afraid of anyone close to them.
- End by asking if there are any questions about expression of sexual feelings, contraception, safe sex practices, or risky behavior.
- Refer those with problems to their doctor, or a gynecologist, urologist, or sex therapist.

Musculoskeletal Assessment

ASSESSING RISK OF FALLING

Many factors must be examined and combined to determine the **fall risk** status of a patient. They include age, sensory deficits, mobility problems, neurological disorders, past history of falling, cognitive impairment, and depression. Some medications, such as those associated with postural hypotension and psychotropic medications, may increase the danger of falls. The presence of dizziness, acute or chronic illness, poor physical status, elimination requirements, medications, and environmental concerns contribute to the risk for falls.

Multiple factors increase risk, so careful history and physical exam are necessary as part of assessment. When the presence of risk factors shows a risk for falls, this information should be communicated to other caregivers by wristband, colored markers on doors, care plans, or other effective means. The factors are then modified as much as possible. The patient should be re-evaluated as their condition changes or after a fall to determine the cause.

> **Review Video: <u>Muscular System</u>**
> Visit mometrix.com/academy and enter code: 967216
>
> **Review Video: <u>Skeletal System</u>**
> Visit mometrix.com/academy and enter code: 256447

ASSESSING PATIENTS WITH DISABILITIES

A patient with **disabilities** may find it very difficult to obtain screening for health problems due to inaccessibility:

- Work with the patient to resolve barriers to obtain weight, mammography, bone density tests, and pap/pelvic exams on a regular basis.
- Ask how to best assist the patient during the assessment.
- Observe the patient carefully for nonverbal communication, such as grimacing.
- If sensation is affected, warn the patient before touching any part of the body.
- Always address all areas of the patient's history, including sexual history.
- Use an interpreter that is not a family member if needed.
- Give the patient extra time to respond to questions when there is aphasia or other communication problems.
- Address the impact of the disability on the ability to perform ADLs, health status in general, access to healthcare, financial status, emotional status, work, community roles, and family wellbeing.

Integumentary Assessment

GENERAL SKIN ASSESSMENT

Skin color varies according to ethnicity. Color changes should be assessed to determine if they are local or extend over the entire body, and if they are permanent or transient. Pallor may indicate stress, impaired oxygenation, and vasoconstriction. Erythema may indicate vasodilation, local inflammation, and blushing. Cyanosis indicates impaired oxygenation, and jaundice indicates increased bilirubin.

Temperature is typically assessed by touching the skin with the back of the hand. Skin should be warm and equal bilaterally. Hypothermia may indicate impaired circulation, intravenous infusion, and immobilized limb (such as in a cast). Hyperthermia may indicate fever, infection, and excessive exercise.

> **Review Video: Skin Assessment**
> Visit mometrix.com/academy and enter code: 794925

EFFECTS OF AGE ON SKIN

Age is an important consideration when evaluating the skin because the characteristics of the skin change as people age.

- An **infant's** skin is thinner than an adult's because, while the epidermis is developed, the dermis layer is only about 60% of that of an adult and continues to develop after birth. The skin of premature infants is especially friable, allowing for transepidermal water loss and evaporative heat loss.
- During **adolescence**, the hair follicles activate, the thickness of the dermis decreases about 20%, and epidermal turnover time increases, so healing slows.
- As people **continue to age**, Langerhans' cells decrease in number, making the skin more prone to cancer, and the inflammatory reactions decrease. The sweat glands, vascularity, and subcutaneous fat all decrease, interfering with thermoregulation and contributing to dryness and irritation of the skin. The epidermal-dermal junction flattens, resulting in skin that is prone to tearing. The elastin in the skin degrades with age and solar exposure. The thinning of the hypodermis can lead to pressure ulcers.

> **Review Video: Integumentary System**
> Visit mometrix.com/academy and enter code: 655980

BRADEN SCALE

The Braden scale is a risk assessment tool that has been validated clinically as predictive of the risk of patient's developing pressure sores. It was developed in 1988 by Barbara Braden and Nancy Bergstrom and is in wide use. The scale scores six different areas with five areas scored 1-4 points, and one area 1-3 points. The lower the score, the greater the risk.

Area	Score of 1	Score of 2	Score of 3	Score of 4
Sensory perception	Completely limited	Very limited	Slightly limited	No impairment
Moisture	Constantly moist	Very moist	Occasionally moist	Rarely moist
Activity	Bed	Chair	Occasional walk	Frequent walk
Mobility	Immobile	Limited	Slightly limited	No limitations
Nutritional pattern	Very poor	Inadequate	Adequate	Excellent
Friction and shear	Problem	Potential problem	No apparent problem	

EVALUATING WOUNDS FOR ETIOLOGY

Wounds should be evaluated for **etiology** during the initial assessment to ensure proper treatment. Wounds can arise from a number of different causes:

- **Pressure**: Wounds that occur over bony prominences, such as the heels and coccyx, may be related to pressure, shear, or friction. The skin should be carefully examined for discolorations or changes in texture that might indicate compromise.
- **Arterial**: Arterial insufficiency is associated with a decrease in pedal pulses, and cool atrophic (shiny, dry) skin. It may result in small punctate-type ulcers, frequently on the dorsum of foot.
- **Venous stasis**: A decrease in venous circulation often results in hemoglobin leaking into the tissues of the lower leg, giving a brown discoloration. Tissue is often edematous, and ulcers are most common near the medial malleolus.
- **Diabetic neuropathy/ischemia**: Neuropathy can result in a lack of sensation to pain so that injuries to the feet may go unnoticed. Diabetes may also cause damage to small vessels, resulting in ischemia that can lead to ulcerations.
- **Trauma**: Injuries resulting from accidents or other types of trauma may vary considerably with some resulting in extensive damage to bones, tissues, organs, and circulation. Additionally, the wounds may be contaminated. Each wound must be assessed individually for multiple factors.
- **Burns**: Burn wounds may be chemical or thermal and should be assessed according to the area, the percentage of the body burned, and the depth of the burn. First-degree burns are superficial and affect the epidermis only. Second-degree burns extend through the dermis. Third degree burns affect underlying tissue, including vasculature, muscles, and nerves.
- **Infection**: An infected surgical or wound site can result in pain, edema, cellulitis, drainage, erosion of the sutures and ulceration of the tissue. Surgical sites must be assessed carefully and laboratory findings reviewed.

ELEMENTS OF WOUND ASSESSMENT

LOCATION AND SIZE

Wound location should be described in terms of anatomic position using landmarks (such as sternal notch, umbilicus, lateral malleolus), correct medical terminology, and directional terms:

- Anterior (in front)
- Posterior (behind)
- Superior (above)
- Inferior (below)

Wound size should be carefully described through actual measurement rather than association (the size of a dime). Measurements should be done with a disposable ruler in millimeters or centimeters. The current standard for measurement:

$$\text{Length} \times \text{width} \times \text{depth} = \text{dimension}$$

However, a clear description requires more detail. The measurement should be done at the greatest width and greatest length. More than two measurements may be needed if the wound is very irregularly shaped. The depth of the wound should be measured by inserting a sterile applicator and grasping or marking the applicator at skin level and then measuring the length below. Ideally, the wound should be photographed as well, following protocols for photography.

WOUND BED TISSUE

Wound bed tissue should be described as completely as possible, including color and general appearance:

- **Granulation tissue** is slightly granular in appearance and deep pink to bright red and moist, bleeding easily if disturbed.
- **Clean non-granular tissue** is smooth and deep pink or red and is not healing.
- **Hypergranulation** is excessive, soft, flaccid granulating tissue that is raised above the level of the periwound tissue, preventing proper epithelization, and may reflect excess moisture in the wound.
- **Epithelization** should appear at wound edges first and then eventually cover the wound. It is dry and light pink or violet in color.
- **Slough** is necrotic tissue that is viscous, soft, and yellow-gray in appearance and adheres to the wound.
- **Eschar** is hard dark brown or black leathery necrotic tissue that accumulates with death of the tissue.

WOUND MARGINS

Wound margins and the tissue surrounding the wound should be described carefully and with correct terminology:

- **Color** should be described using color descriptions and such terms as blanched, erythematous (red), or ecchymosed (purple, green, yellow).
- **Skin texture** may be normal, indurated (hardened), or edematous (swollen). Note if there is cellulitis or maceration evident.
- **Wound edges** may be diffuse (without clear margins), well defined, or rolled. A healing ridge may be evident if granulation has begun. Note if the wound is closed (as with a surgical incision) or open (as with dehiscence or ulcerations). Note if wound edges are attached or unattached (indicating undermining or tunneling).
- **Tunneling or undermining** should be assessed by probing the wound margins with a moist sterile cotton applicator, using clock face locators (toward the head is 12 o'clock, for example). Tunneling may be described as extending from 3 o'clock to 4 o'clock. A large area is usually described as undermining. The size should be measured or estimated as closely as possible.

47

DISTRIBUTION, DRAINAGE, AND ODOR

Distribution of lesions should be clearly delineated if there is more than one lesion over an area. The arrangement of the lesions can be helpful for diagnosis and treatments.

- Linear (in a line)
- Satellites (small lesions around a larger one)
- Diffuse (scattered freely over an area)

Drainage may vary considerably from nothing at all to copious outpourings of discharge.

- Serous drainage is usually clear to slightly yellow.
- Serosanguineous drainage is a combination of serous drainage and blood.
- Sanguineous drainage is bloody.
- Purulent discharge may be thick and milky, yellow, brownish, or green, depending upon the infective agent.

Odor requires more subjective assessment, but the odor and type of discharge together can provide useful information. Some infective agents, such as *Pseudomonas*, produce distinctive odors, which may be described in various ways: musty, foul, sweet.

ASSESSMENT CHARACTERISTICS OF ARTERIAL, NEUROPATHIC, AND VENOUS ULCERS

The assessment process is important in delineating between the arterial, neuropathic, or venous origin of the ulcer. Characteristics of each must be known and closely examined:

Location

- **Arterial**: Ends of toes, pressure points, traumatic nonhealing wounds
- **Neuropathic**: Plantar surface, metatarsal heads, toes, and sides of feet
- **Venous**: Between knees and ankles, medial malleolus

Wound Bed

- **Arterial**: Pale, necrotic
- **Neuropathic**: Red (or ischemic)
- **Venous**: Dark red, fibrinous slough

Exudate

- **Arterial**: Slight amount, infection common
- **Neuropathic**: Moderate to large amounts, infection common
- **Venous**: Moderate to large amounts

Wound Perimeter

- **Arterial**: Circular, well-defined
- **Neuropathic**: Circular, well-defined, often with callous formation
- **Venous**: Irregular, poorly-defined

Pain

- **Arterial**: Very painful
- **Neuropathic**: Pain often absent because of reduced sensation
- **Venous**: Pain varies

Skin

- **Arterial**: Pale, friable, shiny, and hairless, with dependent rubor and elevational pallor
- **Neuropathic**: Ischemic signs (as in arterial) may be evident with comorbidity
- **Venous**: Brownish discoloration of ankles and shin, edema common

Pulses

- **Arterial**: Weak or absent
- **Neuropathic**: Present and palpable, diminished in neuroischemic ulcers
- **Venous**: Present and palpable

Pain Assessment

PATHOPHYSIOLOGY OF PAIN

NOCICEPTORS

Nociceptors are the primary neurons, or **sensory receptors**, responding to stimuli in the skin, muscle, and joints, as well as the stomach, bladder, and uterus. These neurons have specialized responses for mechanical, thermal, or chemical stimuli. The **neuron stimulation** is a direct result of tissue injury and follows four stages: **transduction** where a change occurs, **transmission** where the impulse is transferred along the neural path, **modulation** or translation of the signal, and **perception** by the patient. When injury occurs, the nociceptors initiate the process that begins **depolarization of the peripheral nerve**. Nociceptors may consist of either A-fiber axons or C-fiber axons. The message travels along the neural pathway and creates a perception of pain. A-fiber axons carry these pain messages at a much faster rate than C-fiber axons.

NOCICEPTIVE PAIN

Nociceptive pain is an umbrella term for pain caused by **stimulation of the neuroreceptor**. This stimulation is a direct result of tissue injury. The severity of pain is proportionate to the extent of the injury. Nociceptive pain can be subdivided into two classifications: somatic and visceral pain. **Somatic pain** is located in the cutaneous tissues, bone joints, and muscle tissues. **Visceral pain** is specific to internal organs protected by a layer of viscera, such as the cardiovascular, respiratory, gastrointestinal, or genitourinary systems. Both types are treatable with opioids.

VISCERAL PAIN

Visceral pain is associated with the internal organs. It can be very different depending on the affected organ. Not all internal organs are sensitive to pain (some lack **nociceptors**, such as the spleen, kidney, and pancreas), and may withstand a great deal of damage without causing pain. Other internal organs, such as the stomach, bladder, and ureters, can create significant pain from even the slightest damage. Visceral pain generally has a **poorly defined area**. It is also capable of referring pain to other remote locations away from the area of injury. It is described as a squeezing or cramping: a deep ache within the internal organs. The patient may complain of a generalized sick feeling or have nausea and vomiting. Visceral pain generally responds well to treatment with **opioids**.

SOMATIC PAIN

Somatic pain refers to messages from pain receptors located in the **cutaneous or musculoskeletal tissues**. When the pain occurs within the musculoskeletal tissue, it is referred to as **deep somatic pain**. Metastasizing cancers commonly cause deep somatic pain. **Surface pain** refers to pain concentrated in the **dermis and cutaneous layers** such as that caused by a surgical incision. Deep somatic pain is generally described as a dull, throbbing ache that is well focused on the area of trauma. It responds well to **opioids**. Surface somatic pain is also directly focused on the injury. It is frequently described as sharper than deep somatic pain. It may also present as a burning or pricking sensation.

NEUROPATHIC PAIN

Neuropathic pain results from injury to the **nervous system**. This can result from cancer cells compressing the nerves or spinal cord, from actual cancerous invasion into the nerves or spinal cord, or from chemical damage to the nerves caused by chemotherapy and radiation. Other causes include diabetes- and alcohol-related damage, trauma, neuralgias, or other illnesses affecting the neural path either centrally or peripherally. When the nerves become damaged, they are unable to carry accurate information. This results in more severe, distinct **pain messages**. The nerves may also relay pain messages long after the original cause of the pain is resolved. It can be described as sharp, burning, shooting, shocking, tingling, or electrical in nature. It may travel the length of the nerve path from the spine to a distal body part such as a hand, or down the buttocks to a foot. NSAIDs and opioids are generally ineffective against neuropathic pain, though adjuvants may enhance the therapeutic effect of opioids. Nerve blocks may also be used.

ADVERSE SYSTEMIC EFFECTS OF PAIN

Acute pain causes adverse systemic effects that can negatively affect many body systems.

- **Cardiovascular**: Tachycardia and increased blood pressure is a common response to pain, causing increased cardiac output and systemic vascular resistance. In those with pre-existing cardiovascular disease, such as compromised ventricular function, cardiac output may decrease. The increased myocardial need for oxygen may cause or worsen myocardial ischemia.
- **Respiratory**: Increased need for oxygen causes an increase in minute ventilation and splinting due to pain, which may compromise pulmonary function. If the chest wall movement is constrained, tidal volume falls, impairing the ability to cough and clear secretions. Bed rest further compromises ventilation.
- **Gastrointestinal**: Sphincter tone increases and motility decreases, sometimes resulting in ileus. There may be an increased secretion of gastric acids, which irritates the gastric lining and can cause ulcerations. Nausea, vomiting, and constipation may occur. Reflux may result in aspiration pneumonia. Abdominal distension may occur.
- **Urinary**: Increased sphincter tone and decreased motility result in urinary retention.
- **Endocrine**: Hormone levels are affected by pain. Catabolic hormones such as catecholamine, cortisol, and glucagon increase, and anabolic hormones such as insulin and testosterone decrease. Lipolysis increases along with carbohydrate intolerance. Sodium retention can occur because of increased ADH, aldosterone, angiotensin, and cortisol. This in turn causes fluid retention and a shift to extracellular space.
- **Hematologic**: There may be reduced fibrinolysis, increased adhesiveness of platelets, and increased coagulation.
- **Immune**: Leukocytosis and lymphopenia may occur, increasing risk of infection.
- **Emotional**: Patients may experience depression, anxiety, anger, decreased appetite, and sleep deprivation. This type of response is most common in those with chronic pain, who usually have different systemic responses from those with acute pain.

CORE PRINCIPLES OF PAIN ASSESSMENT AND MANAGEMENT

According to the Joint Commission, assessing pain should be a priority in patient care, and organizations must establish **policies** for assessment and treatment of pain and must educate staff members about these policies. The Joint Commission considers a **plan of care** regarding pain control an essential patient right. Hospitals should be consistent in the use of the same assessment tools throughout the organization, specific to different patient populations (for example, pediatrics and geriatrics). The latest standards (2018) of evidence-based practice include the following:

- Organizations must establish a clinical leadership team to oversee pain management and safe prescription of opioids.
- Patients must be involved in planning and setting goals and should receive education regarding safe use of opioid and non-opioid medications.
- Patients should be screened for pain in all assessments, including visits to the emergency department.
- Patients at high risk for opioid misuse or adverse effects must be identified and monitored.
- Healthcare providers should have access to prescription drug monitoring safety databases, such as the prescription databases provided by most states.
- Organizations must provide performance improvement educational programs regarding pain assessment and management and must collect and analyze data on its pain assessment and management.

AREAS ADDRESSED WHEN ASSESSING PAIN

Information concerning a patient's pain can be gathered from a variety of sources, including observations, interviews with the patient and family, medical records, and observations of other health care providers.

However, it is important to remember that each patient's pain is **subjective** and **personal**. Pain is defined as whatever the patient says it is. Having the patient give parameters of quality, location, duration, speed of onset, and intensity can all be beneficial in forming a treatment plan based on the patient's needs. Pain is also influenced by psychological, social, and spiritual factors. Behavioral, psychological, and subjective assessment information such as physical demeanor and vital signs can be helpful in further defining a patient's pain parameters.

PHYSICAL SIGNS OF PAIN

The best assessment of the patient's pain is **the patient's own report**. All other information is assessed as supporting this report. However, when this method is restricted or unavailable, **physical signs and symptoms** can help the nurse's assessment capabilities. It is important to be familiar with the patient's **baseline** or resting information to give a clear picture of the changes the body may go through when experiencing significant pain. Systolic blood pressure, heart rate, and respirations may all increase above the patient's normal parameters. Tightness or tension may be felt in major muscle groups. Posturing can also occur: the patient may guard areas of the body, curl themselves up into a fetal position, or hold only certain body portions rigid. Calling out, increased volume in speech, and moaning can also be indicators. Facial expressions, such as flat affect or grimacing, and distraction from their surroundings also indicate a significant increase in stressful stimuli.

IMPORTANCE OF PAIN ASSESSMENTS IN ADVANCED DISEASE

As many as 90% of all **advanced disease patients** will experience some level of pain. The hospice and palliative care philosophy focuses on the relief of pain and provision for comfort measures for all patients who desire it to improve quality of life. Each patient has the right to accept or refuse treatment for their pain. This becomes difficult when the patient is unable to **communicate** their desires and pain level. It can be assumed that if a patient was experiencing pain when able to communicate, they will continue to experience pain when the ability to communicate has been compromised—pain will be present even in an unconscious state. Changes from previous behavioral, psychological, and subjective and objective assessment data provide the supporting information for continued pain assessments in a nonverbal patient.

PAIN ASSESSMENT TOOLS
ABCDE MNEMONIC APPROACH TO PAIN ASSESSMENT

The Agency for Healthcare Policy and Research recommends use of the **ABCDE method** for assessing and managing pain:

- **Asking** the patient about the extent of pain and assessing systematically.
- **Believing** that the degree of pain the patient reports is accurate.
- **Choosing** the appropriate method of pain control for the patient and circumstances.
- **Delivering** pain interventions appropriately and in a timely, logical manner.
- **Empowering** patients and family by helping them to have control of the course of treatment.

The **5 key elements of pain assessment** include:

- **Quality**: Words are used to describe pain, such as *burning*, *stabbing*, *deep*, *shooting*, and *sharp*. Some may complain of pressure, squeezing, and discomfort rather than pain.
- **Intensity**: Use of a 0-10 scale or other appropriate scale to quantify the degree of pain.
- **Location**: Where does the patient indicate pain?
- **Duration**: Is it constant; does it come and go; is there breakthrough pain?
- **Aggravating/alleviating factors**: What increases the intensity of pain and what relieves the pain?

UNIDIMENSIONAL TOOLS FOR PAIN ASSESSMENT

Unidimensional tools for pain assessment focus on one aspect only: the patient's level of pain. Tools include:

- **Visual analog/numeric rating scale**: A 1-10 rating scale presented visually or verbally from which the patient chooses a number to describe the degree of pain the patient is experiencing. Zero represents no pain, 1 very mild pain, and 10 the most severe pain the patient can imagine.
- **Descriptive**: Pain is described in simple terms that a patient can choose from: mild, moderate, or severe. This may be especially helpful for patients from other countries or cultures where the 1-10 scale is not generally used.
- **FACES**: A chart shows a facial expression scale of simple drawings showing faces with different emotions, such as happiness, fear, and pain. Used primarily for children over age 3 and for nonverbal adults, although both a child's and an adult's version are available. A revised version applies numeric values to expressions so that pain can be assessed according to a numeric rating scale as well.

> **Review Video: How to Accurately Assess Pain**
> Visit mometrix.com/academy and enter code: 693250
>
> **Review Video: Assessment Tools for Pain**
> Visit mometrix.com/academy and enter code: 634001

MULTIDIMENSIONAL TOOLS FOR PAIN ASSESSMENT

Multidimensional tools used for pain assessment include:

- **Multidimensional pain inventory**: The patient begins by identifying a significant other and then answering 20 questions (rating scale 0-6) about the current rate of pain, the degree of interference in daily life, the ability to work, satisfaction from social/recreational activities, support level of the significant other, mood, pain during the previous week, changes brought about by pain, concerns of the significant other, ability to deal with pain, irritability, and anxiety.
- **Brief pain inventory**: Patients are assessed on the severity of pain (on a 1-10 scale), location of pain, impact of pain on daily function, pain medication, and amount of pain relief in the past 24 hours or the past week. They are asked if the pain interferes with general activity, walking, normal work, mood, interpersonal relations, sleep, or enjoyment of life.
- **McGill pain questionnaire**: The patient marks areas of internal and external pain on body diagrams and selects appropriate adjectives for 20 different sections regarding sensory, affective, and evaluative perceptions. For example, the questionnaire allows the patient to indicate if the pain is "flickering, quivering, pulsing, throbbing, beating, or pounding." The patient also rates present pain intensity (PPI) from 0 (none) to 5 (excruciating).

ASSESSMENT TOOLS FOR COGNITIVELY IMPAIRED OR NONVERBAL PATIENTS

The following are types of assessment tools available for use with cognitively impaired or nonverbal patients:

- **Discomfort Scale for Dementia of the Alzheimer Type (DS-DAT)**: For use with elderly persons experiencing dementia, decreased cognition, and decreased verbalization
- **Assessment of Discomfort in Dementia Protocol (ADD)**: Particularly designed for use with patients exhibiting difficult behaviors
- **Checklist of Nonverbal Pain Indicators (CNPI)**: Pain measurement with cognitive impairment
- **Noncommunicative Patient's Pain Assessment Instrument (NOPPAIN)**: Specifically for use by nursing assistants
- **Pain Assessment for the Dementing Elderly (PADE)**: Assessing physical pain behaviors
- **Pain Assessment Tool in Confused Older Adults (PATCOA)**: Focuses on the observation of nonverbal cues
- **Pain Assessment in Advanced Dementia (PAINAD)**: Adapted from the DS-DAT

- **Pain Assessment Checklist for Seniors with Limited Ability to Communicate (PACSLAC)**: To assess common and subtle symptoms
- **Abbey Pain Scale**: For late-stage dementia in nursing home environments

NEUROPATHIC PAIN SCALE

The neuropathic pain scale (NPS) is the first tool designed specifically to assess the types of pain associated with neuropathy. The NPS comprises 10 sections with 9 assessed with a 0 to 10 (not unpleasant to intolerable) scale:

- Intensity of pain
- Sharpness of pain
- Heat of pain
- Dullness of pain
- Coldness of pain
- Skin sensitivity to touch, clothing
- Itchiness
- Overall unpleasantness of pain
- Intensity of deep and surface pain

The 10th section asks for narrative descriptions of the **time quality** of pain. The patient chooses from three options:

- Feeling background pain all of the time with occasional flare-ups
- Feeling a single type of pain all the time
- Feeling a single type of pain sometimes while having some pain-free periods. The patient then is asked to describe the pain experienced

BARRIERS TO OPTIMAL PAIN ASSESSMENTS

Barriers to optimal pain assessments include:

- **Professional**: Health care providers may lack knowledge about pain assessment and management of different patient populations or may carry out assessments based on personal perceptions rather than validated pain assessment instruments. Some may be concerned about managing adverse effects or the patient's development of tolerance or addiction. In other cases, healthcare providers may lack empathy for patients' suffering. Lack of cultural awareness may affect interpretation of pain. For example, patients in cultures that encourage expression of pain may be assessed as having more pain than patients from cultures that value stoicism.
- **System**: The organization may lack clear policies regarding pain assessment and management, and may not have established clear guidelines for consistent use of pain assessment instruments. Additionally, supervision and accountability may be inadequate, and the organization may be concerned about costs and reimbursement for treatment.
- **Patient**: For personal or cultural reasons, patients may minimize or overstate the degree of pain, interfering with assessment. Some patients may be concerned about addiction or the effects of drugs on cognition (confusion, disorientation, lethargy) or other side effects (constipation, nausea, itching). Some may want to protect family from knowing the extent of pain.
- **Family**: Cultural biases may influence how the family responds to a patient's pain, and this can influence the patient's response as well. Families may lack understanding of the role of pain assessment and management. Some lack understanding about the difference between addiction and pain control at the end of life.
- **Society**: Concerns about drug abuse and addiction often permeate society and influence societal attitudes toward pain control and appropriate drugs to use. Laws and regulations may make access to certain drugs, such as those derived from marijuana, difficult or impossible to obtain.

INFLUENTIAL FACTORS IN PAIN PERCEPTION

Factors that can influence the perception of pain include:

- **Emotional state/Attitude**: Patients who are extremely upset or anxious may be so overwhelmed they don't feel the pain, or they may experience pain as more severe than those who are relaxed and calm. If patients expect to suffer from pain, they are also more likely to report severe pain than patients who expect that their pain will be controlled.
- **Cultural expectations**: Perception may vary according to cultural beliefs about pain. For example, if a patient believes that pain is punishment, the patient may agonize over past sins. If a patient believes that pain is fate and reflects karma, then the patient may feel that bearing pain is necessary.
- **Pain threshold**: Different patients simply perceive and experience pain to different degrees. What may be a minor pain to one individual may be severe to another.

EFFECTS OF GENDER ON PAIN EXPERIENCE

Gender can affect pain sensitivity, tolerance, distress, and exaggeration of pain, and the patient's willingness to report pain, as well as displayed nonverbal cues concerning the pain experience. Studies indicate that women generally have **lower pain thresholds** and **less tolerance** for noxious stimuli or pain factors that hinder them from doing things they enjoy. Women seek help for pain-related problems sooner than men and respond better to therapy. Women also experience more **visceral pain** than men. Men are more prone to experience **somatic pain** and show more stoicism regarding pain experiences than women. **Neuropathic pain** seems to be experienced equally between men and women. Nurses need to be careful that biases concerning gender experiences with pain do not skew their assessments of pain. However, they need to be aware that pain experiences are always individual and may differ between the sexes.

CULTURAL CONSIDERATIONS FOR PAIN MANAGEMENT

The following are cultural considerations for pain management:

- **American Indian** and **Alaskan natives** may be unwilling to show pain or request medications. Pain is a difficulty that must be endured rather than treated.
- **Asian and Pacific Islanders** may not vocalize pain and may have an interest in pursuing nontraditional and nonpharmacological treatments to help relieve pain.
- **Black and African American** cultures may tend to openly express their pain but still believe that it is to be endured. They may avoid medication because of personal fears of addiction or cultural stigmatism.
- **Hispanic cultures** may value the ability to endure pain and suffering as a personal quality of strength. Expression of pain, especially for a male, may be considered a sign of weakness. They may feel that pain is a form of divine punishment or trial.

PSYCHOLOGICAL FACTORS IN EXPERIENCE OF PAIN

Psychological factors that may influence a patient's experience of pain include:

- **Fear**: The fear of pain and the anticipation of having pain are factors in how much pain a person feels, because the fear stimulates areas of the brain that focus attention on the body so that the patient experiences an increased sensation of pain. Fear also causes muscles to tense, blood pressure to increase, and the heart rate to increase, and all of these can exacerbate the perception of pain. While pain medications may be necessary, practicing relaxation and mindfulness exercises may help to reduce anxiety and have a positive effect.
- **Depression**: The same neurotransmitters that transmit sensations of pain are also those that transmit moods, so many people with depression present first with complaints of pain or discomfort, and this can result in chronic pain if the depression is not resolved. In some cases, pain may lead to depression, but then the depression worsens the pain so it becomes a cycle of worsening discomfort. Patients may benefit from cognitive behavioral therapy or medication such as SSRIs.

55

PAIN DOCUMENTATION IN MEDICAL RECORDS

Recommendations for **pain documentation** in the medical record include:

- Describe the time of onset, the location of pain, the character of the pain, and the degree of pain, using a validated pain assessment instrument (either a self-reporting instrument, such as the visual analog scale, or one based on observation, such as PAINAD).
- Document all interventions, both pharmacological (opioids, adjuvants) and nonpharmacological (positioning, massage, relaxation exercises), including the time, the dosage, and the method of administration.
- Assess and document the initial response to the medication based on the expected response time. For example, an IV medication should take effect almost immediately, but oral medications may take up to 20 minutes to take effect.
- Assess and document the duration of response based on the expected duration of the medication. For example, if a medication response is expected to last for 6 hours, the patient's pain level should be assessed at least every 2 hours and more frequently if the rate of pain increases.
- Describe any adverse effects, such as itching or nausea.

Geriatric Assessment

AGE CATEGORIES OF THE ELDERLY

The elderly population can be divided into three groups. The age group ranging from 65-74 years are considered the **young-old**, from 75-84 are considered the **middle-old**, and 85 and older are considered **old-old**. There are many physical and psychological changes that occur as someone moves through these age groups. As this population increases in size, so does the number of those with physical and mental illnesses.

FACTORS THAT INFLUENCE PRESENTATION OF ILLNESS IN OLDER ADULTS

There are three major factors that influence **how an illness will present in an older patient**. These factors, either alone or in combination with one another, have the potential to make an ordinarily standard clinical presentation confusing for the clinician.

- The first of these factors is **underreporting of illness or the symptoms associated** with illness. There are a number of reasons that illnesses are not reported: the patient may fear hospitalization, institutionalization, or loss of control, or the patient may be convinced that there really is no problem.
- Another factor is the **pattern of distribution of illness** amongst the elderly population. This affects presentation because there are a number of diseases and problems that are prevalent among older adults, including congestive heart failure, arthritis, osteoporosis, and pneumonia; therefore, identifying and differentiating the primary diagnosis may be difficult.
- The last factor is an **altered response to illness**. This can make diagnosis and treatment very difficult because symptoms may be exaggerated by other problems, or they may be nonexistent.

AGE-RELATED CONSIDERATIONS WHEN EVALUATING ADULT PATIENTS

Because each individual patient is exposed to different environmental, psychological, and physical stressors that can affect the aging process, it is important to consider that some patients may experience adverse health problems, while other patients of the same age may not be affected. As individuals age, the amount of wear on the body, as well as the likelihood of pathological changes, increases at different rates for every individual. Factors affecting the aging process include proper nutrition (or the lack thereof), level of physical activity, smoking, alcohol consumption, environmental or occupational exposures, and socioeconomic standing. Also, remember that as an individual ages, a disease or problems with one organ or organ system will have a marked effect on other systems, because the body is not able to compensate as it once was. Symptoms may not be noticeable until other functions begin to decline. Most often, health issues manifest in the elderly as confusion, so close attention must be given to this symptom and investigated when present.

BASIC PATIENT SAFETY ASSESSMENTS WHEN EVALUATING A PATIENT

There are four basic assessments that the nurse should make when **assessing a patient's safety** and identifying possible safety concerns:

- The first of these is the **mobility assessment**; different safety risks apply to patients who are mobile as opposed to those who are not. An immobile patient, for example, has a tendency to form pressure ulcers, or bedsores.
- The next assessment is the evaluation of the patient's **level of awareness**; is the patient able to communicate to the nursing staff when something is wrong? If not, certain measures should be undertaken to ensure that the nursing staff is aware of a change in the patient's condition.
- An extension of this assessment is determining whether the patient is in **critical condition**; these patients must be monitored more closely for changes.
- An assessment of the patient's **mental status** is also important because the patient may not be able to make safe decisions on his or her own.

FUNCTIONAL EVALUATION OF ELDERLY PATIENT

A functional evaluation of the elderly patient examines the patient's ability to carry out activities of daily living (ADL) that are critical in gauging the patient's ability to care for oneself without the need of assistance. Use the **Index of Independence in Activities of Daily Living Scale** to check foundational tasks such as taking a shower, getting dressed, eating, and going to the bathroom. Aged patients will be more likely to overstate what they are able to do and understate their limitations, while the patient's family will likely understate what the patient is able to handle. Assess mental ability with the following exams:

- Short Portable Mental Status Questionnaire (SPMSQ)
- Mini-Mental State Exam (MMSE)

The **Tinetti Balance and Gait Evaluation** exams are also important elements of the functional evaluation of an elderly patient. These tests, along with the simple **Up-and-Go test,** are used to assess the balance and gait issues that elderly patients have. The patient has to complete certain actions, such as sitting down and standing up from a chair, turning around, bending over, etc. The entire assessment takes approximately 15–20 minutes. The **Lawton and Brody: Instrumental Activities of Daily Learning** test is used to check whether the patient can do more complex activities important to daily living, second to the ADL's required for basic function. Examples of IADLs include the ability to go shopping, wash clothes, cook, etc. The **Index of Independence of Activities of Daily Living** is utilized to find what the patient is able do independently on a regular basis.

DEPRESSION AND SUICIDE IN THE ELDERLY

Depression commonly goes unidentified in an aging patient. Cognitive changes are often wrongly identified as dementia, confusion, or natural aging changes, rather than depression. It is important to be cognizant of the prevalence of this issue among the elderly, and treat appropriately.

Suicide rates for elderly patients are higher than any other age group. The compounding stress and emotional burden of losing loved ones, mobility, and independence often contribute to suicidal ideations. Other factors include seemingly unbearable psychological anguish, dissatisfaction, and unmet requirements. Suicide is more commonly seen in elderly males (seven times higher rate), Caucasians, unmarried individuals (divorced, separated, single), individuals who are poor and/or out of work, individuals with mental problems, the very sick, individuals with substance additions, individuals that are grieving (particularly in the first year of loss or retirement), those without friends or community relationships, or those who have tried suicide before. Suicidal thoughts and attempts may be overt or covert.

As with patients of other age ranges, if an elderly patient hints at suicidal ideations or thoughts, this must be addressed directly by the nurse.

INDICATIONS AND ASSESSMENTS FOR DELIRIUM

Delirium (acute confusion) presents in a variety of indications. The patient may experience mental issues, including inattention or short attention span, difficulty remembering, trouble with perception, bafflement, and lack of decision-making. There may be changing moods, faulty ability to manage whims, stress, slight to moderate depression, visual or auditory hallucinations, confabulation, changing intellectual ability that worsens at night (sun-downing) and is more frequently seen in patients that have had prior dementia, psychomotor agitation including inability to sleep, tachycardia, enlarged pupils, and perspiration. The patient may appear restless, overcautious, not cautious enough, or appear lost/stunned. There may be tachycardia, high blood pressure, fever, rapid breathing, and there might be focal neurological indications.

Physical assessments include a complete history, physical examination, check of mind and neurological issues to determine what is causing the problem, foundation of lab work such as CBC, electrocardiogram, chest radiograph, urinalysis, urine toxicology, and other assessments that are deemed necessary, such as EED, CT, or blood work for drugs.

Psychological Assessment

ELEMENTS OF THE PSYCHOSOCIAL ASSESSMENT

A psychosocial assessment should provide additional information to the physical assessment to guide the patient's plan of care and should include:

- Previous hospitalizations and experience with healthcare
- Psychiatric history: Suicidal ideation, psychiatric disorders, family psychiatric history, history of violence and/or self-mutilation
- Chief complaint: Patient's perception
- Complementary therapies: Acupuncture, visualization, and meditation
- Occupational and educational background: Employment, retirement, and special skills
- Social patterns: Family and friends, living situation, typical activities, support system
- Sexual patterns: Orientation, problems, and sex practices
- Interests/abilities: Hobbies and sports
- Current or past substance abuse: Type, frequency, drinking pattern, use of recreational drugs, and overuse of prescription drugs
- Ability to cope: Stress reduction techniques
- Physical, sexual, emotional, and financial abuse: Older adults are especially vulnerable to abuse and may be reluctant to disclose out of shame or fear
- Spiritual/Cultural assessment: Religious/Spiritual importance, practices, restrictions (such as blood products or foods), and impact on health/health decisions

COGNITIVE ASSESSMENT

Individuals with evidence of dementia, delirium, or short-term memory loss should have cognition assessed. The **mini-mental state exam (MMSE)** or the **mini-cog test** are both commonly used. These tests require the individual to carry out specified tasks and are used as a baseline to determine change in mental status.

MMSE:

- Remembering and later repeating the names of 3 common objects
- Counting backward from 100 by 7s or spelling "world" backward
- Naming items as the examiner points to them
- Providing the location of the examiner's office, including city, state, and street address
- Repeating common phrases
- Copying a picture of interlocking shapes
- Following simple 3-part instructions, such as picking up a piece of paper, folding it in half, and placing it on the floor

A score of ≥24/30 is considered a normal functioning level.

Mini-cog:

- Remembering and later repeating the names of 3 common objects
- Drawing the face of a clock, including all 12 numbers and the hands, and indicating the time specified by the examiner

A score of 3-5 (out of 5) indicates a lower chance of dementia but does not rule it out.

CONFUSION ASSESSMENT METHOD

The Confusion Assessment Method is an assessment tool intended to be used by those without psychiatric training in order to assess the progression of delirium in patients. The tool covers 9 factors, some factors have a range of possibilities, and others are rated only as to whether the characteristic is present, not present, uncertain, or not applicable. The tool also provides room to describe abnormal behavior. Factors indicative of delirium include:

- **Onset**: Acute change in mental status
- **Attention**: Inattentive, stable, or fluctuating
- **Thinking**: Disorganized, rambling conversation, switching topics, illogical
- **Level of consciousness**: Altered, ranging from alert to coma
- **Orientation**: Disoriented (person, place, and time)
- **Memory**: Impaired
- **Perceptual disturbances**: Hallucinations, illusions
- **Psychomotor abnormalities**: Agitation (tapping, picking, moving) or retardation (staring, not moving)
- **Sleep-wake cycle**: Awake at night and sleepy in the daytime

The Confusion Assessment Method indicates delirium if there is an acute onset, fluctuating inattention, and disorganized thinking OR altered level of consciousness.

HAMILTON ANXIETY SCALE

The Hamilton Anxiety Scale (HAS or HAMA) is utilized to evaluate the anxiety related symptomatology that may be present in adults as well as children. It provides an evaluation of overall **anxiety** and its degree of severity. This includes **somatic anxiety** (physical complaints) and **psychic anxiety** (mental agitation and distress). This scale consists of 14 items based on anxiety produced symptoms. Each item is ranked 0-4 with 0 indicating no symptoms present and 4 indicating severe symptoms present. This scale is frequently utilized in psychotropic drug evaluations. If performed before a particular medication has been started and then again at later visits, the HAS can be helpful in adjusting medication dosages based in part on the individual's score. It is often utilized as an outcome measure in clinical trials.

BECK DEPRESSION INVENTORY

The Beck Depression Inventory (BDI) is a widely utilized, self-reported, multiple-choice questionnaire consisting of 21 items, which measures the **degree of depression**. This tool is designed for use in adults ages 17-80. It evaluates physical symptoms such as weight loss, loss of sleep, loss of interest in sex, fatigue, and attitudinal symptoms such as irritability, guilt, and hopelessness. The items rank in four possible answer choices based on an increasing severity of symptoms. The test is scored with the answers ranging in value from 0 to 3. The total score is utilized to determine the degree of depression. The usual ranges include: 0-9 no signs of depression, 10-18 mild depression, 19-29 moderate depression, and 30-63 severe depression.

EVALUATION FOR SUICIDAL OR HOMICIDAL THOUGHTS

During a risk assessment two of the most important areas to evaluate are the patient's **risk for self-harm or harm to others**. The staff member performing the assessment should very closely evaluate for any descriptions or thoughts the patient may have concerning these risks. Direct questioning on these subjects should be performed and documented. Close evaluation of any delusional thoughts the patient may be having should be carefully evaluated. Does the patient believe he or she is being instructed by others to perform either of these acts? Safety of the patient and others needs to be a top priority and carefully documented. If the patient indicates that they are having these thoughts or ideas, they must be placed in either suicidal or assault precautions with close monitoring per facility protocol.

SUICIDE RISK ASSESSMENT

A suicide risk assessment should be completed and documented upon admission, with each shift change, at discharge, or any time suicidal ideations are suggested by the patient. This risk assessment should evaluate some of the following criteria:

- Would the patient sign a contract for safety?
- Is there a suicide plan? How lethal is the plan?
- What is the elopement risk?
- How often are the suicidal thoughts, and have they attempted suicide before?

Any associated symptoms of hopelessness, guilt, anger, helplessness, impulsive behaviors, nightmares, obsessions with death, or altered judgment should also be assessed and documented. The higher the score the higher the risk for suicide.

ALCOHOL USE ASSESSMENT

The **Clinical Instrument for Withdrawal for Alcohol (CIWA)** is a tool used to assess the severity of alcohol withdraw. Each category is scored 0-7 points based on the severity of symptoms, except #10, which is scored 0-4. A score <5 indicates mild withdrawal without need for medications; for scores ranging 5-15, benzodiazepines are indicated to manage symptoms. A score >15 indicates severe withdrawal and the need for admission to the unit.

1. Nausea/Vomiting
2. Tremor
3. Paroxysmal Sweats
4. Anxiety
5. Agitation
6. Tactile Disturbances
7. Auditory Disturbances
8. Visual Disturbances
9. Headache
10. Disorientation or Clouding of Sensorium

The **CAGE** tool is used as a quick assessment to identify problem drinkers. Moderate drinking, (1-2 drinks daily or one drink a day for older adults) is usually not harmful to people in the absence of other medical conditions. However, drinking more can lead to serious psychosocial and physical problems. One drink is defined as 12 ounces of beer/wine cooler, 5 ounces of wine, or 1.5 ounces of liquor.

- **C** – *Cutting Down*: "Do you think about trying to cut down on drinking?"
- **A** – *Annoyed at Criticism*: "Are people starting to criticize your drinking?"
- **G** – *Guilty feeling*: "Do you feel guilty or try to hide your drinking?"
- **E** – *Eye opener*: "Do you increasingly need a drink earlier in the day?"

"Yes" on one question suggests the possibility of a drinking problem. "Yes" on ≥2 indicates a drinking problem

SCREENING FOR RISK-TAKING BEHAVIOR

The ability to assess outcomes and respond appropriately to risks are part of the decision-making process. Decision making can be impaired in patients with mental health disorders such as depression, anxiety, bipolar disorder, and personality disorders, as well as in patients who have experienced a brain injury or have a dependence on drugs or alcohol. Health care providers should screen patients for the presence of high-risk behaviors. This may be accomplished through a self-administered questionnaire or through a patient interview with a trained clinician. Examples of **high-risk behaviors** include substance use/abuse, high risk sexual behaviors, high risk driving behaviors such as drinking and driving, speeding or riding with a drunk driver, and violence related behaviors. Patients with an increased response to risk taking may exhibit signs of impulsivity and sensation seeking. Conversely, other patients may exhibit abnormally cautious behavior.

ASSESSMENT OF UNIQUE NEEDS OF VETERANS

Assessment of **veterans** must include not only the standard assessments appropriate for the patient's age and gender but also assessment of combat-associated injuries and illnesses:

- Shrapnel and/or gunshot injuries: Associated physical limitations, pain
- Amputations: Mobility and prosthesis issues; body image issues
- PTSD: Extent, frequency of attacks, limiting factors, triggers
- Depression, suicidal ideation
- Substance abuse: Type and extent

Because a large number of veterans are among the homeless population, the veteran's living arrangements should be explored and appropriate referrals made if the patient is in need of housing. Veterans may be unaware of programs offered through the US Department of Veterans Affairs and should be provided information about these programs as appropriate for the patient's needs.

Abuse and Neglect

INDICATORS OF ABUSE THAT MAY BE IDENTIFIED IN THE PATIENT HISTORY

The healthcare provider should always be aware of the presence of any **indicators** that may present a potential for or an actual situation that involves **abuse**. These indicators may present in the **patient's history**. Some examples of indicators concerning their primary complaint may include the following: vague description about the cause of the problem, inconsistencies between physical findings and explanations, minimizing injuries, long period of time between injury and treatment, and over-reactions or under-reactions of family members to injuries. Other important information may be revealed in the family genome, such as family history of violence, time spent in jail or prison, and family history of violent deaths or substance abuse. The patient's health history may include previous injuries, spontaneous abortions, or history of pervious inpatient psychiatric treatment or substance abuse.

During the collection of the patient history, the financial history, the patient's family values, and the patient's relationships with family members can also reveal actual or potential **abuse indicators**.

- The **financial history** may indicate that the patient has little or no money or that they are not given access to money by a controlling family member. They may also be unemployed or utilizing an elderly family member's income for their own personal expenses.
- **Family values** may indicate strong beliefs in physical punishment, dictatorship within the home, inability to allow different opinions within the home, or lack of trust for anyone outside the family.
- **Relationships** within the family may be dysfunctional. Problems such as lack of affection between family members, co-dependency, frequent arguments, extramarital affairs, or extremely rigid beliefs about roles within the family may be present.

During the collection of the patient history, the sexual, social, and psychological history of the patient should be evaluated for any signs of actual or potential abuse.

- The **sexual history** may reveal problems such as previous sexual abuse, forced sexual acts, sexually transmitted infections (STIs), sexual knowledge beyond normal age-appropriate knowledge, or promiscuity.
- The **social history** may reveal unplanned pregnancies, social isolation as evidenced by lack of friends available to help the patient, unreasonable jealousy of significant other, verbal aggression, belief in physical punishment, or problems in school.
- During the **psychological assessment** the patient may express feelings of helplessness and being trapped. The patient may be unable to describe their future, become tearful, perform self-mutilation, have low self-esteem, and have had previous suicide attempts.

OBSERVATIONS THAT MAY INDICATE ABUSE

During the initial assessment, observations may also be made by the provider that can provide vital information about actual or potential abuse. **General observations** may include finding that the patient history is far different from what is objectively viewed by the provider or that there is a lack of proper clothing or lack of physical care provided. The home environment may include lack of heat, water, or food. It may also reveal inappropriate sleeping arrangements or lack of an environmentally safe housing situation. Observations concerning **family communications** may reveal that the abuser answers all the questions for the whole family or that others look to the controlling member for approval or seem fearful of others. Family members may frequently argue, interrupt each other, or act out negative nonverbal behaviors while others are speaking. They may avoid talking about certain subjects that they feel are secretive.

INDICATORS OF ABUSE THAT MAY BE EVIDENT DURING THE PHYSICAL ASSESSMENT

During the **physical assessment** the provider should always be aware of any **indicators of abuse**. These indicators may include increased anxiety about being examined or in the presence of the abuser; poor hygiene;

looks to abuser to answer questions for them; flinching; over or underweight; presence of bruises, welts, scars or cigarette burns; bald patches on scalp for pulling out of hair; intracranial bleeding; subconjunctival hemorrhages; black eye(s); hearing loss from untreated infection or injury; poor dental hygiene; abdominal injuries; fractures; developmental delays; hyperactive reflexes; genital lacerations or ecchymosis; and presence of STIs, rectal bruising, bleeding, edema, or poor sphincter tone.

DOMESTIC VIOLENCE

Men, women, elderly, children, and the disabled may all be victims of **domestic violence**. The violent person harms physically or sexually and uses threats and fear to maintain control of the victim. The violence does not improve unless the abuser gets intensive counseling. The abuser may promise not to do it again, but the violence usually gets more frequent and worsens over time. The provider should ask all patients in private about abuse, neglect, and fear of a caretaker. If abuse is suspected or there are signs present, the state may require **reporting**:

- Give victims information about community hotlines, shelters, and resources.
- Urge them to set up a plan for escape for themselves and any children, complete with supplies in a location away from the home.
- Assure victims that they are not at fault and do not deserve the abuse.
- Try to empower them by helping them to realize that they do not have to take abuse and can find support to change the situation.

ASSESSMENT OF DOMESTIC VIOLENCE

According to the guidelines of the Family Violence Prevention Fund, **assessment** for domestic violence should be done for all adolescent and adult patients, regardless of background or signs of abuse. While females are the most common victims, there are increasing reports of male victims of domestic violence, both in heterosexual and homosexual relationships. The person doing the assessment should be informed about domestic violence and be aware of risk factors and danger signs. The interview should be conducted in private (special accommodations may need to be made for children <3 years old). The manager's office, bathrooms, and examining rooms should have information about domestic violence posted prominently. Brochures and information should be available to give to patients. Patients may present with a variety of physical complaints, such as headache, pain, palpitations, numbness, or pelvic pain. They are often depressed and may appear suicidal and may be isolated from friends and family. Victims of domestic violence often exhibit fear of spouse/partner, and may report injury inconsistent with symptoms.

STEPS TO IDENTIFYING VICTIMS OF DOMESTIC VIOLENCE

The **Family Violence Prevention Fund** has issued guidelines for identifying and assisting victims of domestic violence. There are 7 steps:

1. **Inquiry**: Non-judgmental questioning should begin with asking if the person has ever been abused—physically, sexually, or psychologically.
2. **Interview**: The person may exhibit signs of anxiety or fear and may blame himself or report that others believe he is abused. The person should be questioned if she is afraid for her life or for her children.
3. **Question**: If the person reports abuse, it's critical to ask if the person is in immediate danger or if the abuser is on the premises. The interviewer should ask if the person has been threatened. The history and pattern of abuse should be questioned, and if children are involved, whether the children are abused. Note: State laws vary, and in some states, it is mandatory to report if a child was present during an act of domestic violence as this is considered child abuse. The provider must be aware of state laws regarding domestic and child abuse, and all healthcare providers are mandatory reporters.
4. **Validate**: The interviewer should offer support and reassurance in a non-judgmental manner, telling the patient the abuse is not his or her fault.

5. **Give information**: While discussing facts about domestic violence and the tendency to escalate, the interviewer should provide brochures and information about safety planning. If the patient wants to file a complaint with the police, the interviewer should assist the person to place the call.
6. **Make referrals**: Information about state, local, and national organizations should be provided along with telephone numbers and contact numbers for domestic violence shelters.
7. **Document**: Record keeping should be legal, legible, and lengthy with a complete report and description of any traumatic injuries resulting from domestic violence. A body map may be used to indicate sites of injury, especially if there are multiple bruises or injuries.

INJURIES CONSISTENT WITH DOMESTIC VIOLENCE

There are a number of characteristic **injuries** that may indicate domestic violence, including ruptured eardrum; rectal/genital injury (burns, bites, or trauma); scrapes and bruises about the neck, face, head, trunk, arms; and cuts, bruises, and fractures of the face. The pattern of injuries associated with domestic violence is also often distinctive. The bathing-suit pattern involves injuries on parts of body that are usually covered with clothing as the perpetrator inflicts damage but hides evidence of abuse. Head and neck injuries (50%) are also common. Abusive injuries (rarely attributable to accidents) are common and include bites, bruises, rope and cigarette burns, and welts in the outline of weapons (belt marks). Bilateral injuries of arms/legs are often seen with domestic abuse. Defensive injuries are indicative of abuse.

Defensive injuries to the back of the body are often incurred as the victim crouches on the floor face down while being attacked. The soles of the feet may be injured from kicking at perpetrator. The ulnar aspect of hand or palm may be injured from blocking blows.

IDENTIFYING AND REPORTING NEGLECT OF THE BASIC NEEDS OF ADULTS

Neglect of the basic needs of adults is a common problem, especially among the elderly, adults with psychiatric or mental health problems, or those who live alone or with reluctant or incapable caregivers. In some cases, **passive neglect** may occur because an elderly or impaired spouse or partner is trying to take care of a patient and is unable to provide the care needed, but in other cases, **active neglect** reflects a lack of caring which may be considered negligence or abuse. Cases of neglect should be reported to the appropriate governmental agency, such as adult protective services. Indications of neglect include the following:

- Lack of assistive devices, such as a cane or walker, needed for mobility
- Misplaced or missing glasses or hearing aids
- Poor dental hygiene and dental care or missing dentures
- Patient left unattended for extended periods of time, sometimes confined to a bed or chair
- Patient left in soiled or urine- and feces-stained clothing
- Inadequate food, fluid, or nutrition, resulting in weight loss
- Inappropriate and unkempt clothing, such as no sweater or coat during the winter and dirty or torn clothing
- A dirty, messy environment

Fluids and Electrolytes

SODIUM

Sodium (**Na**) regulates fluid volume, osmolality, acid-base balance, and activity in the muscles, nerves, and myocardium. It is the primary **cation** (positive ion) in extracellular fluid (ECF), necessary to maintain ECF levels that are needed for tissue perfusion:

- Normal range: 135-145 mEq/L
- Hyponatremia: <135 mEq/L
- Hypernatremia: >145 mEq/L

Hyponatremia may result from inadequate sodium intake, excess sodium loss through diarrhea, vomiting, or NG suctioning, or illness, such as severe burns, fever, SIADH, and ketoacidosis.

- **Symptoms**: Irritability to lethargy and alterations in consciousness, cerebral edema with seizures and coma, dyspnea to respiratory failure.
- **Treatment**: Identify and treat the underlying cause and provide Na replacement.

Hypernatremia may result from renal disease, diabetes insipidus, and fluid depletion.

- **Symptoms**: Irritability to lethargy to confusion to coma; seizures; flushing; muscle weakness and spasms; thirst.
- **Treatment**: Identify and treat the underlying cause, monitor Na levels carefully, and give IV fluid replacement.

POTASSIUM

Potassium (**K**) is the primary **electrolyte** in intracellular fluid (ICF), with about 98% inside cells and only 2% in ECF, although this small amount is important for neuromuscular activity. Potassium influences activity of the skeletal and cardiac muscles. Its level is dependent upon adequate renal functioning because 80% is excreted through the kidneys and 20% through the bowels and sweat:

- Normal range: 3.5-5.5 mEq/L
- Hypokalemia: <3.5 mEq/L. Critical value: <2.5 mEq/L
- Hyperkalemia: >5.5 mEq/L. Critical value: >6.5 mEq/L

A healthy NPO patient will need about 40 mEq of K per day to maintain serum K levels. Expect alterations in renal disease and other disease processes.

Hypokalemia is caused by alkalosis, decreased intake associated with starvation, nephritis, and loss of potassium through diarrhea, vomiting, gastric suction, and diuresis.

- **Symptoms**: Lethargy and weakness; nausea and vomiting; paresthesia and tetany; muscle cramps with hyporeflexia; hypotension; dysrhythmias with EKG changes: PVCs or flattened T-waves.
- **Treatment**: Treatment involves identifying and treating the underlying cause and replacing K. When possible, oral replacement is preferable to IV, as it allows slower adjustment of K levels. When given IV, K should be given no faster than 20 mEq/hour via central line if possible. If given peripherally, 10 mEq/hour is preferable for patient comfort.

Hyperkalemia is caused by renal disease, adrenal insufficiency, metabolic acidosis, severe dehydration, burns, hemolysis, and trauma. It rarely occurs without renal disease but may be induced by treatment (such as NSAIDs and potassium-sparing diuretics). Untreated renal failure results in reduced excretion. Those with Addison's disease and deficient adrenal hormones suffer sodium loss that results in potassium retention.

- **Symptoms**: The primary symptoms relate to the effect on the cardiac muscle: ventricular arrhythmias with increasing changes in EKG lead to cardiac and respiratory arrest, weakness with ascending paralysis and hyperreflexia, diarrhea, and increasing confusion.
- **Treatment**: Treatment includes identifying the underlying cause and discontinuing sources of increased K. Calcium gluconate to decrease cardiac effects. Sodium bicarbonate, insulin, and hypertonic dextrose shift K into the cells temporarily. Cation exchange resin (Kayexalate) to decrease K. Peritoneal dialysis or hemodialysis to remove excess K.

Note: When a tourniquet is on, a patient opening and closing their hand can lead to falsely elevated K levels.

CALCIUM

More than 99% of calcium (**Ca**) is in the skeletal system with 1% in serum, but it is important for transmitting nerve impulses and regulating muscle contraction and relaxation, including the myocardium. Calcium activates enzymes that stimulate chemical reactions and has a role in the coagulation of blood:

- Normal range: 8.2-10.2 mg/dL
- Hypocalcemia: <8.2. Critical value: <7 mg/dL
- Hypercalcemia: >10.2 mg/dL. Critical value: >12 mg/dL

Hypercalcemia may be caused by acidosis, kidney disease, hyperparathyroidism, prolonged immobilization, and malignancies. Crisis carries a 50% mortality rate.

- **Symptoms**: Increasing muscle weakness with hypotonicity; anorexia; nausea and vomiting; constipation; bradycardia and cardiac arrest.
- **Treatment**: Identify and treat underlying cause, loop diuretics, IV fluids, phosphate.

Hypocalcemia may be caused by damage to the parathyroid resulting in hypoparathyroidism (directly decreasing calcium production), vitamin D resistance or inadequacy, or liver/kidney disease.

- **Symptoms**: Muscle cramping or spasms; seizures; numbness or tingling of the feet, hands, or lips; tetany if severe.
- **Treatment**: Identify and treat underlying cause, replace calcium by administering IV calcium gluconate in acute circumstances or increasing oral Vitamin D and calcium in chronic cases.

PHOSPHORUS

Phosphorus, or phosphate, (**PO_4**) is necessary for neuromuscular and red blood cell function, the maintenance of acid-base balance, and provides structure for teeth and bones. About 85% is in the bones, 14% in soft tissue, and <1% in ECF.

- Normal range: 2.4-4.5 mEq/L
- Hypophosphatemia: <2.4mEq/L
- Hyperphosphatemia: >4.5 mEq/L

Hypophosphatemia occurs with severe protein-calorie malnutrition, hyperventilation, severe burns, diabetic ketoacidosis, and excess antacids with magnesium, calcium, or aluminum.

- **Symptoms**: Irritability, tremors, seizures to coma; hemolytic anemia; decreased myocardial function; respiratory failure.
- **Treatment***: Identify and treat underlying cause and replace phosphorus.

Hyperphosphatemia occurs with renal failure, hypoparathyroidism, excessive intake, neoplastic disease, diabetic ketoacidosis, muscle necrosis, and chemotherapy.

- **Symptoms**: Tachycardia; muscle cramping; hyperreflexia and tetany; nausea and diarrhea.
- **Treatment**: Identify and treat underlying cause, correct hypocalcemia, and provide antacids and dialysis.

MAGNESIUM

Magnesium (**Mg**) is the second most common intracellular electrolyte (after potassium) and activates many intracellular enzyme systems. Mg is important for carbohydrate and protein metabolism, neuromuscular function, and cardiovascular function, producing vasodilation and directly affecting the peripheral arterial system:

- Normal range: 1.7-2.2 mg/dL
- Hypomagnesemia critical value: <1.2 mg/dL
- Hypermagnesemia critical value: >4.9 mg/dL

Hypomagnesemia occurs with chronic diarrhea, chronic renal disease, chronic pancreatitis, excess diuretic or laxative use, hyperthyroidism, hypoparathyroidism, severe burns, and diaphoresis.

- **Symptoms**: Neuromuscular excitability or tetany; confusion, headaches, dizziness; seizure and coma; tachycardia with ventricular arrhythmias; respiratory depression.
- **Treatment**: Identify and treat underlying cause, provide magnesium replacement. IV magnesium is a vasodilator, 2 g over 60 mins.

Hypermagnesemia occurs with renal failure or inadequate renal function, diabetic ketoacidosis, hypothyroidism, and Addison's disease.

- **Symptoms**: Muscle weakness, seizures, and dysphagia with decreased gag reflex; tachycardia with hypotension.
- **Treatment**: Identify and treat underlying cause, IV hydration with calcium, and dialysis.

> **Review Video: Fluid and Electrolytes**
> Visit mometrix.com/academy and enter code: 384389

Acid Base Imbalances

INVASIVE BLOOD GAS MONITORING

Invasive blood gas monitoring options include the following:

- **Arterial blood gas (ABG)** is the most informative measurement of blood gas status. If an arterial catheter is in place, it is easily obtained by aspirating 1-2 mL of blood.
- **Venous blood gas (VBG)** is easier to obtain if an arterial catheter is not in place. In order to compare the values in the VBG with an ABG, make the following calculations:
    - Add 0.05 to the pH of the VBG.
    - Subtract 5-10 mmHg from the PCO_2 of the VBG.
- **Capillary blood gas (CBG)** can be obtained with a heel stick, without a venous or arterial line, but the values obtained in a CBG are the least accurate and are rarely useful. This is used most often in neonates.

COMPONENTS OF A BLOOD GAS READING

The following are components of a blood gas reading:

- **pH** measures the circulating acid and base levels. Neutral pH for humans is 7.4. A value below 7.35 indicates acidosis and a value greater than 7.45 indicates alkalosis.
- **pCO_2** is the partial pressure of carbon dioxide and it determines the respiratory component of pH. An elevated pCO_2 lowers the pH. A low pCO_2 raises the pH. The pCO_2 value is dependent on adequate pulmonary ventilation and respiration. Changes in respiratory status quickly alter this value. Normal value range for pCO_2 is 35-45 mmHg.
- **pO_2** is the partial pressure of oxygen, which indicates how well the individual is transporting oxygen from the lungs into the bloodstream. Normal value is 75-100 mmHg.
- **HCO_3^-** is bicarbonate, the metabolic component of pH. This value may slowly change in response to abnormal pH, or a disease process may cause an elevation or depression. Low values decrease the pH and high values raise the pH. Normal value for bicarbonate is 22-26 mEq/L.

METABOLIC AND RESPIRATORY ACIDOSIS
PATHOPHYSIOLOGY

- Metabolic acidosis
    - Increase in fixed acid and inability to excrete acid, or loss of base, with compensatory increase of CO_2 excretion by lungs
- Respiratory acidosis
    - Hypoventilation and CO_2 retention with renal compensatory retention of bicarbonate (HCO_3) and increased excretion of hydrogen

LABORATORY

- Metabolic acidosis
    - Decreased serum pH (<7.35) and PCO_2 normal if uncompensated and decreased if compensated
    - Decreased HCO_3
- Respiratory acidosis
    - Decreased serum pH (< 7.35) and increased PCO_2
    - Increased HCO_3 if compensated and normal if uncompensated

CAUSES

- Metabolic acidosis
  - DKA, lactic acidosis, diarrhea, starvation, renal failure, shock, renal tubular acidosis, starvation
- Respiratory acidosis
  - COPD, overdose of sedative or barbiturate (leading to hypoventilation), obesity, severe pneumonia/atelectasis, muscle weakness (Guillain-Barré), mechanical hypoventilation

SYMPTOMS

- Metabolic acidosis
  - Neuro/muscular: Drowsiness, confusion, headache, coma
  - Cardiac: Decreased BP, arrhythmias, flushed skin
  - GI: Nausea, vomiting, abdominal pain, diarrhea
  - Respiratory: Deep inspired tachypnea
- Respiratory acidosis
  - Neuro/muscular: Drowsiness, dizziness, headache, coma, disorientation, seizures
  - Cardiac: Flushed skin, VF, ↓BP
  - GI: Absent
  - Respiratory: Hypoventilation with hypoxia

METABOLIC AND RESPIRATORY ALKALOSIS

PATHOPHYSIOLOGY

- Metabolic alkalosis
  - Decreased strong acid or increased base with possible compensatory CO_2 retention by lungs
- Respiratory alkalosis
  - Hyperventilation and increased excretion of CO_2 with compensatory HCO_3 excretion by kidneys

LABORATORY

- Metabolic alkalosis
  - Increased serum pH (>7.45)
  - PCO_2 normal if uncompensated and increased if compensated
  - Increased HCO_3
- Respiratory alkalosis
  - Increased serum pH (>7.45)
  - Decreased PCO_2
  - HCO_3 normal if uncompensated and decreased if compensated

CAUSES

- Metabolic alkalosis
  - Excessive vomiting, gastric suctioning, diuretics, potassium deficit, excessive mineralocorticoids and $NaHCO_3$ intake
- Respiratory alkalosis
  - Hyperventilation associated with hypoxia, pulmonary embolus, exercise, anxiety, pain, and fever
  - Encephalopathy, septicemia, brain injury, salicylate overdose, and mechanical hyperventilation

SYMPTOMS

- Metabolic alkalosis
  - Neuromuscular: Dizziness, confusion, nervousness, anxiety, tremors, muscle cramping, tetany, tingling, seizures
  - Cardiac: Tachycardia and arrhythmias
  - GI: Nausea, vomiting, anorexia
  - Respiratory: Compensatory hypoventilation
- Respiratory alkalosis
  - Neuro/muscular: Light-headedness, confusion, lethargy
  - Cardiac: Tachycardia and arrhythmias
  - GI: Epigastric pain, nausea, and vomiting
  - Respiratory: Hyperventilation

Cardiovascular Diagnostics

CARDIAC ENZYMES

CK AND CK-MB

Creatine kinase (CK) and CK-MB levels are evaluated every 6–8 hours in a suspected myocardial injury. Total CK and CK-MB (specific to cardiac cells) initially rise within the first 4–6 hours of an MI. A normal range would be 30 IU/L to 180 IU/L for CK and CK-MB totaling 0–5% of the CK level.

Assuming no further damage is sustained, peak levels (in excess of 6 times the normal range) are reached 12–24 hours after the injury. CK levels will return to normal within 3–4 days of the event. Small spikes in CK level might also occur following invasive cardiac procedures.

TROPONIN I AND T

Troponin, which is found in cardiac and skeletal muscle, is a type of protein. Both troponin I and T (isolates of troponin) are found in the myocardium, but troponin T is also found in skeletal muscle, so it is less specific than troponin I. Troponin I, therefore, may be used to detect a myocardial infarction after non-cardiac surgery and to detect acute coronary syndrome. Troponin is released into the bloodstream when injury to the tissue (such as the myocardium) occurs and causes damage to the cell membranes, as occurs with myocardial injury.

- **Troponin I** (<0.05 ng/mL): Appears in 2-6 hours, peaks at 15-20 hours and returns to normal in 5-7 days. Exhibits a second but lower peak at 60-80 hours (biphasic).
- **Troponin T** (<0.2 ng/mL): Increases 2-6 hours after MI and stays elevated. Returns to normal in 7 days. (Less specific than troponin I)

ECHOCARDIOGRAPHY

Echocardiography is a non-invasive ultrasound technology that is very useful for assessing and diagnosing anatomic heart abnormalities, blood flow, and valvular lesions:

- The **standard "2D Echo"** is used best for basic structural imaging, such as valvular lesions and assessment of pericardial disorders.
- The **transesophageal (TEE)** probe is an improved version of echocardiography, which allows better visualization of the left atrium and more precise evaluation of the valvular structure. TEE is also the best modality for evaluation of the thoracic aorta in the setting of suspected aortic dissection or aneurysm.
- **Doppler imaging** is used to measure blood flow, often in the context of velocity across a valve and a pressure gradient.
- **Bubble study** is an addition to echocardiography allowing the study to determine if there is right to left blood flow through a patent foramen ovale or a more distal intrapulmonary shunt of blood.

STRESS ECHOCARDIOGRAPHY

Basic **cardiac stress testing** consists of exercise EKG testing (EET) and exercise imaging testing. The exercise imaging testing may be broken down into exercise, or "stress" echocardiography, and exercise myocardial perfusion imaging.

Exercise imaging testing is usually performed with echocardiography. Stress echocardiography is performed similarly to exercise EKG testing and also requires that the patient meet at least 85% maximum heart rate in order to attain optimum sensitivity and specificity. (The maximum heart rate formula is 220 minus the person's age.) Of note, chemicals may substitute for exercise during the "stress" portion of the test. This may be performed with dobutamine (beta-1-agonist: cannot be used after beta-blocker administration) or adenosine (causes diffuse coronary dilatation, leading to decreased perfusion pressure and unmasking of defects, and cannot be used with asthma). Stress imaging allows the study to determine the actual area of ischemia and whether or not this is a reversible defect. Additional information obtained during echocardiography is cardiac output and measurement of viability.

Endocrine Diagnostics

GLUCOSE LABORATORY TEST

Glucose is manufactured by the liver from ingested carbohydrates and is stored as glycogen for use by the cells. If intake is inadequate, glucose can be produced from muscle and fat tissue, leading to increased wasting. High levels of glucose are indicative of diabetes mellitus, which predisposes people to skin injuries, slow healing, and infection. **Fasting blood glucose levels** are used to diagnose and monitor this condition:

- Normal values: 70–99 mg/dL
- Impaired: 100–125 mg/dL
- Diabetes: ≥126 mg/dL

There are a number of different conditions that can increase glucose levels, including stress, renal failure, Cushing syndrome, hyperthyroidism, and pancreatic disorders. Medications, such as steroids, estrogens, lithium, phenytoin, diuretics, tricyclic antidepressants, may increase glucose levels. Other conditions, such as adrenal insufficiency, liver disease, hypothyroidism, and starvation can decrease glucose levels.

HEMOGLOBIN A1C LABORATORY TEST

Hemoglobin A1c comprises hemoglobin A with a glucose molecule because hemoglobin holds onto excess blood glucose, so it shows the average blood glucose levels over a 3-month period and is used primarily to monitor long-term diabetic therapy:

- Normal value: <6%
- Elevation: >7%

BASIC THYROID FUNCTION TESTING AND ANTIBODY TESTING

Thyroid stimulating hormone (TSH) is produced by the pituitary as a result of thyrotropin releasing hormone (TRH) from the hypothalamus. TSH stimulates the thyroid to produce T4 (mostly) and T3. T4 is deiodinated to T3 (active hormone), and the free hormone is active while the majority is bound to albumin and thyroxine-binding globulin. The best testing of thyroid function is the free T4 (unbound). Free T4 and TSH testing allows appropriate screening for thyroid disease.

Additionally, certain antibodies are used to screen for thyroid disease. Thyroglobulin antibodies are found in 50% of patients with Graves' disease and about 90% of those with Hashimoto's thyroiditis. Thyroid peroxidase antibodies are detected in >90% of those with Hashimoto's thyroiditis. TSH receptor antibodies (TSHR) may be either thyroid stimulating immunoglobulin (TSI) which stimulate the receptor to produce thyroid hormone (found in Graves' disease), or TSHR-blocking antibodies, which may inhibit production of thyroid hormone.

Lab values to consider include:

- **Thyroid stimulating hormone (TSH)** (0.4-6.15 mIU/L). Increase in TSH indicates hypothyroidism and decrease indicates hyperthyrojdism.
- **Free thyroxine**: (FT4) (0.9-2.4 ng/dL). FT4 is used to confirm TSH abnormalities. Serum T3 (80-180 ng/dL) and T4 (4.5-11.5 mcg/dL). These usually increase together, but T3 more accurately diagnoses hyperthyroidism. T3 resin uptake (25-35%). Increases with hyperthyroidism and decreases with hypothyroidism.

ADDITIONAL ENDOCRINE FUNCTION STUDIES

There is a wide range of endocrine function studies:

- **Pituitary:** Serum levels of pituitary hormones and hormones of target organs, dependent on stimulation by pituitary hormones, are measured to determine abnormalities.
- **Parathyroid:** Parathyroid hormone (PTH) level (10-65 ng/L) and serum calcium levels (8.5-10.2 mg/dL) both increase with hyperparathyroidism. Calcium levels decrease with hypoparathyroidism, and phosphate levels (2.5-4.5 mg/dL) increase.
- **Adrenal**: Catecholamine (urine and serum) levels: Epinephrine (<75 ng/L) and norepinephrine (<100-550 ng/mL) elevate with pheochromocytoma. Electrolyte and glucose levels.
- **ACTH** and **serum cortisol levels** and **ACTH stimulation test** to evaluate for Addison's. Dexamethasone suppression test for Cushing's disease.

Hematologic Diagnostics

RED BLOOD CELLS

Red blood cells (RBCs or erythrocytes) are biconcave disks that contain **hemoglobin** (95% of mass), which carries oxygen throughout the body. The heme portion of the cell contains **iron**, which binds to the oxygen. RBCs live about 120 days, after which they are destroyed and their hemoglobin is recycled or excreted. Normal values of **red blood cell count** vary by gender:

- Males >18 years: 4.7-6.1 million per mm^3
- Females >18 years: 4.2-5.4 million per mm^3

The most common **disorders of RBCs** are those that interfere with production, leading to various types of **anemia**:

- Blood loss
- Hemolysis
- Bone marrow failure

The **morphology** of RBCs may vary depending upon the type of anemia:

- Size: Normocytes, microcytes, macrocytes
- Shape: Spherocytes (round), poikilocytes (irregular), drepanocytes (sickled)
- Color (reflecting concentration of hemoglobin): Normochromic, hypochromic

LABORATORY TESTS

A number of different tests are used to evaluate the condition and production of red blood cells in addition to the red blood cell count.

Hemoglobin: Carries oxygen and is decreased in anemia and increased in polycythemia. Normal values:

- Males >18 years: 14.0-17.46 g/dL
- Females >18 years: 12.0-16.0 g/dL

Hematocrit: Indicates the proportion of RBCs in a liter of blood (usually about 3 times the hemoglobin number). Normal values:

- Males >18 years: 40-50%
- Females >18 years: 35-45%

Mean corpuscular volume (MCV): Indicates the size of RBCs and can differentiate types of anemia. For adults, <80 is microcytic and >100 is macrocytic. Normal values:

- Males >18 years: 84-96 μm^3
- Females >18 years: 76-96 μm^3

Reticulocyte count: Measures marrow production and should rise with anemia. Normal values: 0.5-1.5% of total RBCs.

WBC COUNT AND DIFFERENTIAL

White blood cell (leukocyte) count is used as an indicator of bacterial and viral infection. WBC count is reported as the total number of all white blood cells.

- Normal WBC for adults: 4,800-10,000
- Acute infection: 10,000+; 30,000 indicates a severe infection
- Viral infection: 4,000 and below

The **differential** provides the percentage of each different type of leukocyte. An increase in the white blood cell count is usually related to an increase in one type, and often an increase in immature neutrophils (bands), referred to as a "shift to the left," is an indication of an infectious process:

- Normal immature neutrophils (bands): 1-3%, increases with infection
- Normal segmented neutrophils (segs) for adults: 50-62%, increases with acute, localized, or systemic bacterial infections
- Normal eosinophils: 0-3%, decreases with stress and acute infection
- Normal basophils: 0-1%, decreases during acute stage of infection
- Normal lymphocytes: 25-40%, increases in some viral and bacterial infections
- Normal monocytes: 3-7%, increases during recovery stage of acute infection

C-REACTIVE PROTEIN AND ERYTHROCYTE SEDIMENTATION RATE

C-reactive protein is an acute-phase reactant produced by the liver in response to an inflammatory response that causes neutrophils, granulocytes, and macrophages to secrete cytokines. Thus, levels of C-reactive protein rise when there is inflammation or infection. It is helpful to measure the response to treatment for pyoderma gangrenosum ulcers:

- Normal values: 2.6-7.6 µg/dL

Erythrocyte sedimentation rate (sed rate) measures the distance erythrocytes fall in a vertical tube of anticoagulated blood in one hour. Because fibrinogen, which increases in response to infection, also increases the rate of the fall, the sed rate can be used as a non-specific test for inflammation when infection is suspected. The sed rate is sensitive to osteomyelitis and may be used to monitor treatment response. Values vary according to gender and age:

- <50: Males 0-15 mm/hr; females 0-20 mm/hr
- >50: Males 0-20 mm/hr; females 0-30 mm/hr

ELEMENTS OF THE COAGULATION PROFILE

The coagulation profile measures clotting mechanisms, identifies clotting disorders, screens preoperative patients, and diagnoses excessive bruising and bleeding. Values vary depending on lab:

- **Prothrombin time (PT)**: 10-14 seconds
  - Increases with anticoagulation therapy, vitamin K deficiency, decreased prothrombin, DIC, liver disease, and malignant neoplasm. Some drugs may shorten PT.
- **Partial thromboplastin time (PTT)**: 25-35 seconds
  - Increases with hemophilia A and B, von Willebrand disease, vitamin deficiency, lupus, DIC, and liver disease.
- **Activated partial thromboplastin time (aPTT)**: 21-35 seconds
  - Similar to PTT, but decreases in extensive cancer, early DIC, and after acute hemorrhage. Used to monitor heparin dosage.
- **Thrombin clotting time (TCT) or Thrombin time (TT)**: 7-12 seconds
  - Used most often to determine the dosage of heparin. Prolonged with multiple myeloma, abnormal fibrinogen, uremia, and liver disease.
- **Bleeding time**: 2-9.5 minutes
  - (Using the IVY method on the forearm) Increases with DIC, leukemia, renal failure, aplastic anemia, von Willebrand disease, some drugs, and alcohol.
- **Platelet count**: 150,000-400,000 per µL
  - Increased bleeding <50,000 (transfusion required) and increased clotting >750,000.

Neurological Diagnostics

LUMBAR PUNCTURE

The lumbar puncture (spinal tap) is done between the 3rd and 4th or between the 4th and 5th lumbar vertebrae. The patient is in the lateral recumbent position with knees drawn toward the chest during the procedure. A local anesthetic is applied to prevent pain when the needle is inserted into the subarachnoid space to withdraw CSF and measure CSF pressure, which should be 70-200 mmH$_2$O.

Queckenstedt's test: Compress jugular veins on each side of the neck during the procedure. Note pressure and then release the veins and note pressure in 10-second intervals. Pressure should rise quickly with compression and fall quickly with release. Slower or no response indicates blockage of subarachnoid pathways.

Normal values (CSF analysis):

- Clear and colorless
- Protein: 15-45 mg/dL
- Glucose: 60-80 mg/dL
- Lactic acid: <25.2 mg/dL
- Culture: Negative
- RBCs: 0
- WBCs: 0.5/mL

Avoiding Complications After Lumbar Puncture and Use of Epidural Blood Patch

After a lumbar puncture, the patient should remain in the prone position for at least 3 hours to ensure that the needle puncture sites through the dural and arachnoid areas remain separate in order to reduce the chance of CSF leakage. If >20 mL of CSF is removed, then the patient should remain prone for 2 hours, side-lying (flat) for 2-3 hours, and supine or prone for 6 additional hours. Relieving intracranial pressure by withdrawing CSF may cause herniation of the brain, so lumbar puncture should be done with care in the presence of increased ICP. The most common complaint is of spinal headache, which may occur within a few hours or several days of the procedure. Increased fluid intake may reduce risk of headache. If headache occurs, it may be treated with analgesics, fluids, and bed rest; however, if the headache is severe or persistent, an **epidural blood patch** may be done, with venous blood withdrawn and then injected into the epidural space at the site of the puncture to seal the leaking opening.

Gastrointestinal Diagnostics

LIVER FUNCTION STUDIES

Liver function studies are described below:

- **Bilirubin:** Determines the ability of the liver to conjugate and excrete bilirubin, direct 0.0–0.3 mg/dL, total 0.0–0.9 mg/dL, and urine bilirubin, which should be 0
- **Total protein:** Normal: 6.0–8.0 g/dL (Albumin: 4.0–5.5 g/dL, Globulin: 1.7–3.3 g/dL); normal albumin/globulin (A/G) ratio: 1.5:1 to 2.5:1, measured by serum protein electrophoresis
- **Prothrombin time (PT):** 100% or clot detection in 10-14 seconds; PT increases with liver disease
  - International normalized ratio (PT result/normal average): <2 for those not receiving anticoagulation, 2-3 for those receiving anticoagulation, critical value >3 in patients receiving anticoagulation therapy
- **Alkaline phosphatase:** 36–93 units/L in adults (normal values vary with method); indicates biliary tract obstruction if no bone disease
- **AST (SGOT):** 10–40 units (increases with liver cell damage)
- **ALT (SGPT):** 5–35 units (increases with liver cell damage)
- **GGT, GGTP:** 5–55 μ/L females, 5–85 μ/L males (increases with alcohol abuse)
- **LDH:** 100–200 units (increases with alcohol abuse)
- **Serum ammonia:** 150–250 mg/dL (increases with liver failure)
- **Cholesterol:** Increases with bile duct obstruction and decrease with parenchymal disease

NUTRITIONAL LAB MONITORING

TOTAL PROTEIN AND ALBUMIN

Total protein levels can be influenced by many factors, including stress and infection, but it may be monitored as part of an overall nutritional assessment. Protein is critical for general health and wound healing, and because metabolic rate increases in response to a wound, protein needs increase:

- Normal values: 6–8 g/dL
- Diet requirements for wound healing: 1.25–1.5 g/kg/day

Albumin is a protein that is produced by the liver and is a necessary component for cells and tissues. Levels decrease with renal disease, malnutrition, and severe burns. Albumin levels are the most common screening to determine protein levels. Albumin has a half-life of 18–20 days, so it is sensitive to long-term protein deficiencies more than short-term.

- Normal values: 3.5–5.5 g/dL
- Mild deficiency: 3.0–3.5 g/dL
- Moderate deficiency: 2.5–3.0 g/dL
- Severe deficiency: <2.5 g/dL

Levels below 3.2 correlate with increased morbidity and death. Dehydration (poor intake, diarrhea, or vomiting) elevates levels, so adequate hydration is important to ensure meaningful results.

PREALBUMIN

Prealbumin (transthyretin) is most commonly monitored for acute changes in nutritional status because it has a half-life of only 2–3 days. Prealbumin is a protein produced in the liver, so it is often decreased with liver disease. Oral contraceptives and estrogen can also decrease levels. Levels may rise with Hodgkin's disease or the use of steroids or NSAIDS. Prealbumin is necessary for transportation of both thyroxine and vitamin A throughout the body, so if **prealbumin levels** fall, both thyroxine and vitamin A utilization are also affected:

- Normal values: 16–40 mg/dL
- Mild deficiency: 10–15 mg/dL
- Moderate deficiency: 5–9 mg/dL
- Severe deficiency: <5 mg/dL

Prealbumin is a good measurement because it quickly decreases when nutrition is inadequate and rises quickly in response to increased protein intake. Protein intake must be adequate to maintain levels of prealbumin. Death rates increase with any decrease in prealbumin levels.

TRANSFERRIN

Transferrin, which transports about one-third of the body's iron, is a protein produced by the liver. It transports **iron** from the intestines to the bone marrow where it is used to produce **hemoglobin**. The half-life of transferrin is about 8–10 days. It is sometimes used as a measure of nutritional status; however, transferrin levels are sensitive to many factors. Levels rapidly decrease with protein malnutrition. Liver disease and anemia can also depress levels, but a decrease in iron, commonly found with inadequate protein, stimulates the liver to produce more transferrin, which increases transferrin levels but also decreases production of albumin and prealbumin. Transferrin levels may also increase with pregnancy, use of oral contraceptives, and polycythemia. Thus, **transferrin levels** alone are not always reliable measurements of nutritional status:

- Normal values: 200–400 mg/dL
- Mild deficiency: 150–200 mg/dL
- Moderate deficiency: 100–150 mg/dL
- Severe deficiency: <100 mg/dL

EGD

Esophagogastroduodenoscopy (EGD) with a flexible fiberscope equipped with a lighted fiberoptic lens allows direct inspection of the mucosa of the esophagus, stomach, and duodenum. The scope has a still or video camera attached to a monitor for viewing during the procedure. The scope may be used for biopsies or therapeutically to dilate strictures or treat gastric or esophageal bleeding. The patient is positioned on the left side (head supported) to allow saliva drainage. Conscious sedation (midazolam, propofol) is commonly used along with a topical anesthetic spray or gargle to facilitate placing the lubricated tube through the mouth into the esophagus. Atropine reduces secretions. A bite guard in the mouth prevents the patient from biting the scope. The airway must be carefully monitored through the procedure (which usually takes about 30 minutes), including oximeter to measure oxygen saturation. While perforation, bleeding, or infection may occur, most complications are cardiopulmonary in nature and relate to drugs (conscious sedation) used during the procedure, so reversal agents (flumazenil, naloxone) should be available.

> **Review Video: GI Diagnostic Procedures**
> Visit mometrix.com/academy and enter code: 645436

Genitourinary Diagnostics

RENAL FUNCTION STUDIES

Renal function studies are described below:

- **Osmolality (urine):** Normal: 350-900 mOsm/kg/day. Shows early changes when the kidney has difficulty concentrating urine.
- **Osmolality (serum):** Normal: 275-295 mOsm/kg. Gives a picture of the amount of solute in the blood.
- **Uric acid:** Normal: 3.0-7.2 mg/dL. Increases with renal failure.
- **Creatinine clearance (24-hour):** Normal: 75-125 mL/min. Evaluates the amount of blood cleared of creatinine in 1 minute. Approximates the GFR.
- **Serum creatinine:** Normal: 0.6-1.2 mg/dL. Increase with decreased renal function, urinary tract obstruction, and nephritis.
- **Urine creatinine:** Normal: 11-26 mg/kg/day. Product of muscle breakdown. Increase with decreased renal function.
- **Blood urea nitrogen (BUN):** Normal: 7-8 mg/dL (8-20 mg/dL if age >60). An increase indicates impaired renal function, as urea is the end product of protein metabolism.
- **BUN/creatinine ratio:** Normal: 10:1. Increases with hypovolemia. With intrinsic kidney disease, the ratio is increased.
- **Urinalysis:** Tests various qualities of a urine sample that are reflective of kidney function and other disease processes.

URINALYSIS

Urinalysis components and normal findings are described below:

- **Color:** Pale yellow/amber and darkens when urine is concentrated or other substances (such as blood or bile) are present.
- **Appearance:** Clear but may be slightly cloudy.
- **Odor:** Slight. Bacteria may give urine a foul smell, depending upon the organism. Some foods, such as asparagus, change the odor.
- **Specific gravity:** Normal: 1.005-1.025. May increase if protein levels increase or if there is fever, vomiting, or dehydration.
- **pH:** Usually ranges from 4.5-8 with an average of 5-6.
- **Sediment:** Red cell casts from acute infections, broad casts from kidney disorders, and white cell casts from pyelonephritis. Leukocytes >10 per mL^3 are present with urinary tract infections.
- **Glucose, ketones, protein, blood, bilirubin, and nitrate:** Negative. Urine glucose may increase with infection (with normal blood glucose). Frank blood may be caused by some parasites and diseases but also by drugs, smoking, excessive exercise, and menstrual fluids. Increased red blood cells may result from lower urinary tract infections.
- **Urobilinogen:** 0.1-1.0 units.

IVP AND RADIONUCLEOTIDE RENAL SCAN

Intravenous pyelogram (IVP) is done to identify structural defects and tumors and to observe urinary structures. The patient is administered an IV contrast medium and may be administered antihistamine or corticosteroid before the test to minimize allergic response. Serum creatinine and BUN are done prior to the IVP to ensure that the contrast medium can be excreted. During the procedure, radiographs are taken once every minute for five minutes and then again after 15 minutes (giving the contrast medium time to pass into the bladder). A post-voiding radiograph shows how efficiently the bladder is able to empty. Fluid intake should be increased post-procedure to flush contrast.

Radionucleotide renal scan with dimercaptosuccinic acid (DMSA) requires IV administration of a radioactive element followed by a series of CT scans taken over 20 minutes to 4 hours. The scan is used to assess function and perfusion of the kidney and can detect lesions, atrophy, and scars and differentiate among different causes for hydronephrosis. The patient must be well-hydrated and may need to be catheterized to measure the output of urine.

RENAL BIOPSY

Renal biopsy to remove a small segment of cortical tissue helps to identify the extent of **kidney disease** with acute renal failure, transplant rejection, glomerulopathies, and persistent hematuria or proteinuria. Preoperative coagulation studies determine the risk of bleeding. The biopsy is done percutaneously per needle biopsy (guided by fluoroscopy or ultrasound) or surgically through a small flank incision. A urine specimen must be obtained so it can be compared with a post-procedure specimen. **Post-procedure**:

- Maintain the patient in a supine position immediately after the procedure for 4-6 hours and on bed rest overnight.
- Monitor urine for hematuria and compare it with the preop specimen.
- Monitor VS every 5-15 minutes for the first hour and then less frequently. To minimize bleeding, maintain blood pressure <140/90.
- Note anorexia, vomiting, and abdominal discomfort that may suggest bleeding.
- Note pain: Severe colicky pain may indicate a clot in the ureter.
- Monitor urinalysis and CBC post-procedure.
- Maintain fluid intake at 3,000 mL/day in absence of renal insufficiency.
- Provide blood component therapy and surgical repair if bleeding occurs.

RENAL ULTRASOUND

Renal ultrasound is a non-invasive method of viewing the **urinary structures**. Most patients that present with kidney disease of unknown origin should undergo a renal ultrasound to assess for possible obstruction. An ultrasound uses ultrasonic sound waves transmitted by a transducer, which picks up reflected sound waves that a computer converts to electronic images. An ultrasound can show fluid accumulation, the movement of blood through the kidney, masses, malformations (congenital abnormalities), changes in size of the kidney or other structures, and obstructions, such as renal calculi. An ultrasound is usually done before a renal biopsy, and may be done with a needle biopsy to guide the placement of the needle. Patient preparation includes drinking two 8-ounce glasses of water one hour before the examination to ensure that the bladder is full. The patient should be reminded not to urinate before the ultrasound. The patient usually remains in a supine position throughout the procedure but may be asked to turn to the side. No special precautions are necessary post-procedure.

Planning, Implementation and Evaluation

Nursing Care Plan

PLANNING OF NURSING CARE FOR PATIENTS

The patient's needs as defined by the **nursing diagnoses** are first prioritized with the help of the patient and family:

- **Critical needs** are met immediately and then other needs are ranked according to the patient's priorities and Maslow's Hierarchy of Needs.
- When diagnoses are prioritized, **desirable outcomes** for each diagnosis are defined. Outcomes include desirable changes in patient behavior and are the backbone of the care plan. Outcomes are used to determine whether the nursing care has met its objectives.
- **Goals** for each nursing diagnosis are devised with patient and family input. Immediate, intermediate, and long-term goals that combine to meet the desired outcome are defined along with a timetable. Intermediate and long-term goals usually pertain to the prevention of complications and patient and family teaching concerning self-care and rehabilitation needs.

Each goal is then completed by a list of specific **actions** needed to achieve the goal. These actions include nursing interventions and may also include coordination of actions by other healthcare personnel.

> **Review Video: Plan of Care**
> Visit mometrix.com/academy and enter code: 300570

RESOURCES FOR CARE PLANNING

Various resources provide lists of nursing diagnoses, interventions, and expected outcomes to help guide the nurse care planning process:

- The **North American Nursing Diagnosis Association (NANDA)** compiles a list of the most commonly used nursing diagnoses and refines them so that they are acceptable for study and nursing research. This list is updated biannually and is useful when developing care plans.
- **Nursing-Sensitive Outcomes Classification (NOC)** lists nursing outcomes for specific needs. Each outcome has an associated scale of achievement and can be used to evaluate patient progress in achieving the outcome desired.
- **Nursing Interventions Classification (NIC)** consists of interventions appropriate for specific nursing needs. These interventions can be individualized for each patient's needs.

NANDA, NIC, and NOC utilize the **Taxonomy of Nursing Practice** to classify nursing diagnoses, outcomes, and interventions. The Taxonomy of Nursing Practice divides patient problems into four domains:

- **The functional domain** includes classes consisting of patient movement, relief of symptoms, developmental status, nutrition, ADLs, sexuality, belief systems, and sleep.
- **The physiological domain** consists of bodily needs for proper functioning divided into classes concerning the cardiovascular, respiratory, gastrointestinal, genitourinary, neurological, metabolic, immune, reproductive, musculoskeletal, and integumentary systems. The effects of medications and other substances on system functioning are included.

- **The psychosocial domain** contains classes concerning emotional health (coping mechanisms, mental state, self-image, and self-esteem), mental health (knowledge and behaviors), and social status (communication with others, relationships, and support network).
- **The environmental domain** is concerned with patient populations, public and individual health and safety in the environment, healthcare delivery, and management of risks.

By using the taxonomy, all three tools describe the same problems in the same way in language that is specific and refined, yet universal.

UTILIZING CLINICAL PATHWAYS IN CARE PLANNING

Clinical pathways are written tools that direct the treatment of a specific group of patients according to diagnosis. They provide a way to standardize medical and nursing care according to evidence-based practice guidelines, predict the cost of the care, and ensure quality, timeliness, and cost-effectiveness of care. Each plan consists of the DRG or group that it addresses, time segments with specific activities, and desired outcomes for each time segment. They include a place to record activities that deviate from the pathway. Nursing care is charted according to the pathway, which serves as the patient's plan of care. Nurses are responsible for helping to formulate and change clinical pathways. They initiate the pathways when the patient presents for treatment and ensure that the care is given for each time segment. They also use the pathways to monitor patients as case managers for hospitals or insurance companies. The patient may receive a copy that the nurse then discusses to make the patient aware of the treatment course and desired goals.

INCORPORATING PATIENT AND FAMILY RIGHTS INTO PLAN OF CARE

In order for patient and family rights to be incorporated into the plan of care, the care plan needs to be designed as a **collaborative effort** that encourages participation of patients and family members. There are a number of different programs that can be useful, such as including patients and families on advisory committees. Additionally, assessment tools, such as surveys for patients and families, can be utilized to gain insight in the issues that are important to them. While infants and small children and sometimes the elderly cannot speak for themselves, the "patient" is generally understood to include not only the immediate family but also other groups or communities who have an interest in the care of the individual. Because many hospital stays are now short-term, programs that include follow-up interviews and assessments are especially valuable in determining if the needs of the patient were addressed in the care plan.

PSYCHOSOCIAL FACTORS THAT AFFECT CARE PLANNING

There are many psychosocial factors that affect patient care. A patient's **psychological state** influences how that patient interacts with others, including nurses and hospital staff, and can also affect compliance and positive health outcomes. For instance, anxiety or depression can make a patient incapable of performing the instructions necessary for completing a full recovery; the psychological problem would need to be addressed in the patient's care plan.

Social and culture factors also shape a patient's **perception** of health and disease, communication style, and decision-making methods. It is important to understand that differences in ethnicity, race, sex, gender, religion, age, socioeconomic status, family dynamics, sexual orientation, and life experiences mean that patients experience illness and healing differently. Being sensitive to these differences can lead to more effective patient care across the spectrum.

CONSIDERATION OF COMORBIDITIES IN CARE PLANNING

Comorbidity, also known as multimorbidity, refers to the coexistence of multiple chronic or acute medical diseases within one patient. Comorbid conditions are associated with poorer outcomes, the need for more complex medical or surgical management, and elevated healthcare costs. It is now the norm, as opposed to the exception, that patients have multiple comorbid medical conditions. Some examples would be an obese patient with concomitant diabetes, heart disease, and osteoarthritis; a multi-system trauma patient with diabetes, chronic obstructive pulmonary disease, and cardiovascular disease; or a cancer patient with anxiety, depression, and multiple pulmonary emboli.

IMPLEMENTATION OF A NURSING PLAN

The patient's nursing care plan is implemented as soon as the patient has been stabilized. During stabilization, nursing care is guided by standards of practice and logarithms that define care for life-threatening situations. Once the patient is stabilized, **interventions** are guided by the patient's individualized plan of care:

- The nurse has the responsibility of performing the planned nursing interventions and of delegating and coordinating care given by others to meet the patient's needs.
- All care is documented along with patient response.
- Additional patient information, changes in condition, patient priorities, and needs guide the nurse in continuously modifying the care plan.
- Orders are analyzed, clarified, and questioned as needed to meet collaborative patient needs.
- Patient input is necessary to the evaluation of nursing care and revision of the care plan as needed. Patient response to interventions, treatments, and procedures is assessed and care is given accordingly.
- The results of labs and tests are also used to determine actions according to the care plan.

Postoperative Complications

PONV

Postoperative nausea and vomiting (PONV) varies with the type of anesthetic agent used. It occurs in about 20-30% of post-anesthesia patients and may be delayed up to 24 hours. Inhalational agents have a higher incidence of PONV than intravenous, and the incidence is lower with epidural or subarachnoid administration, although it may indicate the onset of hypotension. PONV correlates with the duration of surgery, with longer surgeries causing increased PONV. If high doses of narcotics, propofol, or nitrous oxide are used, PONV is often a problem. PONV is most common in young women and also relates to menstruation. It is also increased in those with a history of smoking or motion sickness. Some surgical procedures correlate with PONV: strabismus repair, ear surgery, laparoscopy, tonsillectomy, orchiopexy, and gynecological procedures to retrieve ova. PONV may be associated with postoperative pain, so managing pain is an important factor in preventing PONV.

RISKS FOR ASPIRATION

Risks for aspiration include:

- **Feeding tubes**: Aspiration pneumonia is a common complication, and because of reduced cough reflex there may be no obvious signs of it. Older age, cognitive impairment, poor oral hygiene, altered level of consciousness, neurological deficits, and history of GERD are all risk factors. Feedings should be given with client sitting up at least 45° if possible, and the client should remain sitting for at least an hour after feedings.
- **Sedation**: Sedation impairs the ability to swallow, increasing risk of aspiration. Risk is lower if the client has been NPO so that the stomach is empty but may still occur with gastric secretions. Oral fluids should be withheld until the client is fully alert.
- **Swallowing difficulties**: Clients with dysphagia, especially those with older age and/or stroke, Parkinson's disease, or muscular dystrophies, are at risk for aspiration. Additionally, clients with mouth sores, esophageal blockage (cancer, stenosis), or a history of radiotherapy or chemotherapy for cancers of the neck or throat are also at increased risk. Clients may need to be on a dysphagia diet, such as with soft foods and thickened liquids, and should eat with supervision while sitting upright.

RISKS FOR INSUFFICIENT VASCULAR PERFUSION

Risk for insufficient vascular perfusion include the following:

- **Immobilized limb**: Usually the result of trauma, which may involve the muscles, bones, ligaments, tendons, vasculature, and nerves—all of which may result in insufficient vascular perfusion—so the limb must be assessed frequently for delayed capillary filling, pallor, edema, and sensory changes. Muscle mass may decrease rapidly even with isometric exercises, and the movement needed to promote adequate venous return is missing. In the case of extended generalized immobility, the client should be put on DVT prophylactic precautions such as a subcutaneous blood thinner (Heparin) and sequential compression devices or compression stockings to prevent clotting and promote perfusion.
- **Post-operative status**: Many conditions associated with surgical repair may result in insufficient vascular perfusion—hypoventilation, hyper- or hypovolemia, mechanical obstruction of blood flow, hypoxemia, and decreased hemoglobin resulting from bleeding. Capillary refill may exceed three seconds, and the client may exhibit dysrhythmias, dyspnea, abnormal ABGs, behavior changes, altered mental status, cooling and pallor of skin, weak/absent pulses, cyanosis, and edema as well as oliguria/anuria.
- **Diabetes**: Often associated with atherosclerosis, neuropathy, hypertension, and peripheral arterial disease, diabetes increases the risk of ulcers because of impaired perfusion.

INDICATIONS OF OUTPUT CHANGES FROM BASELINE

Indications of output changes from baseline include:

- **NG tube**: Drainage per the NG tube should be light yellow/green but volume may vary so it's necessary to monitor both volume and electrolytes to determine what is normal for the client. Reddish or coffee-ground drainage may indicate bleeding, which may increase volume.
- **Emesis**: Clients should not have emesis, so the volume of any emesis must be recorded and steps taken to determine cause and treat.
- **Stool**: Fecal output may range from 3-4 occurrences daily to one every 2-3 days, so the client's normal output should be assessed through history. If diarrhea occurs, then the frequency and volume must be noted as the client may develop dehydration. Constipation lasting longer than several days can be common post-operatively or with a patient on narcotic pain medication, and may require a stool softener. This client should also be monitored for the possibility of an ileus.
- **Urine**: Normal urinary output depends on age, condition, and intake, but is typically 800-2000 mL per day with an intake of 2000 mL. Intake and output should be monitored carefully to establish an output that is normal for the client so that variations can be detected.

PROCEDURES THAT REQUIRE SPECIFIC POSITIONING POST-OPERATIVELY

Procedures that require specific post-operative positioning to prevent complications include:

- **Angiography**: If an extremity is used, place restraint to keep the extremity straight for 6-8 hours.
- **Bronchoscopy**: Place in in semi-Fowler's position to prevent aspiration.
- **Myelogram**: With air contrast, place in Trendelenburg position; with oil contrast, place flat for 6-8 hours; with water-based contrast, place with head of bed elevated for 8 hours.
- **Liver biopsy**: Position on right side with pillow placed beneath the puncture site.
- **Arteriovenous fistula formation**: Elevate extremity.
- **Abdominal aneurysm**: Elevate head of bed to ≤45°.
- **Ear irrigation**: Position client on affected side to promote drainage.
- **Lumbar puncture**: Keep flat for 4-12 hours.
- **Appendectomy**: Place in Fowler's position.
- **Cataract removal**: Place in semi-Fowler's or Fowler's position on back or opposite side of surgery.
- **Kidney transplant**: Place in Semi-Fowler's position on back or turned to opposite side of surgery.
- **Mitral valve replacement**: Place in semi-Fowler's position.
- **Thyroidectomy**: Place in high Fowler's or semi-Fowlers.
- **Tonsillectomy**: Prone or side-lying.
- **Amputation of leg (AK, BK)**: Elevate limb for 24 hours. Place in prone position at least two times daily.
- **Insertion nasogastric tube**: Keep head elevated to at least 30°.

INSERTION AND REMOVAL OF NG/OG TUBE

Procedure for insertion and removal of nasogastric or orogastric tube:

1. Gather PPE and equipment (stethoscope, lubricant, syringe, tape, suction if ordered, and pH strips) and carry out hand hygiene.
2. Assess nostrils for patency (if NG tube), abdomen for bowel sounds, and level of consciousness for ability to follow directions.
3. Position client at 45-90° if possible.
4. Measure NG/OG tube from tip of nose to ear and from ear to xiphoid process and mark tube.
5. Apply clean non-sterile gloves. Flush tube with water or lubricate 3-4 inches with water-soluble lubricant. Curl tube in circles around fingers and then release to ensure proper curvature.

6. Ask client to drop chin down and breathe orally if NG tube. Insert NG tube (curved side down) into nostril and guide downward. Guide OG tube along back of tongue and downward with client breathing through nose. Twist tubes slightly if resistance encountered.
7. Ask client to sip water (if allowed) or dry swallow while tube is advanced nasally or to swallow only if using OG tube.
8. Secure with tape and aspirate contents for pH testing (should be <5).
9. Verify placement with x-ray. If properly placed, measure length of NG/OG tube from where it leaves the nostril/mouth to end.

To remove NG/OG, gather supplies, carry out hand hygiene, and clear the NG/OG tube by injecting 10-20 mL of air. Then remove any tape and clips, ask the client to take and hold a deep breath, and gently pull out the tube in one steady motion.

Maintaining Patency of Tubes

Procedures for maintaining patency of tubes include:

- **NG tube**: Flush with 30-50 mL of water or NS every 4-6 hours and before and after feeding or medications. Ensure tubing is not kinked if attached to drainage and check clamp.
- **Chest tube**: Ensure that tubes are not kinked or dislodged and that clamp is open and fluid has not collected in dependent loops. Keep chest drainage unit below level of client's chest. Ensure water levels are correct. Aggressive milking/stripping can result in negative pressure and damage to tissue and should be avoided. If clots are evident, gently squeezing and releasing the tube hand by hand along the length may prevent occlusion.
- **Percutaneous endoscopic gastrostomy tube**: Care is similar to that for the NG tube with tube flushed before and after feedings, medications, and every 4-6 hours.

Thromboembolism

Thromboembolism includes both the formation of a thrombus (such as in the heart with A-fib and in the deep veins with immobilization) and embolism in which a clot breaks off and travels through the circulatory system. While thromboembolism may cause a heart attack or stroke, the most common presentation is a pulmonary embolism resulting from deep vein thrombosis.

Signs and symptoms: A thrombus is generally asymptomatic. Pain may be present at the thrombus site, which may be swollen and erythematous, typically in the lower extremity. When the patient develops pulmonary embolism, the usual presentation is acute onset of dyspnea. Some patients may have frothy sputum, cough, fever, and/or hemoptysis as well.

Diagnosis: Laboratory tests (CBC, troponins, D-dimer, ABGs, and BNP), ultrasound, spiral CT, pulmonary angiography, and ventilation/perfusion scanning.

Treatment: Anticoagulants, thrombolytic therapy, oxygen, and thrombectomy.

Prevention: Smoking cessation, regular exercise, discontinuation of birth control pills, early ambulation after surgery, SCDs/compression hose, control of high blood pressure, treatment for peripheral arterial disease, and avoiding prolonged sitting.

> **Review Video: <u>DVT - Prevention and Treatment</u>**
> Visit mometrix.com/academy and enter code: 234086

EFFECTS OF MULTIPLE INTERVENTIONS ON POSTOPERATIVE RISK
GENERAL SURGERY PATIENT WITH CO-MORBIDITIES

Multiple interventions in a patient with co-morbidities can increase the risk of postoperative complications. For example, a patient with diabetes who undergoes multiple interventions or surgical procedures may be at an increased risk for cardiac arrest; myocardial infarction; pressure sores, ulcers, or gangrene as a result of peripheral neuropathy; stroke; postoperative wound infection; wound dehiscence; contracting a hospital-acquired infection; worsening glycemic control from the stress of multiple interventions or infection; postoperative sepsis; and multi-organ failure.

ELDERLY PATIENTS

Many elderly patients have between two and four co-morbid conditions, all of which need to be addressed and treated. However, care must be taken to ensure that an intervention for one condition does not lead to adverse complications, particularly when prescribing multiple drugs. Common effects of multiple interventions in elderly patients with co-morbid conditions include an increased fall risk secondary to osteoarthritis and frailty, nosocomial infections secondary to decreased immune function, decubital ulcers as a result of impaired mobility or dementia, adverse medication reactions as a result of a decreased ability to metabolize medications, neurological complications, gastrointestinal bleeding, and delirium.

POST-PROCEDURE COMPLICATIONS AFTER CARDIAC CATHETERIZATION

Post-procedure complications of cardiac catheterization include:

- **Catheterization**: Dysrhythmias (ventricular arrhythmias, atrial fibrillation, conduction abnormalities, and bradycardia) may develop during or after cardiac catheterization caused by irritation of cardiac tissue. Incidence may vary depending on where the tip of the catheter lies. Risks are highest for clients with a history of congenital heart disease and a history of ECG abnormalities. In most cases, these abnormalities revert to a normal sinus rhythm, but they may require immediate intervention. Some may experience an allergic response to contrast medium.
- **Surgical/insertion site**: Bleeding (hematoma/retroperitoneal bleeding), arterial tearing (development of pseudoaneurysm), clot dislodgement (resulting in myocardial infarction or stroke), arterial occlusion (especially of radial artery), and infection (at insertion site or endocarditis) may occur at the insertion site. The surgical site should be assessed frequently (per facility protocol) for any signs of bleeding.

STAGES OF BLOOD LOSS/HYPOVOLEMIA

Stage	Blood loss	Indications
1	15% 750 mL	Client may appear pale but vital signs, urinary output, and capillary refill may remain within normal limits.
2	15-30% 1500 mL	Pallor may increase with skin becoming cool and clammy. Diastolic blood pressure may increase and heart rate may increase to >100 beats per minute. The client may appear anxious. Capillary refill is delayed but urinary output remains at 20-30 mL per hour.
3	30-40% 1500-2000 mL	Client becoming increasingly confused with altered mental status and diaphoresis. Systolic BP drops to below 100 and tachycardia increases to >120 beats per minute. Client is dyspneic with respirations >30 per minute. Capillary refill remains delayed but urinary output remains about 20 mL per hour.
4	>40% >2000 mL	Client increasingly lethargic and may become comatose, remains diaphoretic but skin mottling may be evident. Pulse is thready at >140 beats per minutes and systolic BP falls to below 70. Respirations are very shallow and rapid. Capillary refill is absent and urinary output is negligible or absent.

91

POTENTIAL SOURCES OF INFECTION FOR TRANSPLANT PATIENTS

Infections pose a serious threat to **transplant patients**, especially during the first year. While opportunistic infections have decreased, nosocomial infections have increased, most related to bacterial infections. Transplant patients consistently show higher rates of infection than other patients due to their needs for immunosuppressants to prevent rejection. There are numerous potential sources:

- **Donor-infected organs** can transmit HBV, HBC, herpesvirus, HIV, and human T-cell leukemia virus type I. Additionally, donors who are immunocompromised prior to harvesting of the organs may have nosocomial bacterial or fungal infections that can be transmitted. Organs can also become infected during harvesting.
- **Health care workers** may transmit pathogens through droplets, airborne particles, or contact, frequently transmitting pathogens on their hands or clothing.
- **Blood and blood products** can transmit CMV, but transmission is rare. HCV transmission has been reduced to <1%.
- **Environmental reservoir sources** can include the water system, demolition activities, equipment, and surfaces. Some pathogens, such as MRSA and VRE, may be endemic to the hospital environment.

COMMON VIRAL PATHOGENS IN TRANSPLANT PATIENTS

Several **viral infections** are more likely to occur in transplant patients due to their immunocompromised state:

- **Cytomegalovirus (CMV)**: The most common pathogen related to transplant infections, affecting 40%-90% of recipients.
- **Herpes simplex virus**: Reactivated/new; may disseminate to liver.
- **Human herpesvirus-6**: Mostly reactivation, newer strain.
- **Varicella-zoster virus**: New; may disseminate to viscera.
- **Hepatitis B and C viruses**: Causes liver failure; also affects kidney transplant patients.
- **BK virus (BKV)**: Causes renal dysfunction; transmission unknown.
- **Adenoviruses (AdV)**: Bone marrow transplant; can become systemic.

Prevention is as follows:

- **Serologic matching** can prevent primary transmission but the limited supply of organs may make this impractical.
- **Early diagnosis** with serum assay for targeted treatment.
- **Antiviral prophylaxis** in high-risk patients can be effective.
- **Immunization** has proven to be safe and highly effective, reducing the incidence of infection and the severity.
- **Immunoglobulin** is given to susceptible transplant patients exposed to certain viruses.
- **Reduction in immunosuppressive medications** if possible.
- **High-dose acyclovir** for some viruses may reduce severity of infection.
- Targeting patients at the highest risk of disease through **surveillance** and using proper transmission-based precautions are the most practical methods of infection control.

COMMON BACTERIAL INFECTIONS AFTER TRANSPLANT SURGERY

Staphylococcus aureus is the most common cause of bacterial infection in liver, heart, kidney, and pancreas transplant patients. According to the CDC, as many as 33% of individuals carry *Staphylococcus aureus* in their nares, without any other signs of illness, and approximately 5% of individuals in the hospital carry MRSA (methicillin-resistant *Staphylococcus aureus*). Because it is spread through direct contact, nosocomial infection is common. Specific risk factors for the post-transplant patient in the hospital setting include open wounds and intravenous access. Diligent hand hygiene must be performed by all health care providers and visitors.

Vancomycin-resistant enterococci (VRE) causes 10-15% of liver failures, according to recent studies. Nosocomial transmission occurs frequently, especially with prolonged hospitalization and ICU stay. VRE colonization puts patients at continued risk of infection and poses a reservoir for nosocomial infections.

Nocardia is found in soil and decaying vegetation, and transmission is through inhalation. Lung, heart, and intestinal transplants have the highest rates of infection. Mortality rates are high for those who are infected. Risk factors include high-dose cortisone, high levels of immunosuppressants, and CMV infection within six months.

Infection control strategies include:

- **Handwashing** and basic clean technique are still the best methods of infection control in these patients.
- **Environmental monitoring** should be used.
- **Antibiotic prophylaxis** is effective.

ASPERGILLUS FUNGAL INFECTION AFTER TRANSPLANT SURGERY

Aspergillus infections primarily involve pneumonia and sinusitis, but 25-35% disseminate systemically, and *Aspergillus* pneumonia infections have mortality rates up to 85%. *Aspergillus* is a serious fungal infection in immunocompromised transplant patients, especially lung transplant patients with 8% infection rates within 9 months of surgery. Liver transplant patients have infection rates of 1-4% but disease occurs earlier, within 2-4 weeks. Heart transplant infection rates are 1-6% with disease within 1-2 months. *Aspergillus* affects renal transplants the least with <1% infection rates. Prophylaxis with antifungals has not proven to be effective.

Infection control strategies include:

- **Monitoring environment and improving air filtration** with HEPA filtration or use of laminar air flow rooms for patients at high risk.
- **Construction precautions** to prevent dust and debris from circulating in patient care areas.
- **Standard precautions** include high-resolution CT scans for early diagnosis rather than chest x-rays so treatment with voriconazole (drug of choice) can begin.

INFECTION CONTROL STRATEGIES FOR SPINAL CORD INJURIES

Infection control strategies for neurology/spinal cord injuries target the most common types of infection:

- **Urinary tract infection**: Patients should be monitored for fever and/or changes in spasms or voiding habits that may indicate infection. When possible, intermittent catheterization (sterile rather than clean while in the hospital) should be used rather than continuous. Antibiotic prophylaxis has not proven to be effective but bacterial interference, colonizing of the urinary tract with nonpathogenic *E. coli* 83972, has shown promising results.
- **Decubital ulcers**: Procedures for regular monitoring of skin condition, turning patients, and avoiding friction to prevent pressure from developing are critical. Both staff and patients must be educated about prevention, skin care, and cleanliness. Nutrition and hydration must be adequate to maintain integrity of the skin.
- **Respiratory infections**: Proper use of ventilation equipment must be monitored. Assisted coughing, such as through respiratory therapy and postural drainage, can reduce infections. Prophylactic antibiotics are not recommended, but patients should receive immunizations for pneumonia.

Cardiovascular Pathophysiology

ACUTE CORONARY SYNDROMES

Acute coronary syndrome (ACS) is the impairment of blood flow through the coronary arteries, leading to ischemia of the cardiac muscle. Angina frequently occurs in ACS, manifesting as crushing pain substernally, radiating down the left arm or both arms. However, in females, elderly, and diabetics, symptoms may appear less acute and include nausea, shortness of breath, fatigue, pain/weakness/numbness in arms, or no pain at all (*silent ischemia*). There are multiple **classifications of angina**:

- **Stable angina**: Exercise-induced, short lived, relieved by rest or nitroglycerin. Other precipitating events include decrease in environmental temperature, heavy eating, strong emotions (such as fright or anger), or exertion, including coitus.
- **Unstable angina** (preinfarction or crescendo angina): A change in the pattern of stable angina, characterized by an increase in pain, not responding to a single nitroglycerin or rest, and persisting for >5 minutes. May cause a change in EKG, or indicate rupture of an atherosclerotic plaque or the beginning of thrombus formation. Treat as a medical emergency, indicates impending MI.
- **Variant angina** (Prinzmetal's angina): Results from spasms of the coronary arteries. Associated with or without atherosclerotic plaques and is often related to smoking, alcohol, or illicit stimulants, but can occur cyclically and at rest. Elevation of ST segments usually occurs with variant angina. Treatment is nitroglycerin or calcium channel blockers.

> **Review Video: Coronary Artery Disease**
> Visit mometrix.com/academy and enter code: 950720

MYOCARDIAL INFARCTIONS
NSTEMI AND STEMI

Non–ST-segment elevation MI (NSTEMI): ST elevation on the electrocardiogram (ECG) occurs in response to myocardial damage resulting from infarction or severe ischemia. The absence of ST elevation may be diagnosed as unstable angina or NSTEMI, but cardiac enzyme levels increase with NSTEMI, indicating partial blockage of coronary arteries with some damage. Symptoms are consistent with unstable angina, with chest pain or tightness, pain radiating to the neck or arm, dyspnea, anxiety, weakness, dizziness, nausea, vomiting, and heartburn. Initial treatment may include nitroglycerin, β-blockers, antiplatelet agents, or antithrombotic agents. Ongoing treatment may include β-blockers, aspirin, statins, angiotensin-converting enzyme inhibitors, angiotensin-receptor blockers, and clopidogrel. Percutaneous coronary intervention is not recommended.

ST-segment elevation MI (STEMI): This more severe type of MI involves complete blockage of one or more coronary arteries with myocardial damage, resulting in ST elevation. Symptoms are those of acute MI. As necrosis occurs, Q waves often develop, indicating irreversible myocardial damage, which may result in death, so treatment involves immediate reperfusion before necrosis can occur.

> **Review Video: Myocardial Infarction**
> Visit mometrix.com/academy and enter code: 148923

Q-WAVE AND NON-Q-WAVE MYOCARDIAL INFARCTIONS

Formerly classified as transmural or non-transmural, myocardial infarctions are now classified as Q-wave or non-Q-wave:

- **Q-Wave**
  - Characterized by a series of abnormal Q waves (wider and deeper) on ECG, especially in the early morning (related to adrenergic activity).
  - Infarction is usually prolonged and results in necrosis.
  - Coronary occlusion is complete in 80-90% of cases.
  - Q-wave MI is often, but not always, transmural.
  - Peak CK levels occur in about 27 hours.
- **Non-Q-Wave**
  - Characterized by changes in ST-T wave with ST depression (usually reversible within a few days).
  - Usually reperfusion occurs spontaneously, so infarct size is smaller. Contraction necrosis related to reperfusion is common.
  - Non-Q-wave MI is usually non-transmural.
  - Coronary occlusion is complete in only 20-30%.
  - Peak CK levels occur in 12-13 hours.
  - Reinfarction is common.

LOCATIONS AND TYPES

Myocardial infarctions are also classified according to their location and the extent of injury. Q-wave infarctions involve the full thickness of the heart muscle, often producing a series of Q waves on ECG. While an MI most frequently damages the left ventricle and the septum, the right ventricle may be damaged as well, depending upon the area of the occlusion:

- **Anterior** (V_2 to V_4): Occlusion in the proximal left anterior descending (LAD) or left coronary artery. Reciprocal changes found in leads II, III, aV_F.
- **Lateral** (I, aV_L, V_5, V_6): Occlusion of the circumflex coronary artery or branch of left coronary artery. Often causes damage to anterior wall as well. Reciprocal changes found in leads II, III, aV_F.
- **Inferior/diaphragmatic** (II, III, aV_F): Occlusion of the right coronary artery and causes conduction malfunctions. Reciprocal changes found in leads I and aV_L.
- **Right ventricular** (V_{4R}, V_{5R}, V_{6R}): Occlusion of the proximal section of the right coronary artery and damages in the right ventricle and the inferior wall. No reciprocal changes should be noted on an ECG.
- **Posterior** (V_8, V_9): Occlusion in the right coronary artery or circumflex artery and may be difficult to diagnose. Reciprocal changes found in V_1-V_4.

CLINICAL MANIFESTATIONS AND DIAGNOSIS

Clinical manifestations of myocardial infarction may vary considerably. More than half of all patients present with acute MIs with no prior history of cardiovascular disease.

Signs/symptoms: Angina with pain in chest that may radiate to neck or arms, palpitations, hypertension or hypotension, dyspnea, pulmonary edema, dependent edema, nausea/vomiting, pallor, skin cold and clammy, diaphoresis, decreased urinary output, neurological/psychological disturbances: anxiety, light-headedness, headache, visual abnormalities, slurred speech, and fear.

Diagnosis is based on the following:

- ECG obtained immediately to monitor heart changes over time. Typical changes include T-wave inversion, elevation of ST segment, abnormal Q waves, tachycardia, bradycardia, and dysrhythmias.
- Echocardiogram: decreased ventricular function is possible, especially for transmural MI.

- Labs:
  - **Troponin**: Increases within 3–6 hours, peaks 14–20; elevated for up to 1-2 weeks.
  - **Creatinine kinase (CK-MB)**: Increases 4–8 hours and peaks at about 24 hours (earlier with thrombolytic therapy or PTCA).
  - **Ischemia Modified Albumin (IMA)**: Increase within minutes, peak 6 hours and return to baseline; verify with other labs.
  - **Myoglobin**: Increases in 0.5–4.0 hours, peaks 6–7 hours. While an increase is not specific to an MI, a failure to increase can be used to rule out an MI.

PAPILLARY MUSCLE RUPTURE

Papillary muscle rupture is a rare but often deadly complication of myocardial ischemia/infarct. It most commonly occurs with inferior infarcts. The papillary muscles are part of the cardiac wall structure. Attached to the lower portion of the ventricles, they are responsible for the opening and closing of the tricuspid and mitral valve and preventing prolapse during systole. Rupture of the papillary muscle can occur with myocardial infarct or ischemia in the area of the heart surrounding the papillary muscle. Since the papillary muscles support the mitral valve, rupture will cause severe mitral regurgitation that may result in cardiogenic shock and subsequent death. Rupture of the papillary muscle may be partial or complete and is considered a life-threatening emergency.

Signs and symptoms: Acute heart failure, pulmonary edema, and cardiogenic shock (tachycardia, diaphoresis, loss of consciousness, pallor, tachypnea, mental status changes, weak or thready pulse, and decreased urinary output).

Diagnosis: Transesophageal echocardiography (TEE) to visualize the papillary muscles, color flow Doppler, echocardiogram, and physical assessment. In patients with papillary muscle rupture, a holosystolic murmur starting at the apex and radiating to the axilla may be present.

Treatment: Emergent surgical intervention to repair the mitral valve.

In the cases of complete rupture, patients often experience the rapid development of cardiogenic shock and subsequent death.

AORTIC ANEURYSMS

TYPES

A **dissecting aortic aneurysm** occurs when the wall of the aorta is torn and blood flows between the layers of the wall, dilating and weakening it until it risks rupture (which has a 90% mortality). Aortic aneurysms are more than twice as common in males as females, but females have a higher mortality rate, possibly due to increased age at diagnosis.

Abdominal aortic aneurysms (AAA) are usually related to atherosclerosis, but may also result from Marfan syndrome, Ehlers-Danlos disease, and connective tissue disorders. Rupture usually does not allow time for emergent repair, so identifying and correcting before rupture is essential. Different classification systems are used to describe the type and degree of dissection. Common classification:

- **DeBakey classification** uses anatomic location as the focal point:
  - Type I begins in the ascending aorta but may spread to include the aortic arch and the descending aorta (60%). This is also considered a proximal lesion or Stanford type A.
  - Type II is restricted to the ascending aorta (10-15%). This is also considered a proximal lesion or Stanford type A.
  - Type III is restricted to the descending aorta (25-30%). This is considered a distal lesion or Stanford type B.
- Types I and II are thoracic, and type III is abdominal.

DIAGNOSIS AND TREATMENT

Aortic aneurysms are often asymptomatic, but when symptomatic, patients present with substernal pain, back pain, dyspnea and/or stridor (from pressure on trachea), cough, distention of neck veins, palpable and pulsating abdominal mass, edema of neck and arms.

Diagnosis: x-ray, CT, MRI, Cardiac catheterization, TEE/transthoracic echocardiogram.

Treatment includes:

- **Anti-hypertensives** to reduce systolic BP, such as β-blockers (esmolol) or Alpha-β-blocker combinations (labetalol) to reduce force of blood as it leaves the ventricle to reduce pressure against the aortic wall. IV vasodilators (sodium nitroprusside) may also be needed.
- **Intubation and ventilation** may be required if the patient is hemodynamically unstable.
- **Analgesia/sedation** to control anxiety and pain.
- **Surgical repair**: Types I and II are usually repaired surgically because of the danger of rupture and cardiac tamponade. Type III (abdominal) is often followed medically and surgically only if the aneurysm is >5.5cm or rapidly expanding. There are two types of surgical repair:
  - **Open**: Patient is placed on cardiopulmonary bypass, and through an abdominal incision the damaged portion is removed, and a graft is sutured in place.
  - **Endovascular**: A stent graft is fed through the arteries to line the aorta and exclude the aneurysm.

Complications: Myocardial infarction, renal injury, and GI hemorrhage/ischemic bowel, which may occur up to years after surgery. Endo-leaks can occur with a stent graft, increasing risk of rupture.

AORTIC RUPTURE

Aortic rupture is a catastrophic breakage of the aorta, generally as the result of trauma or rupture of an aortic aneurysm. **Aortic rupture** (spontaneous) most commonly occurs in the abdominal aorta. The patient typically experiences a severe tearing pain and loses consciousness from hypovolemic shock as the blood pours out of the aorta. Tachycardia occurs and the patient may exhibit cyanosis. An ecchymotic area may appear in the flank area because of retroperitoneal pooling of blood. Diagnostic tests include ultrasound or CT. Survival depends on the size of the tear, the amount of blood loss, and the length of time until surgical repair. About 90% of patients die prior to surgery. An aortic occlusion balloon to stem bleeding may be placed temporarily in order to stabilize the patient. Surgical repair may be via an open procedure or endovascular therapy. Risk factors include male gender, older age, smoking, history of MI, family history of abdominal aortic aneurysm, peripheral arterial disease, and hypertension.

CARDIOGENIC SHOCK

In cardiogenic shock, the heart fails to pump enough blood to provide adequate circulation and oxygen to the body. The primary cause of cardiogenic shock is acute myocardial infarction, especially an anterior wall MI. Other causes include papillary muscle/ventricular septal rupture, pericarditis/myocarditis, prolonged tachyarrhythmia, and hypotensive medications.

Signs/Symptoms: Hypotension, altered mental status secondary to decreased cerebral circulation, oliguria, tachypnea or tachycardia, cool extremities, jugular venous distension, and pulmonary edema possible.

Diagnosis: ABGs: metabolic acidosis, hypoxia, hypocapnia; lactic acidosis, BNP, BUN and K elevated; EKG: arrhythmias, specifically SVT/V-tach, Sinus bradycardia, AV block and IVCDs possible; however, the EKG may be normal.

- Pulmonary artery catheter (Swan-Ganz catheter) values: CI <1.8 L/min, PCWP >18 mmHg, SBP <90, MAP <60, Increased CVP and PAP

Treatment includes:

- Dobutamine IV to increase cardiac contractility
- Norepinephrine IV if SBP <70
- Morphine can be given for pain; while potential for hypotension, it will decrease SNS response and decrease HR and MVO_2
- Treat underlying cause (e.g., papillary rupture = valve replacement)
- Intra-aortic balloon pump (IABP): Increases cardiac blood flow
- Re-vascularization if secondary to acute MI (CABG or PCI)

OBSTRUCTIVE SHOCK

Obstructive shock occurs when the preload (diastolic filling of the RV) of the heart is obstructed in one or several ways. There can be obstruction to the great vessels of the heart (such as from pulmonary embolism), there can be excessive afterload because the flow of blood out of the heart is obstructed (resulting in decreased cardiac output), or there can be direct compression of the heart, which can occur when blood or air fills the pericardial sac with cardiac tamponade or tension pneumothorax. Other causes include aortic dissection, vena cava syndrome, systemic hypertension, and cardiac lesions. Obstructive shock is often categorized with cardiogenic shock because of their similarities. **Signs and symptoms** of obstructive shock may vary depending on the underlying cause but typically include:

- Decrease in oxygen saturation
- Hemodynamic instability with hypotension and tachycardia, muffled heart sounds
- Chest pain
- Neurological impairment (disorientation, confusion)
- Dyspnea
- Impaired peripheral circulation (cool extremities, pallor)
- Generalized pallor and cyanosis

Treatment depends on the cause and may include oxygen, pericardiocentesis, needle thoracostomy or chest tube, and fluid resuscitation.

CARDIOMYOPATHY

DILATED CARDIOMYOPATHY

Dilated cardiomyopathy (DCM) occurs when some precipitating factor leads to decreased cardiac perfusion. The resulting ischemic cardiac tissue is replaced with scar tissue, and the healthy cells are forced to over-compensate, causing hypertrophy and over stretching. Eventually, the muscle cells become stretched beyond compensation, and dilated and weak chamber results, unable to properly contract. This causes a decrease in stroke volume and cardiac output, with the end result being enlargement of the mitral and tricuspid valves and severe valve regurgitation. While DCM is the most common form of cardiomyopathy, causes include:

- **Vascular**: Cardiac ischemia, hypertension, atherosclerosis
- **Metabolic**: Diabetes, uremia, thyrotoxicosis, and acromegaly, muscular dystrophy
- **Genetics** (familial DCM), and childbirth (peripartum DCM)
- **Viral infections**, particularly adenovirus, Varicella zoster, HIV, and Hepatitis C may cause DCM
- **Alcohol poisoning or cocaine addiction**
- **Radiation or heavy metal poisoning**, specifically cobalt

Signs/Symptoms: Dyspnea, SOB, tachycardia, S3/S4 heart sounds, holosystolic murmur, wheezes/crackles, pleural effusions, edema, JVD, ascites

Diagnosis: EKG (tachycardia/T wave changes), chest x-ray (cardiomegaly), 2D Echocardiogram (valve regurgitation/EF).

Treatment includes:

- Treat underlying cause if possible; supportive care
- Heart transplant if patient is a candidate and damage is permanent

HYPERTROPHIC CARDIOMYOPATHY

Hypertrophic cardiomyopathy (HCM) is a genetic disorder that causes idiopathic thickening of the heart muscle, primarily involving the ventricular septum and portions of the left ventricle. Patients with HCM produce abnormal sarcomeres and misalignment of muscle cells (myocardial disarray). Basically, HCM is characterized by ventricular hypertrophy, an asymmetrical septum, forceful systole, cardiac dysrhythmias, and myocardial disarray. Because the abnormal cells develop over time, it is common for HCM to remain undiagnosed until middle or late adulthood.

Signs/Symptoms: Exertional or atypical chest pain, dyspnea at rest, syncope, frequent palpitations (common due to reoccurring dysrhythmias).

Diagnosis: 2D echo (structure and EF), EKG (pathological Q waves and dysrhythmias), x-ray (cardiomegaly), Family history (especially cardiac death, reoccurring dysrhythmias, or myocardial hypertrophy).

Treatment includes:

- **Surgery**: Septal myectomy is gold standard: high mortality (3-10%), but increases cardiac output and quality of life.
- **Alcohol-based septal ablation**: Ethanol 100% injected into a branch of the LAD, creating a controlled area of infarction and consequently thinning the septum.

RESTRICTIVE CARDIOMYOPATHY

Restrictive cardiomyopathy (RCM) occurs when the ventricles become stiff and noncompliant, resulting in decreased end-diastolic cardiac refill volume. The ventricular stiffening is caused by the infiltration of fibroelastic tissue into the cardiac muscle (such as in amyloidosis or sarcoidosis). Atrial enlargement can be seen in most cases of RCM as a result of the increased effort required to push blood from the atria into the ventricles. It is not uncommon for a patient to be in atrial fibrillation secondary to atrial enlargement. In advanced cases, ventricular dysrhythmias may also be seen.

Signs/Symptoms: Exercise intolerance/fatigue, edema, crackles, elevated CVP, S3/S4, murmur, SOB at rest

Diagnosis: 2D echo (enlarged atria, decreased compliance of ventricle), hemodynamic monitoring (increased right atrial pressure and pulmonary wedge pressure, and SVR), x-ray (cardiomegaly), EKG (atrial fibrillation), endomyocardial biopsy (to differentiate from constrictive pericarditis).

Treatment includes:

- **Medications**: β-blockers increase ventricular filling; antiarrhythmics may be ordered
- **Surgical**: Heart transplant, if patient is a candidate

DYSRHYTHMIAS

SINUS BRADYCARDIA

There are 3 primary types of **sinus node dysrhythmias**: sinus bradycardia, sinus tachycardia, and sinus arrhythmia. **Sinus bradycardia (SB)** is caused by a decreased rate of impulse from sinus node. The pulse and ECG usually appear normal except for a slower rate.

SB is characterized by a regular pulse <50-60 bpm with P waves in front of QRS, which are usually normal in shape and duration. PR interval is 0.12-0.20 seconds, QRS interval is 0.04-0.11 seconds, and P:QRS ratio of 1:1. SB may be caused by several factors:

- May be normal in athletes and older adults; generally not treated unless symptomatic
- Conditions that lower the body's metabolic needs, such as hypothermia or sleep
- Hypotension and decrease in oxygenation
- Medications such as calcium channel blockers and β-blockers
- Vagal stimulation that may result from vomiting, suctioning, defecating, or certain medical procedures (carotid stent placement, etc.)
- Increased intracranial pressure
- Myocardial infarction

Treatment: involves eliminating cause if possible, such as changing medications. Atropine 0.5-1.0 mg may be given IV to block vagal stimulation or increase rate if symptomatic.

SINUS TACHYCARDIA

Sinus tachycardia (ST) occurs when the sinus node impulse increases in frequency. ST is characterized by a regular pulse >100 with P waves before QRS but sometimes part of the preceding T wave. QRS is usually of normal shape and duration (0.04-0.11 seconds) but may have consistent irregularity. PR interval is 0.12-0.20 seconds and P:QRS ratio of 1:1.

The rapid pulse decreases diastolic filling time and causes reduced cardiac output with resultant hypotension. Acute pulmonary edema may result from the decreased ventricular filling if untreated. ST may be **caused** by a number of factors:

- Acute blood loss, shock, hypovolemia, anemia
- Sinus arrhythmia, hypovolemic heart failure
- Hypermetabolic conditions, fever, infection

- Exertion/exercise, anxiety, stress
- Medications, such as sympathomimetic drugs

Treatment: eliminating precipitating factors, calcium channel blockers and β-blockers to reduce heart rate.

SUPRAVENTRICULAR TACHYCARDIA

Supraventricular tachycardia (SVT) (>100 BPM) may have a sudden onset and result in congestive heart failure. Rate may increase to 200–300 BMP, which will significantly decrease cardiac output due to decreased filling time. SVT originates in the atria rather than the ventricles but is controlled by the tissue in the area of the AV node rather than the SA node. Rhythm is usually rapid but regular. The P wave is present but may not be clearly defined as it may be obscured by the preceding T wave, and the QRS complex appears normal. The PR interval is 0.12-0.20 seconds and the QRS interval is 0.04-0.11 seconds with a P:QRS ratio of 1:1.

SVT may be episodic with periods of normal heart rate and rhythm between episodes of SVT, so it is often referred to as paroxysmal SVT (PSVT).

Treatment: Adenosine, digoxin (Lanoxin), Verapamil (Calan, Verelan), vagal maneuvers, cardioversion.

SINUS ARRHYTHMIA

Sinus arrhythmia (SA) results from irregular impulses from the sinus node, often paradoxical (increasing with inspiration and decreasing with expiration) because of stimulation of the vagal nerve during inspiration and rarely causes a negative hemodynamic effect. These cyclic changes in the pulse during respiration are quite common in both children and young adults and often lesson with age but may persist in some adults. Sinus arrhythmia can, in some cases, relate to heart or valvular disease and may be increased with vagal stimulation for suctioning, vomiting, or defecating. Characteristics of SA include a regular pulse 50-100 BPM, P waves in front of QRS with duration (0.04-0.11 seconds) and shape of QRS usually normal, PR interval of 0.12-0.20 seconds, and P:QRS ratio of 1:1.

Treatment is usually not necessary unless it is associated with bradycardia.

PREMATURE ATRIAL CONTRACTION

There are 3 primary types of **atrial dysrhythmias**: premature atrial contraction, atrial flutter, and atrial fibrillation. Premature atrial contraction (PAC) is essentially an extra beat precipitated by an electrical impulse to the atrium before the sinus node impulse. The extra beat may be caused by alcohol, caffeine, nicotine, hypervolemia, hypokalemia, hypermetabolic conditions, atrial ischemia, or infarction. Characteristics include an irregular pulse because of extra P waves, the shape and duration of QRS is usually normal (0.04-0.11 seconds) but may be abnormal, PR interval remains between 0.12-0.20, and P:QRS ratio is 1:1. Rhythm is irregular with varying P-P and R-R intervals.

PACs can occur in an essentially healthy heart and are not usually cause for concern unless they are frequent (>6 per hr) and cause severe palpitations. In that case, atrial fibrillation should be suspected.

ATRIAL FLUTTER

Atrial flutter (AF) occurs when the atrial rate is faster, usually 250-400 beats per minute, than the AV node conduction rate so not all of the beats are conducted into the ventricles. The beats are effectively blocked at the AV node, preventing ventricular fibrillation although some extra ventricular impulses may pass though. AF is caused by the same conditions that cause A-fib: coronary artery disease, valvular disease, pulmonary disease, heavy alcohol ingestion, and cardiac surgery. AF is characterized by atrial rates of 250-400 with ventricular rates of 75-150, with ventricular rate usually being regular. P waves are saw-toothed (referred to as F waves), QRS shape and duration (0.04-0.11 seconds) are usually normal, PR interval may be hard to calculate because of F waves, and the P:QRS ratio is 2:1 to 4:1. Symptoms include chest pain, dyspnea, and hypotension.

Treatment includes:

- Emergent cardioversion if condition is unstable
- Medications to slow ventricular rate and conduction through AV node: non-dihydropyridine calcium channel blockers (Cardizem, Calan) and beta blockers
- Medications to convert to sinus rhythm: Corvert, Tikosyn, Amiodarone; also used in practice: Cardioquin, Norpace, Cordarone

ATRIAL FIBRILLATION

Atrial fibrillation (A-fib) is rapid, disorganized atrial beats that are ineffective in emptying the atria, so that blood pools in the chambers. This can lead to thrombus formation and emboli. The ventricular rate increases with a decreased stroke volume, and cardiac output decreases with increased myocardial ischemia, resulting in palpitations and fatigue. A-fib is caused by coronary artery disease, valvular disease, pulmonary disease, heavy alcohol ingestion, infection, and cardiac surgery; however, it can also be idiopathic. A-fib is characterized by a very irregular pulse with atrial rate of 300-600 and ventricular rate of 120-200, shape and duration (0.04-0.11

seconds) of QRS is usually normal. Fibrillatory (F) waves are seen instead of P waves. The PR interval cannot be measured and the P:QRS ratio is highly variable.

Treatment is the same as atrial flutter.

> **Review Video: EKG Interpretation: Afib and Aflutter**
> Visit mometrix.com/academy and enter code: 263842

PREMATURE JUNCTIONAL CONTRACTION

The area around the AV node is the junction, and dysrhythmias that arise from that area are called junctional dysrhythmias. Premature junctional contraction (PJC) occurs when a premature impulse starts at the AV node before the next normal sinus impulse reaches the AV node. PJC is similar to premature atrial contraction (PAC) and generally requires no treatment although it may be an indication of digoxin toxicity. The ECG may appear basically normal with an early QRS complex that is normal in shape and duration (0.04-0.11 seconds). The P wave may be absent or it may precede, be part of, or follow the QRS with a PR interval of 0.12 seconds. The P:QRS ratio may vary from <1:1 to 1:1 (with inverted P wave). The underlying rhythm is usually regular at a heart rate of 60-100. Significant symptoms related to PJC are rare.

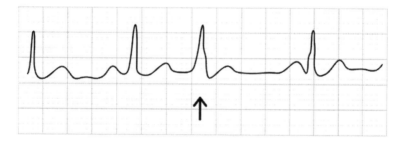

JUNCTIONAL RHYTHMS

Junctional rhythms occur when the AV node becomes the pacemaker of the heart. This can happen because the sinus node is depressed from increased vagal tone or a block at the AV node prevents sinus node impulses from being transmitted. While the sinus node normally sends impulses 60-100 beats per minute, the AV node junction usually sends impulses at 40-60 beats per minute. The QRS complex is of usual shape and duration (0.04-0.11 seconds). The P wave may be inverted and may be absent, hidden or after the QRS. If the P wave precedes the QRS, the PR interval is <0.12 seconds. The P:QRS ratio is <1:1 or 1:1. The junctional escape rhythm is a protective mechanism preventing asystole with failure of the sinus node. An **accelerated**

junctional rhythm is similar, but the heart rate is 60-100. **Junctional tachycardia** occurs with heart rate of >100.

AV NODAL REENTRY TACHYCARDIA

AV nodal reentry tachycardia occurs when an impulse conducts to the area of the AV node and is then sent in a rapidly repeating cycle back to the same area and to the ventricles, resulting in a fast ventricular rate. The onset and cessation are usually rapid. AV nodal reentry tachycardia (also known as paroxysmal atrial tachycardia or supraventricular tachycardia if there are no P waves) is characterized by atrial rate of 150-250 with ventricular rate of 75-250, P wave that is difficult to see or absent, QRS complex that is usually normal and a PR interval of <0.12 if a P wave is present. The P:QRS ratio is 1-2:1. Precipitating factors include nicotine, caffeine, hypoxemia, anxiety, underlying coronary artery disease and cardiomyopathy. Cardiac output may be decreased with a rapid heart rate, causing dyspnea, chest pain, and hypotension.

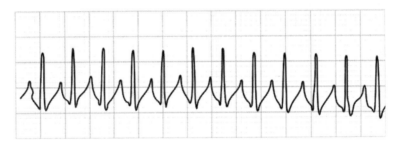

Treatment includes:

- Vagal maneuvers (carotid sinus massage, gag reflex, holding breath/bearing down)
- Medications (adenosine, verapamil, or diltiazem)
- Cardioversion if other methods unsuccessful

PREMATURE VENTRICULAR CONTRACTIONS

Premature ventricular contractions (PVCs) are those in which the impulse begins in the ventricles and conducts through them prior to the next sinus impulse. The ectopic QRS complexes may vary in shape, depending upon whether there is one site (unifocal) or more (multifocal) that stimulates the ectopic beats. PVCs usually cause no morbidity unless there is underlying cardiac disease or an acute MI. PVCs are characterized by an irregular heartbeat, QRS that is ≥0.12 seconds and oddly shaped. PVCs are often not treated in otherwise healthy people. PVCs may be precipitated by electrolyte imbalances, caffeine, nicotine, or alcohol. Because PVCs may occur with any supraventricular dysrhythmia, the underlying rhythm must be noted as well as the PVCs. If there are more than six PVCs in an hour, that is a risk factor for developing ventricular tachycardia.

Bigeminy is a rhythm where every other beat is a PVC. **Trigeminy** is a rhythm where every third beat is a PVC.

Ventricular bigeminy is a rhythm where every other beat is a PVC. **Ventricular trigeminy** is a rhythm where every third beat is a PVC.

Treatment: Lidocaine (affects the ventricles, may cause CNS toxicity with nausea and vomiting), Procainamide (affects the atria and ventricles and may cause decreased BP and widening of QRS and QT); treat underlying cause.

VENTRICULAR TACHYCARDIA

Ventricular tachycardia (VT) is greater than 3 PVCs in a row with a ventricular rate of 100-200 beats per minute. Ventricular tachycardia may be triggered by the same factors as PVCs and often is related to underlying coronary artery disease. The rapid rate of contractions makes VT dangerous as the ineffective beats may render the person unconscious with no palpable pulse. A detectable rate is usually regular and the QRS complex is ≥0.12 seconds and is usually abnormally shaped. The P wave may be undetectable with an irregular PR interval if P wave is present. The P:QRS ratio is often difficult to ascertain because of the absence of P waves.

Treatment is as follows:

- With pulse: Synchronized cardioversion, adenosine
- No pulse: Same as ventricular fibrillation

NARROW COMPLEX AND WIDE COMPLEX TACHYCARDIAS

Tachycardias are classified as narrow complex or wide complex. Wide and narrow refer to the configuration of the QRS complex.

- **Wide complex tachycardia (WCT)**: About 80% of cases of WCT are caused by ventricular tachycardia. WCT originates at some point below the AV node and may be associated with palpitations, dyspnea, anxiety, diaphoresis, and cardiac arrest. Wide complex tachycardia is diagnosed with more than 3 consecutive beats at a heart rate >100 BPM and QRS duration ≥0.12 seconds.

- **Narrow complex tachycardia (NCT)**: NCT is associated with palpitations, dyspnea, and peripheral edema. NCT is generally supraventricular in origin. Narrow complex tachycardia is diagnosed with ≥3 consecutive beats at heart rate of >100 BPM and QRS duration of <0.12 seconds.

VENTRICULAR FIBRILLATION

Ventricular fibrillation (VF) is a rapid, very irregular ventricular rate >300 beats per minute with no atrial activity observable on the ECG, caused by disorganized electrical activity in the ventricles. The QRS complex is not recognizable as ECG shows irregular undulations. The causes are the same as for ventricular tachycardia and asystole. VF is accompanied by lack of palpable pulse, audible pulse, and respirations and is immediately life threatening without defibrillation.

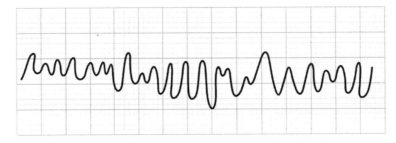

Treatment includes:

- Emergency defibrillation, the cause should be identified and treated
- Epinephrine 1 mg q 3-5minutes then amiodarone 300mg (2nd dose: 150mg) IV push

Review Video: **EKG Interpretation: Ventricular Arrythmias**
Visit mometrix.com/academy and enter code: 933152

IDIOVENTRICULAR RHYTHM

Ventricular escape rhythm (idioventricular) occurs when the Purkinje fibers below the AV node create an impulse. This may occur if the sinus node fails to fire or if there is blockage at the AV node so that the impulse does not go through. Idioventricular rhythm is characterized by a regular ventricular rate of 20-40 BPM. Rates >40 BPM are called accelerated idioventricular rhythm. The P wave is missing and the QRS complex has a very bizarre and abnormal shape with duration of ≥0.12 seconds. The low ventricular rate may cause a decrease in cardiac output, often making the patient lose consciousness. In other patients, the idioventricular rhythm may not be associated with reduced cardiac output.

VENTRICULAR ASYSTOLE

Ventricular asystole is the absence of audible heartbeat, palpable pulse, and respirations, a condition often referred to as "cardiac arrest." While the ECG may show some P waves initially, the QRS complex is absent although there may be an occasional QRS "escape beat" (agonal rhythm). Cardiopulmonary resuscitation is required with intubation for ventilation and establishment of an intravenous line for fluids. Without immediate treatment, the patient will suffer from severe hypoxia and brain death within minutes. Identifying the cause is critical for the patient's survival. Consider the "Hs & Ts": hypovolemia, hypoxia, hydrogen ions (acidosis), hypo/hyperkalemia, hypothermia, tension pneumothorax, tamponade (cardiac), toxins, and thrombosis (pulmonary or coronary). Even with immediate treatment, the prognosis is poor and ventricular asystole is often a sign of impending death.

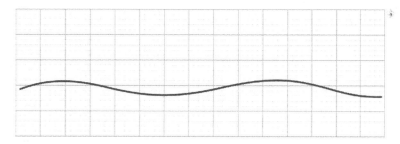

Treatment includes:

- CPR only; Asystole is not a shockable rhythm therefore defibrillation is not indicated
- Epinephrine 1 mg q 3-5 minutes

SINUS PAUSE

Sinus pause occurs when the sinus node fails to function properly to stimulate heart contractions, so there is a pause on the ECG recording that may persist for a few seconds to minutes, depending on the severity of the dysfunction. A prolonged pause may be difficult to differentiate from cardiac arrest. During the sinus pause, the P wave, QRS complex and PR and QRS intervals are all absent. P:QRS ratio is 1:1 and the rhythm is irregular. The pulse rate may vary widely, usually 60-100 BPM. Patients with frequent pauses may complain of dizziness or syncope. The patient may need to undergo an electrophysiology study and medication reconciliation to determine the cause. If measures such as decreasing medication are not effective, a pacemaker is usually indicated (if symptomatic).

FIRST-DEGREE AV BLOCK

First-degree AV block occurs when the atrial impulses are conducted through the AV node to the ventricles at a rate that is slower than normal. While the P and QRS are usually normal, the PR interval is >0.20 seconds, and the P:QRS ratio is 1:1. A narrow QRS complex indicates a conduction abnormality only in the AV node, but a widened QRS indicates associated damage to the bundle branches as well. *Chronic* first-degree block may be caused by fibrosis/sclerosis of the conduction system related to coronary artery disease, valvular disease, cardiac myopathies and carries little morbidity, thus is often left untreated. *Acute* first-degree block, on the other hand, is of much more concern and may be related to digoxin toxicity, β-blockers, amiodarone, myocardial infarction, hyperkalemia, or edema related to valvular surgery.

Treatment: involves eliminating cause if possible, such as changing medications. Atropine 0.5-1.0 mg may be given IV if rate falls.

SECOND-DEGREE AV BLOCK

Second-degree AV block occurs when some of the atrial beats are blocked. Second-degree AV block is further subdivided according to the patterns of block.

TYPE I

Mobitz type I block (Wenckebach) occurs when each atrial impulse in a group of beats is conducted at a lengthened interval until one fails to conduct (the PR interval progressively increases), so there are more P waves than QRS complexes, but the QRS complex is usually of normal shape and duration. The sinus node functions at a regular rate, so the P-P interval is regular, but the R-R interval usually shortens with each impulse. The P:QRS ratio varies, such as 3:2, 4:3, 5:4. This type of block by itself usually does not cause significant morbidity unless associated with an inferior wall myocardial infarction.

TYPE II

In Mobitz type II, only some of the atrial impulses are conducted unpredictably through the AV node to the ventricles, and the block always occurs below the AV node in the bundle of His, the bundle branches, or the Purkinje fibers. The PR intervals are the same if impulses are conducted, and the QRS complex is usually widened. The P:QRS ratio varies 2:1, 3:1, and 4:1. Type II block is more dangerous than Type I because it may progress to complete AV block and may produce Stokes-Adams syncope. Additionally, if the block is at the Purkinje fibers, there is no escape impulse. Usually, a transcutaneous cardiac pacemaker and defibrillator should be at the patient's bedside. **Symptoms** may include chest pain if the heart block is precipitated by myocarditis or myocardial ischemia.

THIRD-DEGREE

With third-degree AV block, there are more P waves than QRS complexes, with no clear relationship between them. The atrial rate is 2-3 times the pulse rate, so the PR interval is irregular. If the SA node malfunctions, the AV node fires at a lower rate, and if the AV node malfunctions, the pacemaker site in the ventricles takes over at a bradycardic rate; thus, with complete AV block, the heart still contracts, but often ineffectually. With this type of block, the atrial P (sinus rhythm or atrial fibrillation) and the ventricular QRS (ventricular escape rhythm) are stimulated by different impulses, so there is AV dissociation.

The heart may compensate at rest but can't keep pace with exertion. The resultant bradycardia may cause congestive heart failure, fainting, or even sudden death, and usually conduction abnormalities slowly worsen. **Symptoms** include dyspnea, chest pain, and hypotension, which are treated with IV atropine. Transcutaneous pacing may be needed. Complete persistent AV block normally requires implanted pacemakers, usually dual chamber.

> **Review Video: AV Heart Blocks**
> Visit mometrix.com/academy and enter code: 487004

BUNDLE BRANCH BLOCKS

A **right bundle branch block (RBBB)** occurs when conduction is blocked in the right bundle branch that carries impulses from the Bundle of His to the right ventricle. The impulse travels through the left ventricle instead, and then reaches the right ventricle, but this causes a slight delay in contraction of the right ventricle. A RBBB is characterized by normal P waves (as the right atrium still contracts appropriately), but the QRS complex is widened and notched (referred to as an "RSR pattern" that resembles the letter "M") in lead V1, which is a reflection of the asynchronous ventricular contraction. The PR interval is normal or prolonged, and the QRS interval is > 0.12 seconds. P:QRS ratio remains 1:1 with regular rhythms.

A **left bundle branch block (LBBB)** occurs when there is a delay in conduction between the left atrium and left ventricle. It is also characterized by normal or inverted P waves, but the QRS complex may be widened with a deep S wave and an interval of >0.12 seconds (in lead V1) that resembles a "W." The PR interval may be normal or prolonged. The P:QRS ratio is 1:1 and the rhythm is regular.

HEART FAILURE

Heart failure (formerly congestive heart failure) is a cardiac disease that includes disorders of contractions (systolic dysfunction) or filling (diastolic dysfunction) or both and may include pulmonary, peripheral, or systemic edema. The most common causes are coronary artery disease, systemic or pulmonary hypertension, cardiomyopathy, and valvular disorders. The incidence of chronic heart failure correlates with age. The 2 main types of HF are systolic and diastolic. HF is classified according to symptoms and prognosis:

- **Class I**: The patient is essentially asymptomatic during normal activities with no pulmonary congestion or peripheral hypotension. There is no restriction on activities, and prognosis is good.
- **Class II**: Symptoms appear with physical exertion but are usually absent at rest, resulting in some limitations of activities of daily living (ADLs). Slight pulmonary edema may be evident by basilar rales. Prognosis is good.
- **Class III**: Obvious limitations of ADLs and discomfort on any exertion. Prognosis is fair.
- **Class IV**: Symptoms at rest. Prognosis is poor.

Treatment may include:

- Careful monitoring of **fluid balance** and **weight** to determine changes in fluid retention
- **Low sodium diet**
- **Restriction of activity**
- **Medications** may include diuretics, vasodilators, or ACE inhibitors to decrease the heart's workload, digoxin may be given to increase contractibility
- **Anticoagulant therapy** if distended atria, enlarged ventricles, or atrial fibrillation to decrease the danger of thromboembolic

---

Review Video: <u>Congestive Heart Failure</u>
Visit mometrix.com/academy and enter code: 924118

SYSTOLIC HEART FAILURE

Systolic heart failure is the typical "left-sided" failure and reduces the amount of blood ejected from the ventricles during contraction (decreased ejection fraction). This stimulates the SNS to produce catecholamines to support the myocardium, which eventually causes down regulation, the destruction of beta and adrenergic receptor sites, and ultimately further myocardial damage. Because of reduced perfusion, the R-A-A pathway (renin, angiotensin I&II, aldosterone) is initiated by the kidneys, causing sodium and fluid retention. The end result of these processes is increased preload and afterload, thus increased workload on the ventricles. They begin to lose contractibility and blood begins to pool inside, stretching the myocardium (ventricular remodeling). The heart compensates by thickening the muscle (hypertrophy) without an adequate increase in capillary blood supply, leading to ischemia.

Symptoms: Activity intolerance, dyspnea/orthopnea (sleeping in a recliner is a classic symptom), cough (frothy sputum), edema, heart sounds S3 and S4, hepatomegaly, JVD, LOC changes, and tachycardia.

Treatment includes:

- Medication
- **Surgery**: Heart transplant (if a candidate)
- **Lifestyle modification**: Low-sodium diet, supplemental oxygen, daily weights (report >3 lb/day or 5 lb/week weight gain to physician)

DIASTOLIC HEART FAILURE

Diastolic heart failure may be difficult to differentiate from systolic heart failure based on clinical symptoms, which are similar. With diastolic heart failure, the myocardium is unable to sufficiently relax to facilitate filling of the ventricles. This may be the end result of systolic heart failure as myocardial hypertrophy stiffens the muscles, and the causes are similar. Diastolic heart failure is more common in females >75. Typically, intra-cardiac pressures at rest are within normal range but increase markedly on exertion. Because the relaxation of the heart is delayed, the ventricles do not expand enough for the fill-volume, and the heart cannot increase stroke volume during exercise, so symptoms (dyspnea, fatigue, pulmonary edema) are often pronounced on exertion. Ejection fractions are usually >40-50% with increase in left ventricular end-diastolic pressure (LVEDP) and decrease in left ventricular end-diastolic volume (LVEDV).

The major goal with all types of heart failure is to prevent further damage and remodeling, prevent exacerbations, and improve the patient's long-term prognosis.

ACUTE HEART FAILURE

Acute decompensated heart failure occurs when the body cannot compensate for the heart's inability to provide adequate perfusion. Cardiac output is no longer sufficient to meet the metabolic demands of the body. Acute heart failure occurs suddenly and can be precipitated by dysrhythmias, illness, noncompliance with medications, acute ischemia, fluid overload or hypertensive crisis. Acute heart failure is most commonly related to left ventricular systolic or diastolic dysfunction. It requires immediate treatment to restore adequate perfusion and is often life-threatening.

Signs and symptoms: Dyspnea, cough, edema, ascites and elevated jugular venous pressure, fatigue, cool extremities, hypotension and altered mental status

Diagnostic testing: Chest x-ray, electrocardiogram, physical exam; labs—basic metabolic panel, BUN, creatinine, and B-natriuretic peptide (BNP)

Treatment: Rapid assessment and stabilization of the patient. The physical assessment should include a thorough evaluation of the patient's respiratory status and supplemental oxygen and potentially ventilator support may be necessary. Medications: Diuretics to decrease fluid volume; vasodilators to decrease pulmonary congestion. Cardiac monitoring, urine output monitoring, sodium restriction, and venous thromboembolism prophylaxis may also be utilized.

ACUTE CARDIAC-RELATED PULMONARY EDEMA

Acute cardiac-related pulmonary edema occurs when heart failure results in fluid overload, leading to third-spacing of fluid into the interstitial spaces of the lungs. Pulmonary edema may result from MI, chronic HF, volume overload, ischemia, or mitral stenosis.

Symptoms include severe dyspnea, cough with blood-tinged frothy sputum, wheezing/rales/crackles on auscultation, cyanosis, and diaphoresis.

Diagnosis: Auscultation, chest x-ray, and echocardiogram.

Treatment includes:

- Sitting position with 100% oxygen by mask to achieve PO_2 >60%
- Non-invasive pressure support ventilation (BiPAP) or endotracheal intubation and mechanical ventilation
- Morphine sulfate 2-8 mg (IV for severe cases), repeated every 2-4 hours as needed—decreases pre-load and anxiety
- IV diuretics (furosemide ≥40 mg or bumetanide ≥1 mg) to provide venous dilation and diuresis
- Nitrates as a bolus with an infusion—decreases pre-load
- Inhaled β-adrenergic agonists or aminophylline for bronchospasm
- Digoxin IV for tachycardia
- ACE inhibitors, nitroprusside to reduce afterload

ENDOCARDITIS

Endocarditis is an infection of the lining of the heart that covers the heart valves and contains Purkinje fibers, known as the endocardium. Risk factors include being over 60 years of age, being male, IV drug use, and dental infections. Staphylococcal aureus is the most common cause of infective endocarditis. Etiology includes subacute bacterial endocarditis (often related to dental procedures), prosthetic valvular endocarditis (following valve replacement), and right sided endocarditis (often related to catheter infections and IV drug use). Organisms enter the bloodstream from portals of entry (surgery, catheterization, IV drug abuse) and migrate to the heart, growing on the endothelial tissue and forming vegetations (verrucae), collagen deposits, and platelet thrombi. With endocarditis, the valves frequently become deformed, but the pathogenic agents may also invade other tissues, such as the chordae tendineae. The lesions may invade adjacent tissue and break off, becoming emboli. The mitral valve is the most common valve affected, followed by aortic, tricuspid, and the pulmonary valve being the least often affected. Positive blood cultures, widened pulse pressures, ECG, murmurs, and vegetations seen on a transesophageal echocardiogram are used to make the diagnosis. After diagnosis is made, antibiotics are used for treatment, and when unsuccessful or when heart failure is present, valve repair may be warranted. Serious complications from endocarditis include emboli, sepsis, and heart failure. Untreated endocarditis is fatal.

DIAGNOSIS AND TREATMENT

Diagnosis of endocarditis is made on the basis of clinical presentation and **diagnostic procedures** that may include:

- **Blood cultures** should be done with 3 sets for both aerobic and anaerobic bacteria. Diagnosis is definitive if 2 cultures are positive, but a negative culture does not preclude bacterial endocarditis.
- **Echocardiogram** may identify vegetation on valves or increasing heart failure
- **ECG** may demonstrate prolonged PR interval
- **Anemia** (normochromic, normocytic)
- Elevated **white blood cell count**
- Elevated **erythrocyte sedimentation rate** (ESR) and **C-reactive protein** (CRP)

Treatment includes general management of symptoms and the following:

- **Antimicrobials** specific to the pathogenic organism, usually administered IV for 4 to 6 weeks
- **Surgical replacement** of aortic and/or mitral valves may be necessary (in 30% to 40% of cases) if there is no response to treatment and/or after infection is controlled if there are severe symptoms related to valve damage

CLINICAL SYMPTOMS

Clinical symptoms of endocarditis usually relate to the response to infection, the underlying heart disease, emboli, or immunological response. Typical **symptoms** include:

- Slow onset with unexplained low-grade and often intermittent **fever**
- **Anorexia** and weight loss, difficulty feeding
- General **lassitude** and malaise
- **Splenomegaly** present in 60% of patients; **hepatomegaly** may also be present
- **Anemia** is present in almost all patients
- Sudden **aortic valve insufficiency** or mitral valve insufficiency
- **Cyanosis** with clubbing of fingers
- **Embolism** of other body organs (brain, liver, bones)
- **Congestive heart failure**
- **Dysrhythmias**
- New or change in **heart murmur**
- **Immunological responses**
- **Janeway lesions**: painless areas of hemorrhage on palms of hands and soles of feet
- **Splinter hemorrhages**: thin, brown-black lines on nails of fingers and toes
- **Petechiae**: pinpoint-sized hemorrhages on oral mucous membranes, as well as hands and trunk

- **Roth spots**: retinal hemorrhagic lesions caused by emboli on nerve fibers
- **Glomerulonephritis**: microscopic hematuria

MYOCARDITIS

Myocarditis is inflammation of the cardiac myocardium (muscle tissue), usually triggered by a viral infection, such as the influenza virus, Coxsackie virus, and HIV. Myocarditis can also be caused by bacteria, fungi, or parasites, or an allergic response to medications. In some cases, it is also a complication of endocarditis. It may also be triggered by chemotherapy drugs and some antibiotics. Myocarditis can result in dilation of the heart, development of thrombi on the heart walls (known as mural thrombi), and infiltration of blood cells around the coronary vessels and between muscle fibers, causing further degeneration of the muscle tissue. The heart may become enlarged and weak, as the ability to pump blood is impaired, leading to congestive heart failure. Symptoms depend upon the extent of damage but may include fatigue, dyspnea, pressure and discomfort in chest or epigastric area, and palpitations.

DIAGNOSIS AND TREATMENT

Diagnosis of myocarditis depends upon the clinical picture, as there is no test specific for myocarditis, although a number of tests may be done to verify the **clinical diagnosis**:

- **Chest radiograph** may indicate cardiomegaly or pulmonary edema.
- **ECG** may show nonspecific changes.
- **Echocardiogram** may indicate cardiomegaly and demonstrate defects in functioning.
- **Cardiac catheterization** and **cardiac biopsy** will yield confirmation in 65% of cases, but not all of the heart muscle may be affected, so a negative finding does not rule out myocarditis.
- **Viral cultures** of nasopharynx and rectal may help to identify organism.
- **Viral titers** may increase as disease progresses.
- **Polymerase chain reaction** (PCR) of biopsy specimen may be most effective for diagnosis.

Treatment:

- As indicated for underlying cause (such as antibiotics)
- Restriction of activities
- Careful **monitoring** for heart failure and medical treatment as indicated (e.g., diuretics, digoxin)
- **Oxygen** as needed to maintain normal oxygen saturation
- **IV gamma globulin** for acute stage

ACUTE PERICARDITIS

Pericarditis is inflammation of the pericardial sac with or without increased pericardial fluid. It may be an isolated process or the effect of an underlying disease. If the underlying cause is autoimmune or related to malignancy of some sort, the patient usually presents with symptoms that relate to that disorder. However, most cases are related to a viral etiology, and therefore usually present with flu-like symptoms. Patients that have idiopathic pericarditis or viral pericarditis have a good prognosis with medication alone.

Signs/Symptoms: Sharp chest pain, worsened with inspiration and relieved by leaning forward or sitting up (most common symptom; "Mohammad's Sign"), pericardial effusion, respiratory distress, auscultated friction rub, ST elevation/PR depression (progresses to flattened T, inverted T, then return to normal); risk of pericardial effusion.

Diagnosis: Echocardiogram, ECG, pericardiocentesis or pericardial biopsy, cardiac enzymes (may be mildly elevated), WBC/ESR/CRP all elevated.

Treatment includes:

- **Medications**: NSAIDs for pain/inflammation, Colchicine 0.5 mg twice a day for six months is often prescribed in adjunct to NSAID therapy, as it decreases the incidence of recurrence
- **Surgery**: Pericardiectomy only in extreme cases

MITRAL STENOSIS

Mitral stenosis is a narrowing of the mitral valve that allows blood to flow from the left atrium to the left ventricle. Pressure in the left atrium increases to overcome resistance, resulting in enlargement of the left atrium and increased pressure in the pulmonary veins and capillaries of the lung (pulmonary hypertension). Mitral stenosis can be caused by infective endocarditis, calcifications, or tumors in the left atrium.

Signs/Symptoms: Exertional dyspnea, orthopnea/nocturnal dyspnea, right-sided heart failure, loud S_1 and S_2, and mid-diastolic murmur.

Diagnosis: Cardiac catheterization, chest x-ray, echocardiogram, ECG.

Treatment includes:

- **Medications**: Antiarrhythmic, anticoagulant, and antihypertensive medications
- **Surgical**: Open/closed commissurotomy, balloon valvuloplasty, and mitral valve replacement

MITRAL VALVE INSUFFICIENCY

Mitral valve insufficiency occurs when the mitral valve fails to close completely so that there is backflow into the left atrium from the left ventricle during systole, decreasing cardiac output. It may occur with mitral stenosis or independently. Mitral valve insufficiency can result from damage caused by rheumatic fever, myxomatous degeneration, infective endocarditis, collagen vascular disease (Marfan's syndrome), or cardiomyopathy/left heart failure. There are **three phases** of the disease:

- **Acute**: May occur with rupture of a chordae tendineae or papillary muscle causing sudden left ventricular flooding and overload.
- **Chronic compensated**: Enlargement of the left atrium to decrease filling pressure, and hypertrophy of the left ventricle.
- **Chronic decompensated**: Left ventricle fails to compensate for the volume overload; decreased stroke volume and increased cardiac output.

Symptoms: Orthopnea/dyspnea, split S_2/S_3/S_4 heart sounds, systolic murmur, palpitations, right-sided heart failure, fatigue, angina (rare).

Diagnosis: Cardiac catheterization, chest x-ray, echocardiogram, ECG.

Treatment includes:

- **Medications**: Antiarrhythmic, anticoagulant, and antihypertensive medications.
- **Surgical**: Annuloplasty or valvuloplasty, and mitral valve replacement.

AORTIC STENOSIS

Aortic stenosis is a stricture (narrowing) of the aortic valve that controls the flow of blood from the left ventricle. This causes the left ventricular wall to thicken as it increases pressure to overcome the valvular resistance, increasing afterload and increasing the need for blood supply from the coronary arteries. This condition may result from a birth defect or childhood rheumatic fever, and tends to worsen over the years as the heart grows.

Symptoms: Angina, exercise intolerance, dyspnea, split S_1 and S_2, systolic murmur at base of carotids, hypotension on exertion, syncope, left-sided heart failure; sudden death can occur.

Diagnosis: Cardiac catheterization, chest x-ray, echocardiogram, ECG.

Treatment includes:

- **Medications**: Antiarrhythmic, anticoagulant, and antihypertensive medications
- **Surgical**: Balloon valvuloplasty, and aortic valve replacement

PULMONIC STENOSIS

Pulmonic stenosis is a stricture of the pulmonary blood that controls the flow of blood from the right ventricle to the lungs, resulting in right ventricular hypertrophy as the pressure increases in the right ventricle and decreased pulmonary blood flow. The condition may be asymptomatic or symptoms may not be evident until adulthood, depending upon the severity of the defect. Pulmonic stenosis may be associated with a number of other heart defects.

Symptoms: May be asymptomatic; dyspnea on exertion, systolic heart murmur, right-sided heart failure.

Diagnosis: Cardiac catheterization, chest x-ray, echocardiogram, ECG.

Treatment includes:

- **Medications**: Antiarrhythmic, anticoagulant, and antihypertensive medications
- **Surgical**: Balloon valvuloplasty, valvotomy, valvectomy with or without transannular patch, and pulmonary valve replacement

CAROTID ARTERY STENOSIS

The common carotid artery branches from the subclavian artery and then bifurcates into the external carotid and internal carotid arteries. This point of bifurcation is a common site for the development of plaques, causing **carotid artery stenosis** that interferes with cranial blood flow. When stenosis develops slowly, collateral vessels may form to aid circulation, but sudden occlusion can cause permanent brain damage and death. Most stenosis is caused by atherosclerosis, with increasing incidence with age. Most ischemia relates to an embolism or thrombus formation.

Symptoms of occlusion are often asymptomatic; however, they include severe pain, anxiety, and those symptoms common to brain attacks (hemiparesis, confusion, aphasia, and diplopia).

Diagnosis: Duplex ultrasound (combining conventional ultrasound with Doppler, determines blood flow and obstruction), CT scan, MRA or angiogram (will indicate degree of blockage).

Treatment may include:

- Medications: Anticoagulants and thrombolytics.
- Carotid endarterectomy (recommended if stenosis >60%): poses the danger of a post-procedure stroke due to plaque dislodgement or increased blood flow to narrowed vessels, so the benefits must be carefully weighed.
- Carotid stents/angioplasty (newer non-invasive approaches).

CARDIAC TAMPONADE

Cardiac tamponade occurs with pericardial effusion, causing pressure against the heart. It may be a complication of trauma, pericarditis, cardiac surgery, pneumothorax, or heart failure. About 50 mL of fluid normally circulates in the pericardial area to reduce friction, and a sudden increase in this volume or air in the pericardial sac can compress the heart, causing a number of cardiac responses such as:

- Increased end-diastolic pressure in both ventricles
- Decrease in venous return
- Decrease in ventricular filling

Symptoms may include pressure or pain in the chest, dyspnea, and pulsus paradoxus >10 mmHg. Beck's triad (increased CVP, distended neck veins, muffled heart sounds, and hypotension) is common. A sudden decrease in chest tube drainage can occur as fluid and clots accumulate in the pericardial sac, preventing the blood from filling the ventricles and decreasing cardiac output and perfusion of the body, including the kidneys (resulting in decreased urinary output). X-ray may show change in cardiac silhouette and mediastinal shift (in 20%). Treatment includes pericardiocentesis with large bore needle or surgical repair to control bleeding and relieve cardiac compression. Risk factors include cardiac surgery, cardiac tumors, MI, and chest trauma.

HYPERTENSIVE CRISES

Hypertensive crises are marked elevations in blood pressure that can cause severe organ damage if left untreated. Hypertensive crises may be caused by endocrine/renal disorders (pheochromocytoma), dissection of an aortic aneurysm, pulmonary edema, subarachnoid hemorrhage, stroke, eclampsia, and medication noncompliance. There are two **classifications**:

- **Hypertensive emergency** occurs when acute hypertension, usually >220 systolic and 120 mmHg diastolic, must be treated immediately to lower blood pressure in order to prevent damage to vital organs.
- **Hypertensive urgency** occurs when acute hypertension must be treated within a few hours but the vital organs are not in immediate danger. Blood pressure is lowered more slowly to avoid hypotension, ischemia of vital organs, or failure of autoregulation.
  - o 1/3 reduction in 6 hours
  - o 1/3 reduction in next 24 hours
  - o 1/3 reduction over days 2-4

Symptoms: Basilar HA, blurred vision, chest pain, N/V, SOB, seizures, ruddy pallor, and anxiety

Diagnostics: ECG, Chest x-ray, CBC, BMP, Urinalysis (+ blood and casts)

Treatment includes:

- Medications: Vasodilators (Cardene, Nitro, etc.) and diuretics
- Nursing Interventions: Raise HOB to 90°, supplemental O_2, frequent neuro checks, teach concerning medication compliance

PERIPHERAL ARTERIAL AND VENOUS INSUFFICIENCY

Characteristics of peripheral arterial and venous insufficiency are listed below:

- **Arterial insufficiency**
  - o **Pain**: Ranging from intermittent claudication to severe and constant shooting pain
  - o **Pulses**: Weak or absent
  - o **Skin**: Rubor on dependency, but pallor of foot on elevation; pale, shiny, and cool skin with loss of hair on toes and foot; nails thick and ridged
  - o **Ulcers**: Painful, deep, circular, often necrotic ulcers on toe tips, toe webs, heels, or other pressure areas
  - o **Edema**: Minimal

- **Venous insufficiency**
  - o **Pain**: Aching/cramping
  - o **Pulses**: Strong/present
  - o **Skin**: Brownish discoloration around ankles and anterior tibial area
  - o **Ulcers**: Varying degrees of pain in superficial, irregular ulcers on medial or lateral malleolus and sometimes the anterior tibial area
  - o **Edema**: Moderate to severe

ACUTE PERIPHERAL VASCULAR INSUFFICIENCY

Acute peripheral arterial insufficiency can occur when sudden occlusion of a blood vessel causes tissue ischemia, ultimately leading to cellular death and necrosis. This can occur as a result of traumatic injury or non-traumatic events such as arterial thrombus or embolism, vasospasm, or severe swelling (compartment syndrome). Risk factors for acute peripheral arterial insufficiency include age, tobacco use, diabetes mellitus, hyperlipidemia, and hypertension.

- **Signs and symptoms**: Classic 6 P's: Pain (extreme, unrelieved by narcotics), pallor, pulselessness, poikilothermia (the inability to regulate body temperature; extremity is room temperature), paresthesias, and paralysis (late).
- **Diagnosis**: Ultrasound, angiography, and physical exam; labs—coagulation studies, CBC, BMP, creatinine phosphokinase
- **Treatment**: Re-establishment of blood flow to the affected area
- **Arterial thrombus or embolism**: Mechanical thrombolysis may be performed to remove the clot occluding the vessel.
  - o **Trauma**: Surgical repair of the severed/injured vessels. Fasciotomy may be performed in the event of compartment syndrome to relieve pressure.
  - o **Other treatment options**: Hyperbaric oxygen therapy, anti-platelet therapy for the prevention of arterial thrombosis and anti-coagulant therapy for the prevention of venous thrombosis

ACUTE VENOUS THROMBOEMBOLISM

Acute venous thromboembolism (VTE) is a condition that includes both deep vein thrombosis (DVT) and pulmonary emboli (PE). VTE may be precipitated by invasive procedures, lack of mobility, and inflammation, so it is a common complication in critical care units. **Virchow's triad** comprises common risk factors: blood stasis, injury to endothelium, and hypercoagulability. Some patients may be initially asymptomatic, but **symptoms** may include:

- Aching or throbbing pain
- Positive Homan's sign (pain in calf when foot is dorsiflexed)
- Unilateral erythema and edema
- Dilation of vessels
- Cyanosis

Diagnosis: ultrasound and/or D-dimer test, which tests the serum for cross-linked fibrin derivatives. A CT scan, pulmonary angiogram, and ventilation-perfusion lung scan may be used to diagnose pulmonary emboli.

Treatment includes:

- Medications: IV heparin, tPA, or other anticoagulation; analgesia for pain
- Surgical: May have to surgically remove clot if large
- Bed rest, elevation of affected limb; stockings on ambulation

Prevention: Use of sequential compression devices (SCDs) or foot pumps, routine anticoagulant use for those at highest risk (Heparin SQ), early and frequent ambulation

Cardiovascular Procedures and Interventions

CARDIOVERSION

Cardioversion sends a timed electrical stimulation to the heart to convert a tachydysrhythmia (such as atrial fibrillation) to a normal sinus rhythm. Usually, anticoagulation therapy is done for at least 3 weeks prior to elective cardioversion to reduce the risk of emboli, and digoxin is discontinued for at least 48 hours prior. During the procedure, the patient is usually sedated and/or anesthetized. Electrodes in the form of gel-covered paddles or pads are placed in the anteroposterior position and then connected by leads to a computerized ECG and cardiac monitor with a defibrillator. The defibrillator is synchronized with the ECG so that the electrical current is delivered during ventricular depolarization (QRS). The timing must be precise in order to prevent ventricular tachycardia or ventricular fibrillation. Sometimes, drug therapy is used in conjunction with cardioversion; for example, antiarrhythmics (Cardizem, Cordarone) may be given before the procedure to slow the heart rate.

Arrhythmia	Beginning Monophasic Shock	Beginning Biphasic Shock
Atrial Fibrillation	50-100 J	25 J
Atrial Flutter	25-50 J	15 J
Ventricular Tachycardia	100-200 J	50 J

EMERGENCY DEFIBRILLATION

Emergency defibrillation delivers a non-synchronized shock that is given to treat acute ventricular fibrillation, pulseless ventricular tachycardia, or polymorphic ventricular tachycardia with a rapid rate and decompensating hemodynamics. **Defibrillation** can be given at any point in the cardiac cycle. It causes depolarization of myocardial cells, which can then repolarize to regain a normal sinus rhythm. Defibrillation delivers an electrical discharge through pads/paddles. In an acute care setting, the preferred position to place the pads is the anteroposterior position. In this position, one pad is placed to the right of the sternum about the second to third intercostal space, and the other pad is placed between the left scapula and the spinal column. This decreases the chances of damaging implanted devices, such as pacemakers, and this positioning has also been shown to be more effective for external cardioversion (if indicated at some point during resuscitation). There are two main types of defibrillator shock waveforms: monophasic and biphasic. Biphasic defibrillators deliver a shock in one direction for half of the shock, and then in the return direction for the other half, making them more effective and able to be used at lower energy levels. Monophasic defibrillation is given at 200-360 J and biphasic defibrillation is given at 100-200 J.

PERICARDIOCENTESIS

Pericardiocentesis is done with ultrasound guidance to diagnose pericardial effusion or with ECG and ultrasound guidance to relieve cardiac tamponade. **Pericardiocentesis** may be done as treatment for cardiac arrest or with presentation of PEA with increased jugular venous pressure. Non-hemorrhagic tamponade may be relieved in 60-90% of cases, but hemorrhagic tamponade requires thoracotomy, as blood will continue to accumulate until the cause of the hemorrhage is corrected. Resuscitation equipment must be available, including a defibrillator, intravenous line in place, and cardiac monitoring.

The **procedure** is as follows:

- Elevate the chest 45° to bring the heart closer to the chest wall, pre-medicate with atropine, and insert a nasogastric tube if indicated.
- Cleanse the skin with chlorhexidine or another appropriate cleanser.
- After insertion of the needle using ultrasound guidance, remove the obturator and attach a syringe for aspiration.
- The needle can often be replaced with a catheter after removal for drainage.
- A post-procedure chest x-ray should be done to check for pneumothorax.

119

Possible Complications: Pneumo/hemothorax, coronary artery rupture, hepatic injury, dysrhythmias, and false negative/positive aspiration.

PACEMAKERS

Pacemakers are used to stimulate the heart when the normal conduction system of the heart is defective. **Pacemakers** may be used temporarily or be permanently implanted. Temporary pacemakers for external cardiac pacing are commonly used in the emergency setting. Temporary pacemakers may be used prophylactically or therapeutically to treat a cardiac abnormality. Clinical uses include:

- To treat persistent **dysrhythmias** not responsive to medications
- To increase **cardiac output** with bradydysrhythmia by increasing rate
- To decrease **ventricular or supraventricular tachycardia** by "overdrive" stimulation of contractions
- To treat **secondary heart block** caused by myocardial infarction, ischemia, and drug toxicity
- To improve **cardiac output** after cardiac surgery
- To provide **diagnostic information** through electrophysiology studies, which induce dysrhythmias for purposes of evaluation
- To provide **pacing** when a permanent pacemaker malfunctions

> **Review Video: Pacemaker Care**
> Visit mometrix.com/academy and enter code: 979075

TRANSCUTANEOUS PACING

Transcutaneous pacing is used temporarily in an emergency situation to treat symptomatic bradydysrhythmias that don't respond to medications (atropine) and result in hemodynamic instability. Generally, the patient is provided oxygen and some sort of mild sedation before the pacing. The placement of pacing pads is usually one pacing pad (negative) on the left chest, inferior to the clavicle, and the other (positive) on the left back, inferior to the scapula, so the heart is sandwiched between the two. Lead wires attach the pads to the monitor. The rate of pacing is usually set around 80 bpm. The current is increased slowly until capture occurs—a spiking followed by QRS sequence—then the current is readjusted downward if possible just to maintain capture, keeping it 5-10 mA above the pacing threshold. Both demand and fixed modes are available, but demand mode is preferred. The patient should be warned that the shocks may induce pain.

EPICARDIAL PACING

Epicardial pacing wires may be attached directly to the exterior atria, ventricles, or both at the conclusion of surgery for CPB or valve repair in the event that postoperative pacing support is required or for those with risk of AV block because of medications used to control atrial fibrillation. Cold cardioplegia may precipitate the transient sinus node or AV node dysfunction. While some surgeons avoid placing epicardial pacing wires because of concerns about bleeding and cardiac tamponade on removal, recommendations include placing at least one ventricular pacing wire. A typical configuration for pacing wires is atrial pacing wires placed in a plastic disk that is sutured low on the right atrium. The two ventricular wires are attached over the right ventricular wall. Atrial pacing wires may be used to record atrial activity and, and with standard ECG, can help to distinguish atrial and junctional arrhythmias and ventricular arrhythmias. Pacing wires can also be used therapeutically to increase the heart rate to about 90 bpm in order to achieve optimal hemodynamics. The epicardial leads are intended for use of 7 days or less and may be less reliable if used for extended periods. The wires are removed by applying gentle traction.

TEMPORARY TRANSVENOUS PACEMAKERS

Transvenous pacemakers, comprised of a catheter with a lead at the end, may be used prophylactically or therapeutically on a temporary basis to treat symptomatic bradycardias or heart blocks when other methods have failed. The catheter has a balloon tip that must be checked for leaks prior to insertion – this is usually done by inflating the catheter tip while submersed in normal saline and checking for bubbles. After the balloon's integrity is verified, the catheter is inserted through the femoral or jugular vein and the balloon is inflated. The catheter is then attached to an external pulse generator, and the settings are adjusted to achieve capture. The balloon is then deflated, and placement can be verified via ultrasound or chest x-ray.

Complications are similar to those of PCI and permanent pacemaker insertion, including infection, hemorrhage, catheter migration, perforation, embolism, thrombosis, and pacemaker syndrome.

TRANSVENOUS PACER SETTINGS

Temporary transvenous pacing utilizes bipolar leads with two tails, positive/proximal and negative/distal, and these must be connected properly to the pulse generator, with the distal end of the pacing lead to the negative terminal and the proximal end to the positive terminal. Once the transvenous pacing wire is inserted and the leads are connected to the pulse generator, it must be set to the patient's needs:

- **Rate**: The beats per minute are usually set between 70 and 80 (allowable range is generally 50-90), but this may vary according to individual needs.
- **Sensitivity**: The myocardial voltage needed for the pacing electrode to detect P or R waves. The sensitivity is usually set at 2 mV and then adjusted as needed to ensure capture. Most pacemakers can sense 0.3-10.0 mV from the atria and 0.8-29.0 mV from the ventricles, but setting it relatively low prevents oversensing.
- **Output**: The current or pulse produced by the pulse generator is usually set at 5 mA. The current is delivered rapidly, in about 0.6 ms.

PROBLEMS RELATED TO TRANSVENOUS PACING

With transvenous pacing (usually per a pulse generator connected to a pacing cable and a pacing wire, which is inserted into the right internal jugular to the right ventricle for ventricular pacing and right atrium for atrial pacing), sensing refers to the ability to detect electrical activity of the heart. Capture occurs when an artificial stimulus (the pulse generator) depolarizes the heart, indicated by a pacer spike followed by the QRS complex. **Problems** include:

Undersensing	**Undersensing:** The sensitivity is too low to detect cardiac depolarizations, and triggers unneeded contractions, competing with the patient's native rhythm. This may be related to the dislodging of the lead, incorrect positioning of the lead, or a low-amplitude cardiac signal.
Oversensing	**Oversensing:** The sensitivity is too high and misinterprets artifacts (such as muscle contractions) and non-depolarization events as contractions and fails to trigger, resulting in decreased cardiac output because of the interruption in contractions. This may result from damage or disconnection of the lead.
Noncapture	**Noncapture:** The pacemaker does not trigger contractions. This may be related to settings, lead disconnection, low battery, or metabolic changes.

PACEMAKER COMPLICATIONS

Pacemakers, transvenous and permanent, are invasive foreign bodies and, as such, can cause a number of different **complications**:

- Infection, bleeding, or hematoma may occur at the entry site of leads for temporary pacemakers or at the subcutaneous area of implantation for permanent generators.
- Puncture of the subclavian vein or internal mammary artery may cause a hemothorax.

- The endocardial electrode may irritate the ventricular wall, causing ectopic beats or tachycardia.
- Dislodgement of the transvenous lead may lead to malfunction or perforation of the myocardium. This is one of the most common early complications.
- Dislocation of leads may result in phrenic nerve or muscle stimulation (which may be evidenced by hiccupping).
- Cardiac tamponade may result when the epicardial wires of temporary pacing are removed.
- General malfunctioning of the pacemaker may indicate dislodgement, dislocation, interference caused by electromagnetic fields, and the need for new batteries or a new generator.
- Pacemaker syndrome

PACEMAKER SYNDROME

Pacemaker syndrome can occur with any type of pacemaker if there is inadequate synchronicity between the contractions of the atria and ventricles, resulting in a decrease in cardiac output and inadequate atrial contribution to the filling of the ventricles. Total peripheral vascular resistance may increase to maintain blood pressure, but hypotension occurs after decompensation.

- **Mild**:
  - Pulsations evident in the neck and abdomen
  - Cardiac palpitations
  - Headache and feeling of anxiety
  - General malaise and unexplained weakness
  - Pain or feeling of fullness in jaw and/or chest
- **Moderate**:
  - Increasing dyspnea on exertion with accompanying orthopnea
  - Dizziness, vertigo, and increasing confusion
  - Feeling of choking
- **Severe**:
  - Increasing pulmonary edema with dyspnea even at rest
  - Crackling rales
  - Syncope
  - Heart failure

AUTOMATIC ICD

The **automatic implantable cardioverter-defibrillator (AICD)** is similar to the pacemaker and is implanted in the same way, with one or more leads to the ventricular myocardium or the epicardium, but it is used to control tachycardia and/or fibrillation. Most AICDs consist of a pacing/sensing electrode, a pulse generator, and defibrillation electrodes. Severe tachycardia may be related to electrical disturbances, cardiomyopathy, or postoperative response to the repair of congenital disease. In some cases, it is not responsive to medications. When the pulse reaches a certain preset rate, then the device automatically provides a small electrical impulse to the atrial or ventricular myocardium to slow the heart. If fibrillation occurs, a higher energy shock is delivered. It takes 5-15 seconds for the device to detect abnormalities in the pulse rate, and more than one shock may be required so fainting can occur. Contemporary devices can function as both a pacemaker and an ICD, which is especially important for those who have episodes of both bradycardia and tachycardia. The use of adjunctive antiarrhythmics or ablation is important to prevent AICD shocks.

Mometrix

ARTERIAL LINE INSERTION

Indications for an **arterial line** include hemodynamic instability, frequent ABG monitoring, placement of IABP, monitoring arterial pressure, and medication administration when venous access cannot be obtained. Sterile technique is utilized for arterial line insertion. Insertions sites include radial (most common), femoral (second choice), brachial, or dorsalis pedis arteries.

Procedure:

- Verify adequate perfusion and position.
  - Radial: Perform modified Allen test and position wrist in dorsiflexion with an arm board.
  - Femoral: Place the patient in a supine position with the leg on the insertion side slightly abducted and extended.
- Prep and drape. Apply 1% lidocaine if the patient is conscious.
- Insert needle.
  - Over-the-needle catheter insertion: Needle is inserted at a 30-45° degree angle and decreased to a 10-15° angle when blood returns, catheter advanced into vessel, needle removed, and catheter connected to transducer.
  - Over-wire catheter insertion: Needle is inserted into the artery at a 30-45° angle until blood returns. A wire is then inserted and advanced through the needle, and needle removed, leaving the wire in place. A catheter is then advanced over the wire, wire removed, and catheter connected to transducer system.
- A small incision is made at insertion site and catheter sutured into place.

Complications include bleeding, coagulopathy, thrombosis (especially with larger catheters or smaller arteries), advanced atherosclerosis, and infection.

> **Review Video: <u>Nursing Care of Arterial Lines</u>**
> Visit mometrix.com/academy and enter code: 561047

123

CENTRAL LINE INSERTION

Central lines allow rapid administration of large volumes of fluid, blood testing, and CVP measuring. Central lines may be placed into the internal jugular vein (right preferred), subclavian vein, or femoral vein (usually avoided). The insertion site is located through an ultrasound. The patient is positioned, supine Trendelenburg (or legs elevated) for interior jugular, using sterile technique. Following skin prep, the CVC kit is placed on a sterile field and opened, the equipment is prepared, and the insertion site is again verified by a probe (covered with sterile cover). Topical anesthetic (lidocaine) is administered and the needle inserted with the triangulation or spear method, always pulling back on the plunger of the syringe so that blood returns when entering the vein. The syringe is removed and the guidewire inserted into needle ≤20 cm. The needle is then removed and the wire position verified with ultrasound. A small incision is made at the insertion site, and a dilator is applied over the wire and inserted about 2.5-3.5 cm. The catheter is placed over the wire and advanced into the vein (13-17 cm). The wire is then removed, the lines are flushed, and the catheter is sutured in place and dressing is applied. Long (24-inch) PICCs may be inserted in the basilic or cephalic veins and advanced into central circulation.

INTRAOSSEOUS INFUSION

Intraosseous (IO) infusion is an alternative to IV access for neonates, pediatric emergencies, and adult emergencies when rapid temporary access is necessary or when peripheral or vascular access can't be achieved. It is often used in pediatric cardiac arrest. Because yellow marrow replaces red marrow, access in those older than 5 is more difficult. Preferred sites are based on age, though across all ages, the **proximal tibia is preferred**. Additional sites include:

- 0-1: Distal femur
- 1-12: Distal tibia or fibula
- 12-18: Distal tibia or fibula, sternum
- 18 and older: Distal tibia or fibula, proximal humerus, sternum

IO infusion is used to administer fluids and anesthesia and to obtain blood samples. Equipment requires a special needle (13-20 gauge) as standard needles may bend. The bone injection gun (BIG) with a loaded spring facilitates insertion. The FAST needle is intended for use in the sternum of adults and prevents accidental puncture of the thoracic cavity. Knowledge of bony landmarks and correct insertion angle and site is important. The position is confirmed by aspiration of 5-10 mL of blood and marrow before infusion.

VASCULAR INTERVENTIONS

Vascular interventions are required when a patient has a condition that is decreasing blood flow to the limbs, causing ischemia-related damage. Conditions that require a vascular intervention include acute occlusion (embolus), severe unresponsive vascular disease, ruptured/dissecting aneurysm, damaged vessels, or congenital defect.

- **Bypass grafts:** The MD uses a harvested vein from another part of the body (saphenous usually) or synthetic graft to bypass the occlusion. Because veins have valves, they must be reversed or stripped of valves prior to attachment; however, synthetic grafts have a higher failure rate. A common peripheral bypass is the femoropopliteal (Fem-pop) bypass, extending from the femoral artery around the blockage to the popliteal artery.
- **Embolectomy:** A catheter is inserted into the blocked artery and threaded through the thrombus. Then a balloon on the tip is inflated, and the physician removes the catheter, removing the clot with it.
- **Aortic aneurysm repair:** This is an intense procedure, requiring an open incision and the patient to be placed on cardiopulmonary bypass. The affected area is resected and replaced with a vascular or Dacron graft.

Nursing considerations: Monitor and control blood pressure carefully to protect the patency and integrity of the grafts. Neurologic and renal function should also be carefully monitored, as emboli could block the renal or cerebral artery. Frequent neuro, urine output, vascular, and dressing checks.

Possible complications: Pulmonary infection, graft-site infection, renal dysfunction, occlusion, hemorrhage, and embolus/thrombus.

PERIPHERAL STENTS

Peripheral vascular stenting may be utilized as an intervention in the treatment of peripheral vascular insufficiency. Often performed in interventional radiology, the interventionalist uses balloon angioplasty to unblock the vessel under fluoroscopic guidance. A small balloon attached to a catheter is inserted into the occluded vessel and inflated to expand the arterial wall and compress the blockage. A small metal tube (stent) is then placed to support the vessel and maintain its patency. Stents are primarily made of stainless steel or a metal alloy. This intervention helps to restore circulation to the affected area and prevent restenosis of the vessel. There are different types of stents available based on the type of vessel affected and the type of lesion. Stenting may be used in both peripheral and coronary arteries.

- **Indications**: Stenting may be the initial choice of intervention in patients with iliac, renal, subclavian, or carotid stenosis. Stenting may be indicated in patients with severe claudication, non-healing ulcers of the extremities, ischemic pain with rest, and in patients who have a high operative risk. Peripheral stenting often results in shorter hospital stays and shorter recovery times in comparison with surgical intervention.
- **Complications**: Complications that may occur in patients undergoing peripheral stenting include bleeding, infection, arterial spasm or rupture, dissection of the vessel, restenosis or thrombus formation within the vessel, and intravascular fracture of the stent.

FEM-POP BYPASS

Femoropopliteal (Fem-Pop) bypass is used for femoral artery disease in order to bypass an occluded femoral artery above or below the knee. Either a man-made or a vein graft (such as the saphenous vein) is used and is sewn above the blocked area to the femoral artery and below to the popliteal artery, allowing the blood to bypass the occluded area. In addition to the incisions in the affected leg, if a vein graft is obtained from the other leg, the patient may also have a long incision where the vein was removed. Edema in the surgical sites is common and may persist for up to 3 months. Femoral popliteal bypass surgery is indicated for peripheral vascular insufficiency that does not respond to medical treatment, causes severe intermittent claudication and/or ischemic resting pain, and results in gangrene or other non-healing wounds, especially if the limb is at risk for amputation because of impaired oxygenation. The limb(s) must be monitored carefully in the postoperative period for color, sensation, warmth, and ability to move.

Cardiovascular Pharmacology

ANTI-HYPERTENSIVE MEDICATIONS

The classes of anti-hypertensive medications are as follows: Diuretics, sympatholytics, vasodilators, calcium channel blockers, and angiotensin-converting enzyme inhibitors (ACE inhibitors).

- Diuretics include hydrochlorothiazide, chlorthalidone, chlorothiazide, indapamide, metolazone, amiloride, spironolactone, triamterene, furosemide, bumetanide, ethacrynic acid, and torsemide.
- Sympatholytics are clonidine, methyldopa, guanabenz, guanadrel, guanethidine, reserpine, labetalol, prazosin, and terazosin.
- Vasodilators include diazoxide, hydralazine, minoxidil, and nitroprusside sodium.
- Calcium channel blockers include amlodipine, nimodipine, isradipine, nicardipine, nifedipine, bepridil, diltiazem, and verapamil.
- ACE inhibitors include benazepril, captopril, enalapril, fosinopril, lisinopril, moexipril, quinapril, ramipril, and losartan.

DIURETICS

Diuretics increase **renal perfusion and filtration**, thereby reducing preload and decreasing peripheral and pulmonary edema, hypertension, CHF, diabetes insipidus, and osteoporosis. There are different types of diuretics: loop, thiazide, and potassium sparing.

LOOP DIURETICS

Loop diuretics inhibit the reabsorption of sodium and chloride (primarily) in the ascending loop of Henle. They also cause increased secretion of other electrolytes, such as calcium, magnesium, and potassium, and this can result in imbalances that cause dysrhythmias. Other side effects include frequent urination, postural hypotension, and increased blood sugar and uric acid levels. They are short-acting so are less effective than other diuretics for control of hypertension.

- **Bumetanide** (Bumex) is given intravenously after surgery to reduce preload or orally to treat heart failure.
- **Ethacrynic acid** (Edecrin) is given intravenously after surgery to reduce preload.
- **Furosemide** (Lasix) is used for the control of congestive heart failure as well as renal insufficiency. It is used after surgery to decrease preload and to reduce the inflammatory response caused by cardiopulmonary bypass (post-perfusion syndrome).

> **Review Video: <u>Diuretics</u>**
> Visit mometrix.com/academy and enter code: 373276

THIAZIDE DIURETICS

Thiazide diuretics inhibit the **reabsorption of sodium and chloride** primarily in the early distal tubules, forcing more sodium and water to be excreted. Thiazide diuretics increase secretion of potassium and bicarbonate, so they are often given with supplementary potassium or in combination with potassium-sparing diuretics. Thiazide diuretics are the first line of drugs for treatment of **hypertension**. They have a long duration of action (12-72 hours, depending on the drug) so they are able to maintain control of hypertension better than short-acting drugs. They may be given daily or 3–5 days per week. There are numerous thiazide diuretics, including:

- Chlorothiazide (Diuril)
- Bendroflumethiazide (Naturetin)
- Chlorthalidone (Hygroton)
- Trichlormethiazide (Naqua)

Side effects include, dizziness, lightheadedness, postural hypotension, headache, blurred vision, and itching, especially during initial treatment. Thiazide diuretics cause sensitivity to sun exposure, so people should be counseled to use sunscreen.

POTASSIUM-SPARING DIURETICS

Potassium-sparing diuretics inhibit the **reabsorption of sodium** in the late distal tubule and collecting duct. They are weaker than thiazide or loop diuretics, but do not cause a reduction in potassium level; however, if used alone, they may cause an increase in potassium, which can cause weakness, irregular pulse, and cardiac arrest. Because potassium-sparing diuretics are less effective alone, they are often given in a combined form with a thiazide diuretic (usually chlorothiazide), which mitigates the potassium imbalance. Typical side effects include dehydration, blurred vision, nausea, insomnia, and nasal congestion, especially in the first few days of treatment.

- **Spironolactone** (Aldactone) is a synthetic steroid diuretic that increases the secretion of both water and sodium and is used to treat congestive heart failure. It may be given orally or intravenously.
- **Eplerenone** is an antimineralocorticoid similar to spironolactone but with fewer side effects.

ANTIDYSRHYTHMIC DRUGS

Antidysrhythmic drugs include a number of drugs that act on the conduction system, the ventricles and/or the atria to control dysrhythmias. There are four classes of drugs that are used as well as some that are unclassified:

- **Class I:** 3 subtypes of sodium channel blockers (quinidine, lidocaine, procainamide)
- **Class II:** β-receptor blockers (esmolol, propranolol)
- **Class III:** Slows repolarization (amiodarone, ibutilide)
- **Class IV:** Calcium channel blockers (diltiazem, verapamil)
- **Unclassified:** Miscellaneous drugs with proven efficacy in controlling arrhythmias (adenosine, electrolyte supplements)

SMOOTH MUSCLE RELAXANTS

Smooth muscle relaxants decrease peripheral vascular resistance, but may cause hypotension and headaches.

- Sodium nitroprusside (Nipride) dilates both arteries and veins; rapid-acting and used for reduction of hypertension and afterload reduction for heart failure.
- Nitroglycerin (Tridil) primarily dilates veins and is used sublingual or IV to reduce preload for acute heart failure, unstable angina, and acute MI. Nitroglycerin may also be used prophylactically after PCIs to prevent vasospasm.
- Hydralazine (Apresoline) dilates arteries and is given intermittently to reduce hypertension.

CALCIUM CHANNEL BLOCKERS

Calcium channel blockers are primarily arterial vasodilators that may affect the peripheral and/or coronary arteries.

- Side effects: Lethargy, flushing, edema, ascites, and indigestion:
- Nifedipine (Procardia) and nicardipine (Cardene) are primarily arterial vasodilators, used to treat acute hypertension. Diltiazem (Cardizem) and Verapamil (Calan, Isoptin) dilate primarily coronary arteries and slow the heart rate, thus are used for angina, atrial fibrillation, and SVT. *Note:* Nifedipine (Procardia) should be avoided in older adults due to increased risk of hypotension and myocardial ischemia.

> **Review Video: Ca Channel Blockers**
> Visit mometrix.com/academy and enter code: 942825

ADDITIONAL VASODILATORS

B-type natriuretic peptide (BNP) (Nesiritide [Natrecor]) is type of vasodilator (non-inotropic), which is a recombinant form of a peptide of the human brain. It decreases filling pressure, vascular resistance, and increases U/O.

- May cause hypotension, headache, bradycardia, and nausea. It is used short term for worsening decompensated CHF; contraindicated in SBP<90, cardiogenic shock, contrictive pericarditis, or valve stenosis.

Alpha-adrenergic blockers block alpha receptors in arteries and veins, causing vasodilation.

- May cause orthostatic hypotension and edema from fluid retention.
- Labetalol (Normodyne) is a combination peripheral alpha-blocker and cardiac β-blocker that is used to treat acute hypertension, acute stroke, and acute aortic dissection.
- Phentolamine (Regitine) is a peripheral arterial dilator that reduces afterload. It is used for HTN crisis in patients with pheochromocytoma, as well as a subcutaneous injection for extravasation of vessicants.

Selective specific dopamine DA-1-receptor agonists:

- Fenoldopam (Corlopam) is a peripheral dilator affecting renal and mesenteric arteries and can be used for patients with renal dysfunction or those at risk of renal insufficiency.

INOTROPIC AGENTS

Inotropic agents are drugs used to increase cardiac output and improve contractibility. IV inotropic agents may increase the risk of death, but may be used when other drugs fail. Oral forms of these drugs are less effective than intravenous. Inotropic agents include:

- **β-Adrenergic agonists:**
  - **Dobutamine** improves cardiac output, treats cardiac decompensation, and increases blood pressure. It helps the body to utilize norepinephrine. Side effects include increased or labile blood pressure, increased heart rate, PVCs, N/V, and bronchospasm.
  - **Dopamine** improves cardiac output, blood pressure, and blood flow to the renal and mesenteric arteries. Side effects include tachycardia or bradycardia, palpitations, BP changes, dyspnea, nausea and vomiting, headache, and gangrene of extremities.
- **Phosphodiesterase III inhibitors:**
  - **Milrinone** (Primacor) increases strength of contractions and cause vasodilation. Side effects include ventricular arrhythmias, hypotension, and headaches.
- **Digoxin (Lanoxin)** increases contractibility and cardiac output and prevents arrhythmias.

MEDICATIONS FOR HEART FAILURE

A patient with heart failure may be prescribed with one or multiple of the drugs below:

- **ACE inhibitors:** Captopril (Capoten), enalapril (Vasotec), and lisinopril (Prinivil). Decrease afterload/preload and reverse ventricular remodeling; they also prevent neuropathy in DM. Contraindicated with renal insufficiency, renal artery stenosis, and pregnancy.
  - Side effects include cough (#1), hyperkalemia, hypotension, angioedema, dizziness, and weakness.
- **Angiotensin receptor blockers (ARBs):** Losartan (Cozaar) and valsartan (Diovan). Decrease afterload/preload and reverse ventricular remodeling, causing vasodilation and reducing blood pressure. They are used for those who cannot tolerate ACE inhibitors.

- Side effects include cough (less common than with ACE inhibitors), hyperkalemia, hypotension, headache, dizziness, metallic taste, and rash.
- **β-Blockers:** Metoprolol (Lopressor), carvedilol (Coreg) and esmolol (Brevibloc). Slow the heart rate, reduce hypertension, prevent dysrhythmias, and reverse ventricular remodeling. Contraindicated in bradyarrythmias, decompensated HF, uncontrolled hypoglycemia/diabetes mellitus, and airway disease.
  - Side effects: bradycardia, hypotension, bronchospasm, may mask signs of hypoglycemia.
- **Aldosterone agonist:** Spironolactone (Aldactone). Decreases preload and myocardial hypertrophy and reduces edema and sodium retention but may increase serum potassium.
- **Furosemide (Lasix)** is used for the control of congestive heart failure as well as renal insufficiency. It is used after surgery to decrease preload and to reduce the inflammatory response caused by cardiopulmonary bypass (post-perfusion syndrome).

DIGOXIN (LANOXIN)

Digitalis drugs, most commonly administered in the form of digoxin (Lanoxin), are derived from the foxglove plant and are used to increase myocardial contractility, left ventricular output, and slow conduction through the AV node, decreasing rapid heart rates and promoting diuresis. Digoxin does not affect mortality, but increases tolerance to activity and reduces hospitalizations for heart failure. Therapeutic levels (0.5-2.0 ng/mL) should be maintained to avoid digitalis toxicity, which can occur even if digoxin levels are within therapeutic range, so observation of symptoms is critical. Because patients with heart failure are often on diuretics which decrease potassium levels, they are at increased risk for toxicity.

Symptoms of toxicity are as follows:

- Early signs: Increasing fatigue, lethargy, depression, and nausea and vomiting; progress to severe diarrhea, blurred vision/yellow or green halos around lights, fatigue/weakness
- Arrythmias: SA or AV block, VT/VF, PVCs, and bradycardia

Treatment consists of the following:

- Monitor serum levels and symptoms.
- Digoxin immune FAB (Digibind) may be used to bind to digoxin and inactivate it if necessary.

GLYCOPROTEIN IIB/IIIA INHIBITORS

Glycoprotein IIB/IIIA Inhibitors are drugs that are used to inhibit platelet binding and prevent clots prior to and following invasive cardiac procedures, such as angioplasty and stent placement. These medications are used in combination with anticoagulant drugs, such as heparin and aspirin for the following:

- Acute coronary syndromes (ACS), such as unstable angina or myocardial infarctions
- Percutaneous coronary intervention (PCI), such as angioplasty and stent placement

These medications are contraindicated in those with a low platelet count or active bleeding:

- **Eptifibatide (Integrilin):** Used with both heparin and aspirin for ACS and PCI and affects platelet binding for 6-8 hours after administration. Should not be used in patients with renal problems.
- **Tirofiban (Aggrastat):** Used with heparin for PCI patients with reduced dosage for those with renal problems and affects platelet binding for only 4-8 hours after administration.

PHARMACOLOGIC MEASURES TO MAXIMIZE PERFUSION

The primary focus of pharmacologic measures to **maximize perfusion** is to reduce the risk of **thromboses**:

- **Antiplatelet agents**, such as aspirin, Ticlid, and Plavix, which interfere with the function of the plasma membrane, interfering with clotting. These agents are ineffective to treat clots but prevent clot formation.
- **Vasodilators** may divert blood from ischemic areas, but some may be indicated, such as Pletal, which dilates arteries and decreases clotting, and is used for control of intermittent claudication.
- **Antilipemic**, such as Zocor and Questran, slow progression of atherosclerosis.
- **Hemorheologic agents**, such as Trental, reduce fibrinogen, reducing blood viscosity and rigidity of erythrocytes; however, clinical studies show limited benefit. It may be used for intermittent claudication.
- **Analgesics** may be necessary to improve quality of life. Opioids may be needed in some cases.
- **Thrombolytics** may be injected into a blocked artery under angiography to dissolve clots.
- **Anticoagulants**, such as Coumadin and Lovenox, prevent blood clots from forming.

ADMINISTRATION OF FIBRINOLYTIC (THROMBOLYTIC) INFUSIONS FOR MI

Fibrinolytic infusion is indicated for acute myocardial infarction under these conditions:

- Symptoms of MI, <6-12 hours since onset of symptoms
- ≥1 mm elevation of ST in ≥2 contiguous leads
- No contraindications and no cardiogenic shock

Fibrinolytic agents should be administered as soon as possible, within 30 minutes is best. All agents convert plasminogen to plasmin, which breaks down fibrin, dissolving clots:

- Streptokinase and anistreplase (1st generation)
- Alteplase or tissue plasminogen activator (tPA) (2nd generation)
- Reteplase and tenecteplase (3rd generation)

Contraindications

- Present or recent bleeding or history of severe bleeding
- History of intracranial hemorrhage
- History of stroke (<3 months unless within 3 hours)
- Aortic dissection or pericarditis
- Intracranial/intraspinal surgery or trauma within 3 months or neoplasm, aneurysm, or AVM

Relative contraindications

- Active peptic ulcer
- >10 minutes of CPR
- Advanced renal or hepatic disease
- Pregnancy
- Anticoagulation therapy
- Acute uncontrolled hypertension or chronic poorly controlled hypertension
- Recent (2–4 weeks) internal bleeding
- Non-compressible vascular punctures

Respiratory Pathophysiology

ACUTE PULMONARY EMBOLISM

Acute pulmonary embolism occurs when a pulmonary artery or arteriole is blocked, cutting off blood supply to the pulmonary vessels and subsequent oxygenation of the blood. While most pulmonary emboli are from thrombus formation, they can also be caused by air, fat, or septic embolus (from bacterial invasion of a thrombus). Common originating sites for thrombus formation are the deep veins in the legs, the pelvic veins, and the right atrium. Causes include stasis related to damage to endothelial wall and changes in blood coagulation factors. Atrial fibrillation poses a serious risk because blood pools in the right atrium, forming clots that travel directly through the right ventricle to the lungs. The obstruction of the artery/arteriole causes an increase in alveolar dead space in which there is ventilation but impairment of gas exchange because of the ventilation/perfusion mismatching or intrapulmonary shunting. This results in hypoxia, hypercapnia, and the release of mediators that cause bronchoconstriction. If more than 50% of the vascular bed becomes excluded, pulmonary hypertension occurs.

SYMPTOMS AND DIAGNOSIS

Clinical manifestations of acute pulmonary embolism (PE) vary according to the size of the embolus and the area of occlusion.

Symptoms include:

- Dyspnea with tachypnea
- Cyanosis; may turn grey or blue from nipple line up (massive PE)
- Anxiety and restlessness, feeling of doom
- Chest pain, tachycardia, may progress to arrhythmias (PEA)
- Fever
- Rales
- Cough (sometimes with hemoptysis)
- Hemodynamic instability

Diagnostic tests are as follows:

- ABG analysis may show hypoxemia (decreased PaO_2), hypocarbia (decreased $PaCO_2$) and respiratory alkalosis (increased pH).
- D-dimer will show elevation with PE but is not definitively diagnostic without a CT scan.
- ECG may show sinus tachycardia or other abnormalities.
- Echocardiogram can show emboli in the central arteries and can assess the hemodynamic status of the right side of the heart.
- Spiral CT may provide definitive diagnosis.
- V/Q scintigraphy can confirm diagnosis.
- Pulmonary angiograms also can confirm diagnosis.

MEDICAL MANAGEMENT

Medical management of pulmonary embolism starts with preventive measures for those at risk, including leg exercises, elastic compression stockings, and anticoagulation therapy. Most pulmonary emboli present as medical emergencies, so the immediate task is to stabilize the patient. **Medical management** may include:

- **Oxygen** to relieve hypoxemia
- **Intravenous infusions:** Dobutamine (Dobutrex) or dopamine (Intropin) to relieve hypotension
- **Cardiac monitoring** for dysrhythmias and issues due to right sided heart failure
- **Medications** as indicated: digitalis glycosides, diuretic, and antiarrhythmics
- Intubation and mechanical ventilation may be required

- **Analgesics** (such as morphine sulfate) or sedation to relieve anxiety
- **Anticoagulants** to prevent recurrence (although it will not dissolve clots already present), including heparin and warfarin (Coumadin)
- **Placement of percutaneous venous filter** (Greenfield) in the inferior vena cava to prevent further emboli from entering the lungs, if anticoagulation therapy is contraindicated
- **Thrombolytic therapy,** recombinant tissue-type plasminogen activator (rt-PA) or streptokinase, for those severely compromised, but these treatments have limited success and pose the danger of bleeding

ACUTE LUNG INJURY AND ACUTE RESPIRATORY DISTRESS SYNDROME

Acute lung injury (ALI) comprises a syndrome of respiratory distress culminating in acute respiratory distress syndrome (ARDS). ARDS is a dangerous, potentially fatal respiratory condition, always caused by an illness or injury to the lungs. Lung injury causes fluid to leak into the spaces between the alveoli and capillaries, increasing pressure on the alveoli, causing them to collapse. With increased fluid accumulation in the lungs, the ability of the lungs to move oxygen into the blood is decreased, resulting in hypoxemia. Lung injury also causes a release of cytokines, a type of inflammatory protein, which then brings neutrophils to the lung. These proteins and cells leak into nearby blood vessels and cause inflammation throughout the body. This immune response, in combination with low levels of blood oxygen, can lead to organ failure. Symptoms are characterized by respiratory distress within 72 hours of surgery or a serious injury to a person with otherwise normal lungs and no cardiac disorder. Untreated, the condition results in respiratory failure, MODS, and a mortality rate of 5-30%.

Symptoms include:

- Refractory hypoxemia (hypoxemia not responding to increasing levels of oxygen)
- Crackling rales/wheezing in lungs
- Decrease in pulmonary compliance which results in increased tachypnea with expiratory grunting
- Cyanosis/skin mottling
- Hypotension and tachycardia
- Symptoms associated with volume overload are missing (3rd heart sound or JVD)
- Respiratory alkalosis initially but, as the disease progresses, replaced with hypercarbia and respiratory acidosis
- Normal x-ray initially but then diffuse infiltrates in both lungs, while the heart and vessels appear normal

MANAGEMENT

The management of acute respiratory distress syndrome (ARDS) involves providing adequate gas exchange and preventing further damage to the lung from forced ventilation.

Treatment includes:

- Mechanical ventilation to maintain oxygenation and ventilation
- Corticosteroids (may increase mortality rates in some patient populations, though this is the most commonly given treatment), nitrous oxide, inhaled surfactant, and anti-inflammatory medications
- Treatment of the underlying condition is the only proven treatment, especially identifying and treating an infection with appropriate antibiotics, as sepsis is most common etiology for ARDS, but prophylactic antibiotics are not indicated.
- Conservative fluid management is indicated to reduce days on the ventilator, but does not reduce overall mortality.

Pharmacologic preventive care: Enoxaparin 40 mg subcutaneously QD, sucralfate 1 g NGT four times daily or omeprazole 40 mg IV QD, and enteral nutrition support within 24 hours of ICU admission or intubation.

VENTILATION MANAGEMENT

Ventilation management in ARDS consists of the following:

- O_2 therapy by nasal prongs, cannula, or mask may be sufficient in very mild cases to maintain oxygen saturation above 90%. Oxygen should be administered at 100% because of the mismatch between ventilation (V) and perfusion (Q), which can result in hypoxia on position change.
- ARDS oxygenation goal is PaO_2 55-80 mmHg or SpO_2 88-95%.
- Endotracheal intubation may be needed if SpO_2 falls or CO_2 levels rise.
- The ARDS Network recommends low tidal volumes (6 mL/kg) and higher PEEP (12 cmH_2O or more).
- The low tidal volume ventilation described above is referred to as lung protective ventilation, and it has been shown to reduce mortality in patients with ARDS.
- Placing patients with severe ARDS in prone position for 18-24 hours per day with chest and pelvis supported and abdomen unsupported allows the diaphragm to move posteriorly, increasing functional residual capacity (FRC) in many patients.

ACUTE RESPIRATORY FAILURE
CARDINAL SIGNS

The cardinal signs of respiratory failure include:

- Tachypnea
- Tachycardia
- Anxiety and restlessness
- Diaphoresis

Symptoms may vary according to the cause. An obstruction may cause more obvious respiratory symptoms than other disorders.

- Early signs may include changes in the depth and pattern of respirations with flaring nares, sternal retractions, expiratory grunting, wheezing, and extended expiration as the body tries to compensate for hypoxemia and increasing levels of carbon dioxide.
- Cyanosis may be evident.
- Central nervous depression, with alterations in consciousness occurs with decreased perfusion to the brain.
- As the hypoxemia worsens, cardiac arrhythmias, including bradycardia, may occur with either hypotension or hypertension.
- Dyspnea becomes more pronounced with depressed respirations.
- Eventually stupor, coma, and death can occur if the condition is not reversed.

HYPOXEMIC AND HYPERCAPNIC RESPIRATORY FAILURE

Hypoxemic respiratory failure occurs suddenly when gaseous exchange of oxygen for carbon dioxide cannot keep up with demand for oxygen or production of carbon dioxide:

- PaO_2 <60 mmHg
- $PaCO_2$ >40 mmHg
- Arterial pH <7.35

Hypoxemic respiratory failure can be the result of low inhaled oxygen, as at high elevations or with smoke inhalation. The following ventilatory mechanisms may be involved:

- Alveolar hypotension
- Ventilation-perfusion mismatch (the most common cause)

133

- Intrapulmonary shunts
- Diffusion impairment

Hypercapnic respiratory failure results from an increase in $PaCO_2$ >45-50 mmHg associated with respiratory acidosis and may include:

- Reduction in minute ventilation, total volume of gas ventilated in one minute (often related to neurological, muscle, or chest wall disorders, drug overdoses, or obstruction of upper airway)
- Increased dead space with wasted ventilation (related to lung disease or disorders of chest wall, such as scoliosis)
- Increased production of CO_2 (usually related to infection, burns, or other causes of hypermetabolism)
- Oxygen saturation normal or below normal

UNDERLYING CAUSES

There are a number of underlying causes for respiratory failure:

- **Airway obstruction:** Obstruction may result from an inhaled object or from an underlying disease process, such as cystic fibrosis, asthma, pulmonary edema, or infection.
- **Inadequate respirations:** This is a common cause among adults, especially related to obesity and sleep apnea. It may also be induced by an overdose of sedation medications such as opioids.
- **Neuromuscular disorders:** Those disorders that interfere with the neuromuscular functioning of the lungs or the chest wall, such as muscular dystrophy or spinal cord injuries can prevent adequate ventilation.
- **Pulmonary abnormalities:** Those abnormalities of the lung tissue, found in pulmonary fibrosis, burns, ARDS, and reactions to drugs, can lead to failure.
- **Chest wall abnormalities:** Disorders that impact lung parenchyma, such as severe scoliosis or chest wounds can interfere with lung functioning.

Nursing interventions to help prevent respiratory issues:

- Turn, position, and ambulate the patient.
- Have the patient cough and breathe deeply.
- Use vibration and percussion treatments.
- Hydrate the patient to help hydrate the airway secretions, and incentive spirometry.

MANAGEMENT

Respiratory failure must be **treated** immediately before severe hypoxemia causes irreversible damage to vital organs.

- **Identifying and treating** the underlying cause should be done immediately because emergency medications or surgery may be indicated. Medical treatments will vary widely depending upon the cause; for example, cardiopulmonary structural defects may require surgical repair, pulmonary edema may require diuresis, inhaled objects may require surgical removal, and infections may require aggressive antimicrobials.
- **Intravenous lines/central lines** are inserted for testing, fluids, and medications.
- **Oxygen therapy** should be initiated to attempt to reverse hypoxemia; however, if refractory hypoxemia occurs, then oxygen therapy alone will not suffice. Oxygen levels must be titrated carefully.
- **Intubation and mechanical ventilation** are frequently required to maintain adequate ventilation and oxygenation. Positive end expiratory pressure (PEEP) may be necessary with refractory hypoxemia and collapsed alveoli.
- **Respiratory status** must be monitored constantly, including arterial blood gases and vital signs.

PNEUMONIA

Pneumonia is inflammation of the lung parenchyma, filling the alveoli with exudate. It is common throughout childhood and adulthood. Pneumonia may be a primary disease or may occur secondary to another infection or disease, such as lung cancer. Pneumonia may be caused by bacteria, viruses, parasites, or fungi. Common causes for community-acquired pneumonia (CAP) include:

- *Streptococcus pneumoniae*
- *Legionella* species
- *Haemophilus influenzae*
- *Staphylococcus aureus*
- *Mycoplasma pneumoniae*
- Viruses

Pneumonia may also be caused by chemical damage. Pneumonia is characterized by **location**:

- **Lobar** involves one or more lobes of the lungs. If lobes in both lungs are affected, it is referred to as bilateral or double pneumonia.
- **Bronchial/lobular** involves the terminal bronchioles, and exudate can involve the adjacent lobules. Usually, the pneumonia occurs in scattered patches throughout the lungs.
- **Interstitial** involves primarily the interstitium and alveoli where white blood cells and plasma fill the alveoli, generating inflammation and creating fibrotic tissue as the alveoli are destroyed.

> **Review Video: Pneumonia**
> Visit mometrix.com/academy and enter code: 628264

HOSPITAL-ACQUIRED PNEUMONIA

Hospital-acquired pneumonia (HAP) is defined as pneumonia that did not appear to be present on admission that occurs at least 48 hours after admission to a hospital. **Healthcare-associated pneumonia (HCAP)** is defined as pneumonia that occurs in a patient within 90 days of being hospitalized for 2 or more days at an acute care hospital or LTAC. **Ventilator-associated pneumonia (VAP)** is one type of hospital acquired pneumonia that a patient acquires more than 48 hours after having an ETT placed. The most common way that the patient is infected is via aspiration of bacteria that is colonized in the upper respiratory tract. It is estimated that close to 75% of patients that are critically ill will be colonized with multidrug resistant bacteria within 48 hours of entering an ICU. Aspiration occurs at a rate of about 45% in patients with no health problems and the rate is much higher in those with HAP, HCAP, and VAP. The frequency of patients developing these types of pneumonia is increasing, with those at highest risk being those with immunosuppression, septic shock, currently hospitalized for more than five days, and those who have had antibiotics for another infection within the previous three months. These types of pneumonia should be considered if a patient already hospitalized has purulent sputum or a change in respiratory status such as deoxygenating, in combination with a worsening or new chest x-ray infiltrate.

Treatment includes:

- Antibiotic therapy
- Using appropriate isolation and precautions with infected patients
- Preventive measures including maintaining ventilated patients in 30° upright positions, frequent oral care for vent patients, and changing ventilator circuits as per protocol

Antibiotic treatment options for HAP, HCAP, and VAP should take into account many factors, including culture data (when available), patient's comorbidities, flora in the unit, any recent antibiotics by the patient, and whether the patient is at high risk for having multidrug resistant bacteria. As most critical care patients are at high risk, due to factors such as being in an ICU setting, ventilators, and comorbidities, antibiotic recommendations to follow are for coverage for patients with risk factors for multidrug resistant bacteria.

One of the following:

- Ceftazidime 2 g every 8 hours IV **OR**
- Cefepime 2 g every 8 hours IV **OR**
- Imipenem 500 mg every 6 hours IV **OR**
- Piperacillin-tazobactam 4.5 g every 6 hours IV

AND one of the following:

- Ciprofloxacin 400 mg every 8 hours IV **OR**
- Levaquin 750 mg every 24 hours IV

ASPIRATION PNEUMONITIS/PNEUMONIA

Aspiration pneumonitis/pneumonia may occur as the result of any type of aspiration, including foreign objects. The aspirated material creates an inflammatory response, with the irritated mucous membrane at high risk for bacterial infection secondary to the aspiration, causing pneumonia. Gastric contents and oropharyngeal bacteria are commonly aspirated. Gastric contents can cause a severe chemical pneumonitis with hypoxemia, especially if the pH is <2.5. Acidic food particles can cause severe reactions. With acidic damage, bronchospasm and atelectasis occur rapidly with tracheal irritation, bronchitis, and alveolar damage with interstitial edema and hemorrhage. Intrapulmonary shunting and V/Q mismatch may occur. Pulmonary artery pressure increases. Non-acidic liquids and food particles are less damaging, and symptoms may clear within 4 hours of liquid aspiration or granuloma may form about food particles in 1-5 days. Depending upon the type of aspiration, pneumonitis may clear within a week, ARDS or pneumonia may develop, or progressive acute respiratory failure may lead to death.

There are a number of risk factors that can lead to **aspiration pneumonitis/pneumonia:**

- Altered level of consciousness related to illness or sedation
- Depression of gag, swallowing reflex
- Intubation or feeding tubes
- Ileus or gastric distention
- Gastrointestinal disorders, such as gastroesophageal reflux disorders (GERD)

Diagnosis is based on clinical findings, ABGs showing hypoxemia, infiltrates observed on x-ray, and elevated WBC if infection is present.

Symptoms: Similar to other pneumonias:

- Cough often with copious sputum
- Respiratory distress, dyspnea
- Cyanosis
- Tachycardia
- Hypotension

Treatment includes:

- Suctioning as needed to clear upper airway
- Supplemental oxygen
- Antibiotic therapy as indicated after 48 hours if symptoms not resolving
- Symptomatic respiratory support

FOREIGN BODY ASPIRATION

Foreign body aspiration can cause obstruction of the pharynx, larynx, or trachea, leading to acute dyspnea or asphyxiation, and the object may also be drawn distally into the bronchial tree. With adults, most foreign bodies migrate more readily down the right bronchus. Food is the most frequently aspirated, but other small objects, such as coins or needles, may also be aspirated. Sometimes the object causes swelling, ulceration, and general inflammation that hampers removal.

Symptoms include:

- **Initial**: Severe coughing, gagging, sternal retraction, wheezing. Objects in the larynx may cause inability to breathe or speak and lead to respiratory arrest. Objects in the bronchus cause cough, dyspnea, and wheezing.
- **Delayed**: Hours, days, or weeks later, an undetected aspirant may cause an infection distal to the aspirated material. Symptoms depend on the area and extent of the infection.

Treatment includes:

- Removal with laryngoscopy or bronchoscopy (rigid is often better than flexible)
- Antibiotic therapy for secondary infection
- Surgical bronchotomy (rarely required)
- Symptomatic support

CHRONIC BRONCHITIS

Chronic bronchitis is a pulmonary airway disease characterized by severe cough with sputum production for at least 3 months a year for at least 2 consecutive years. Irritation of the airways (often from smoke or pollutants) causes an inflammatory response, increasing the number of mucus-secreting glands and goblet cells while ciliary function decreases so that the extra mucus plugs the airways. Additionally, the bronchial walls thicken, alveoli near the inflamed bronchioles become fibrotic, and alveolar macrophages cannot function properly, increasing susceptibility to infections. Chronic bronchitis is most common in those >45 years old and occurs twice as frequently in females as males.

Symptoms include:

- Persistent cough with increasing sputum
- Dyspnea
- Frequent respiratory infections

Treatment includes:

- Bronchodilators
- Long term continuous oxygen therapy or supplemental oxygen during exercise
- Pulmonary rehabilitation to improve exercise and breathing
- Antibiotics during infections
- Corticosteroids for acute episodes

EMPHYSEMA

Emphysema, the primary component of COPD, is characterized by abnormal distention of air spaces at the ends of the terminal bronchioles, with destruction of alveolar walls so that there is less and less gaseous exchange and increasing dead space with resultant hypoxemia, hypercapnia, and respiratory acidosis. The capillary bed is damaged as well, altering pulmonary blood flow and raising pressure in the right atrium (cor pulmonale) and pulmonary artery, leading to cardiac failure. Complications include respiratory insufficiency and failure. There are two primary types of emphysema (and both forms may be present):

- **Centrilobular** (the most common form) involves the central portion of the respiratory lobule, sparing distal alveoli, and usually affects the upper lobes. Typical symptoms include abnormal ventilation-perfusion ratios, hypoxemia, hypercapnia, and polycythemia with right-sided heart failure.
- **Panlobular** involves enlargement of all air spaces, including the bronchiole, alveolar duct, and alveoli, but there is minimal inflammatory disease. Typical symptoms include hyperextended rigid barrel chest, marked dyspnea, weight loss, and active expiration.

COPD

STAGES

Functional dyspnea, body mass index (BMI), and spirometry are used to assess the **stages of chronic obstructive pulmonary disease (COPD)**. Spirometry measures used are the ratio of forced expiratory volume in the first second of expiration (FEV_1) after full inhalation to total forced vital capacity (FVC). Normal lung function decreases after age 35; so normal values are adjusted for height, weight, gender, and age:

- **Stage I** (mild): Minimal dyspnea with or without cough and sputum. FEV_1 is ≥80% of predicted rate and FEV_1:FVC <70%.
- **Stage 2** (moderate): Moderate to severe chronic exertional dyspnea with or without cough and sputum. FEV_1 is 50-80% of predicted rate and FEV_1:FVC <70%.
- **Stage 3** (severe): Same as stage 2 but with repeated episodes with increased exertional dyspnea and condition impacting quality of life. FEV_1 is 30-50% of predicted rate and FEV_1:FVC <70%.
- **Stage 4** (very severe): Severe dyspnea and life-threatening episodes that severely impact quality of life. FEV_1 is 30% of predicted rate or <50% with chronic respiratory failure and FEV_1:FVC <70%.

MANAGEMENT

COPD is not reversible, so management aims at slowing its progression, relieving symptoms, and improving quality of life:

- Smoking cessation is the primary means to slow progression and may require smoking cessation support in the form of classes or medications, such as Zyban, nicotine patches or gum, clonidine, or nortriptyline.
- Bronchodilators, such as albuterol (Ventolin) and salmeterol (Serevent), relieve bronchospasm and airway obstruction.
- Corticosteroids, both inhaled (Pulmicort, Vanceril) and oral (prednisone) may improve symptoms but are used mostly for associated asthma.
- Oxygen therapy may be long term continuous or used during exertion.
- Bullectomy (for bullous emphysema) to remove bullae (enlarged airspaces that do not ventilate).
- Lung volume reduction surgery may be done if involvement in the lung is limited; however, mortality rates are high.
- Lung transplantation is a definitive high-risk option.
- Pulmonary rehabilitation includes breathing exercises, muscle training, activity pacing, and modification of activities.

CHRONIC VENTILATORY FAILURE

Chronic ventilatory failure occurs when alveolar ventilation fails to increase in response to increasing levels of carbon dioxide, usually associated with chronic pulmonary diseases, such as asthma and COPD, drug overdoses, or diseases that impair respiratory effort, such as Guillain-Barré and myasthenia gravis. Normally, the ventilatory system is able to maintain PCO_2 and pH levels within narrow limits, even though PO_2 levels may be more variable, but with ventilatory failure, the body is not able to compensate for the resultant hypercapnia and pH falls, resulting in respiratory acidosis. Symptoms include increasing dyspnea with tachypnea, gasping respirations, and use of accessory muscles. Patients may become confused as hypercapnia causes increased intracranial pressure. If pH is <7.2, cardiac arrhythmias, hyperkalemia, and hypotension can occur as pulmonary arteries constrict and the peripheral vascular system dilates. Diagnosis is per symptoms, ABGs consistent with respiratory acidosis (PCO_2 >50 and pH <7.35), pulse oximetry, and chest x-ray. Treatment can include non-invasive PPV (BiPAP), endotracheal mechanical ventilation, corticosteroids, and bronchodilators.

CHRONIC ASTHMA

The three primary symptoms of chronic asthma are cough, wheezing, and dyspnea. In cough-variant asthma, a severe cough may be the only symptom, at least initially. Chronic asthma is characterized by recurring bronchospasm and inflammation of the airways resulting in airway obstruction. Asthma affects the bronchi and not the alveoli. While no longer considered part of COPD because airway obstruction is not constant and is responsive to treatment, over time fibrotic changes in the airways can result in permanent obstruction, especially if asthma is not treated adequately. **Symptoms** of chronic asthma include nighttime coughing, exertional dyspnea, tightness in the chest, and cough. Acute exacerbations may occur, sometimes related to triggers, such as allergies, resulting in increased dyspnea, wheezing, cough, tachycardia, bronchospasm, and rhonchi. **Treatment** of chronic asthma includes chest hygiene, identification and avoidance of triggers, prompt treatment of infections, bronchodilators, long-acting β-2 agonists, and inhaled glucocorticoids.

STATUS ASTHMATICUS

PATHOPHYSIOLOGY

Status asthmaticus is a severe acute attack of asthma that does not respond to conventional therapy. An acute attack of asthma is precipitated by some stimulus, such as an antigen that triggers an allergic response, resulting in an inflammatory cascade that causes edema of the mucous membranes (swollen airway), contraction of smooth muscles (bronchospasm), increased mucus production (cough and obstruction), and hyperinflation of airways (decreased ventilation and shunting). Mast cells and T lymphocytes produce cytokines, which continue the inflammatory response through increased blood flow coupled with vasoconstriction and bronchoconstriction, resulting in fluid leakage from the vasculature. Epithelial cells and cilia are destroyed, exposing nerves and causing hypersensitivity. Sympathetic nervous system receptors in the bronchi stimulate bronchodilation.

CLINICAL SYMPTOMS

The person with status asthmaticus will often present in acute distress, non-responsive to inhaled bronchodilators. **Symptoms** include:

- Signs of airway obstruction
- Sternal and intercostal retractions
- Tachypnea and dyspnea with increasing cyanosis
- Forced prolonged expirations
- Cardiac decompensation with increased left ventricular afterload and increased pulmonary edema resulting from alveolar-capillary permeability. Hypoxia may trigger an increase in pulmonary vascular resistance with increased right ventricular afterload.
- Pulsus paradoxus (decreased pulse on inspiration and increased on expiration) with extra beats on inspiration detected through auscultation but not detected radially. Blood pressure normally decreases slightly during inspiration, but this response is exaggerated. Pulsus paradoxus indicates increasing severity of asthma.
- Hypoxemia (with impending respiratory failure)
- Hypocapnia followed by hypercapnia (with impending respiratory failure)
- Metabolic acidosis

INDICATIONS FOR MECHANICAL VENTILATION FOR STATUS ASTHMATICUS

Mechanical ventilation (MV) for status asthmaticus should be avoided, if possible, because of the danger of increased bronchospasm as well as barotrauma and decreased circulation. However, there are some absolute indications for the use of intubation and ventilation and a number of other indications that are evaluated on an individual basis.

The following are **absolute indications for MV:**

- Cardiac and/or pulmonary arrest
- Markedly depressed mental status (obtundation)
- Severe hypoxia and/or apnea

The following are **relative indications for MV:**

- Exhaustion/muscle fatigue from exertion of breathing
- Sharply diminished breath sounds and no audible wheezing
- Pulse paradoxus >20-40 mmHg; absent = imminent respiratory arrest
- PaO_2 <70 mmHg on 100% oxygen
- Dysphonia
- Central cyanosis
- Increased hypercapnia
- Metabolic/respiratory acidosis: pH <7.20

In this patient population, ventilator goal is to minimize airway pressures while oxygenating the patient. Vent settings include: low tidal volume (6-8 mL/kg), low respiratory rate (10-14 respirations/minute), and high inspiratory flow rate (80-100 L/min).

> **Review Video: Mechanical Ventilation**
> Visit mometrix.com/academy and enter code: 679637

AIR LEAK SYNDROMES

Air leak syndromes may result in significant respiratory distress. Leaks may occur spontaneously or secondary to some type of trauma (accidental, mechanical, iatrogenic) or disease. As pressure increases inside the alveoli, the alveolar wall pulls away from the perivascular sheath and subsequent alveolar rupture allows air to follow the perivascular planes and flow into adjacent areas. There are two categories:

- **Pneumothorax:**
  - Air in the pleural space causes a lung to collapse.
- **Barotrauma/volutrauma** with air in the interstitial space (usually resolve over time):
  - Pneumoperitoneum is air in the peritoneal area, including the abdomen and occasionally the scrotal sac of male infants.
  - Pneumomediastinum is air in the mediastinal area between the lungs.
  - Pneumopericardium is air in the pericardial sac that surrounds the heart.
  - Subcutaneous emphysema is air in the subcutaneous tissue planes of the chest wall.
  - Pulmonary interstitial emphysema (PIE) is air trapped in the interstitium between the alveoli.

PNEUMOTHORAX

Pneumothorax occurs when there is a leak of air into the pleural space, resulting in complete or partial collapse of a lung.

PNEUMOTHORAX

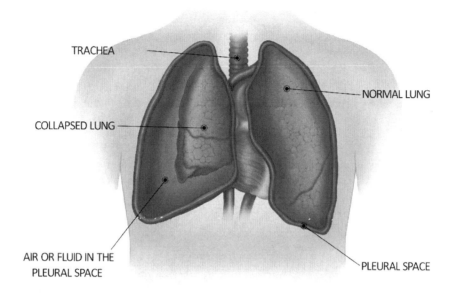

TRACHEA

NORMAL LUNG

COLLAPSED LUNG

AIR OR FLUID IN THE
PLEURAL SPACE

PLEURAL SPACE

Symptoms: Vary widely depending on the cause and degree of the pneumothorax and whether or not there is an underlying disease. Symptoms include acute pleuritic pain (95%), usually on the affected side, and decreased breath sounds. In a *tension pneumothorax,* symptoms include tracheal deviation and hemodynamic compromise.

Diagnosis: Clinical findings; radiograph: 6-foot upright posterior-anterior; ultrasound may detect traumatic pneumothorax.

Treatment: Chest-tube thoracostomy with underwater seal drainage is the most common treatment for all types of pneumothorax.

- Tension pneumothorax: Immediate needle decompression and chest tube thoracostomy
- Small pneumothorax, patient stable: Oxygen administration and observation for 3-6 hours. If no increase is shown on repeat x-ray, patient may be discharged with another x-ray in 24 hours.
- Primary spontaneous pneumothorax: Catheter aspiration or chest tube thoracostomy

PLEURAL EFFUSION AND EMPYEMA

Pleural effusion is the accumulation of fluid in the pleural space, usually secondary to other disease processes, such as heart failure, TB, neoplasms, nephrotic syndrome, and viral respiratory infections. The fluid may be serous, bloody, or purulent (empyema) and transudative or exudative. Signs and symptoms depend on underlying condition but includes dyspnea, from mild to severe. Tracheal deviation away from the affected side may be evident. Diagnosis includes chest x-ray, lateral decubitus x-ray, CT, thoracentesis, and pleural biopsy. Treatment includes treating underlying cause, thoracentesis to remove fluid, insertion of chest tube, pleurodesis, or pleurectomy or pleuroperitoneal shunt (primarily with malignancy).

> **Review Video: Pleural Effusions**
> Visit mometrix.com/academy and enter code: 145719

Empyema is a pleural effusion in which the collection of pleural fluid is thick and purulent, usually as a result of bacterial pneumonia or penetrating chest trauma. Empyema may also occur as a complication of thoracentesis or thoracic surgery. Signs and symptoms include acute illness with fever, chills, pain, cough, and dyspnea. Diagnosis is per chest CT and thoracentesis with culture and sensitivity. Treatment includes antibiotics and drainage of pleural space per needle aspiration, tube thoracostomy, or open chest drainage with thoracotomy.

PULMONARY FIBROSIS

Pulmonary fibrosis is a progressive disease of the lungs in which scarring of the tissue causes the lining of the lungs to thicken. This thickening prevents adequate oxygen exchange from occurring. The cause of pulmonary fibrosis is unknown, however environmental toxins such as asbestos, infections, smoking and occupational exposure to wood or metal dust may be contributing factors. The disease is more prevalent in males and the average age at the time of diagnosis is between 40 and 70. There may also be a genetic predisposition in the development of pulmonary fibrosis. The median survival for patients diagnosed with pulmonary fibrosis is less than five years.

Signs and symptoms: Shortness of breath, dry cough, fatigue, weight loss, and clubbing of the finger tips and nails.

Diagnosis: Physical assessment, chest x-ray and/or computed tomography, pulmonary function tests, arterial blood gases and lung biopsy.

Treatment: There is no cure for pulmonary fibrosis and treatment options are minimal. Anti-inflammatory medications such as corticosteroids may be used for symptom management as well as supplemental oxygen therapy. Lung transplantation may be an option for some patients based on age and advancement of disease. Some patients may be eligible for participation in a clinical trial, as there are research efforts focused on treatment options to halt the progression of the disease.

PULMONARY HYPERTENSION AND PULMONARY ARTERIAL HYPERTENSION

Pulmonary arterial hypertension (PAH) is a progressive disease of the pulmonary arteries that can severely compromise cardiovascular patients. It may involve multiple processes. Usually, the pulmonary vasculature adjusts easily to accommodate blood volume from the right ventricle. If there is increased blood flow, the low resistance causes vasodilation and vice versa. However, sometimes the pulmonary vascular bed is damaged or obstructed, and this can impair the ability to handle changing volumes of blood. In that case, an increase in flow will increase the pulmonary arterial pressure, increasing pulmonary vascular resistance (PVR). This in turn, increases pressure on the right ventricle (RV) with increased RV workload and eventually causes RV hypertrophy with displacement of the intraventricular septum and tricuspid regurgitation (cor pulmonale). Over time, this leads to right heart failure and death. Pulmonary hypertension is usually diagnosed by right-sided heart catheterization and is indicated by systolic pulmonary artery pressure >30 mmHg and mean pulmonary artery pressure >25 mmHg. Non-invasive testing may include echocardiogram to look for cardiac changes.

TYPES

Pulmonary hypertension or pulmonary arterial hypertension (PAH) may be classified as primary (idiopathic) or secondary.

- **Primary (idiopathic) PAH** may result from changes in immune responses, pulmonary emboli, sickle cell disease, collagen diseases, Raynaud's, and the use of contraceptives. The cause may be unknown or genetic.

- **Secondary PAH** may result from pulmonary vasoconstriction brought on by hypoxemia related to COPD, sleep-disordered breathing, kyphoscoliosis, obesity, smoke inhalation, altitude sickness, interstitial pneumonia, and neuromuscular disorders. It may also be caused by a decrease in pulmonary vascular bed of 50-75%, which may result from pulmonary emboli, vasculitis, tumor emboli, and interstitial lung disease, such as sarcoidosis. Primary cardiac disease, such as congenital defects in infants, and acquired disorders, such as rheumatic valve disease, mitral stenosis, and left ventricular failure may also contribute to PAH.

TREATMENT OPTIONS FOR PAH

Medical treatment for pulmonary arterial hypertension (PAH) aims to identify and treat any underlying cardiac or pulmonary disease, control symptoms, and prevent complications:

- **Oxygen therapy** may be needed, especially supplemental oxygen during exercise.
- **Calcium channel blockers** may provide vasodilation for some patients.
- **Pulmonary vascular dilators**, such as IV epoprostenol (Flolan) and subcutaneous treprostinil sodium (Remodulin) and oral bosentan (Tracleer) help to control symptoms and prolong life.
- **Anticoagulants**, such as warfarin (Coumadin) are an important part of therapy because of recurrent pulmonary emboli. Studies have shown that anticoagulation increases survival rates.
- **Diuretics**, such as furosemide (Lasix) may be needed to relieve edema and restrict fluids, especially with right ventricular hypertrophy.

In some patients who cannot be managed adequately through medical treatment, a heart-lung transplant may be considered as the only effective treatment for long-term survival.

Respiratory Procedures and Interventions

NON-INVASIVE VENTILATION

NASAL CANNULA

A nasal cannula can be used to deliver supplemental oxygen to a patient, but it is only useful for flow rates ≤6 L/min as higher rates are drying of the nasal passages. As it is not an airtight system, some ambient air is breathed in as well so oxygen concentration ranges from about 24-44%. The nasal cannula does not allow for control of respiratory rate, so the patient must be able to breathe independently.

NON-REBREATHER MASK

A non-rebreather mask can be used to deliver higher concentrations (60-90%) of oxygen to those patients who are able to breathe independently. The mask fits over the nose and mouth and is secured by an elastic strap. A 1.5 L reservoir bag is attached and connects to an oxygen source. The bag is inflated to about 1 liter at a rate of 8-15 L/min before the mask is applied as the patient breathes from this reservoir. A one-way exhalation valve prevents most exhaled air from being rebreathed.

NON-INVASIVE POSITIVE PRESSURE VENTILATORS

Non-invasive positive pressure ventilators provide air through a tight-fitting nasal or face mask, usually pressure cycled, avoiding the need for intubation and reducing the danger of hospital-acquired infection and mortality rates. It can be used for acute respiratory failure and pulmonary edema. There are 2 types of non-invasive positive pressure ventilators:

- **CPAP (Continuous positive airway pressure)** provides a steady stream of pressurized air throughout both inspiration and expiration. CPAP improves breathing by decreasing preload for patients with congestive heart failure. It reduces the effort required for breathing by increasing residual volume and improving gas exchange.
- **Bi-PAP (Bi-level positive airway pressure)** provides a steady stream of pressurized air as CPAP but it senses inspiratory effort and increases pressure during inspiration. Bi-PAP pressures for inspiration and expiration can be set independently. Machines can be programmed with a backup rate to ensure a set number of respirations per minute.

NEVER place a patient in wrist restraints while wearing these devices. If the patient vomits, they need to be able to remove the mask to prevent aspiration.

FACE MASK

Ensuring that a face mask (Ambu bag) is the correct fit and type is important for adequate ventilation, oxygenation, and prevention of aspiration. Difficulties in management of face mask ventilation relate to risk factors: >55 years, obesity, beard, edentulous, and history of snoring. In some cases, if dentures are adhered well, they may be left in place during induction. The face mask is applied by lifting the mandible (jaw thrust) to the mask and avoiding pressure on soft tissue. Oral or nasal airways may be used, ensuring that the distal end is at the angle of the mandible. There are a number of steps to prevent mask airway leaks:

- Increasing or decreasing the amount of air to the mask to allow better seal
- Securing the mask with both hands while another person ventilates
- Accommodating a large nose by using the mask upside down
- Utilizing a laryngeal mask airway if excessive beard prevents seal

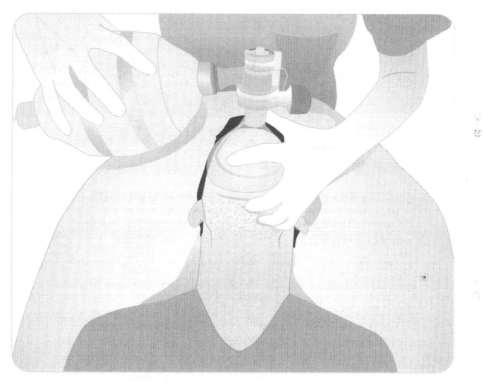

HIGH AND LOW FLOW OXYGEN DELIVERY

High flow oxygen delivery devices provide oxygen at flow rates higher than the patient's inspiratory flow rate at specific medium to high FiO_2, up to 100%. However, a flow of 100% oxygen actually provides only 60-80% FiO_2 to the patient because the patient also breathes in some room air, diluting the oxygen. The actual amount of oxygen received depends on the type of interface or mask. Additionally, the flow rate is actually less than the inspiratory flow rate upon actual delivery. High flow oxygen delivery is usually not used in the sleep center. Humidification is usually required because the high flow is drying.

Low flow oxygen delivery devices provide 100% oxygen at flow rates lower than the patient's inspiratory flow rate, but the oxygen mixes with room air, so the FiO_2 varies. Humidification is usually only required if flow rate is >3L/min. Much oxygen is wasted with exhalation, so a number of different devices to conserve oxygen are available. Interfaces include transtracheal catheters and cannulae with reservoirs.

AIRWAY DEVICES

OROPHARYNGEAL, NASOPHARYNGEAL, AND TRACHEOSTOMY TUBES

Airways are used to establish a patent airway and facilitate respirations:

- **Oropharyngeal**: This plastic airway curves over the tongue and creates space between the mouth and the posterior pharynx. It is used for anesthetized or unconscious patients to keep tongue and epiglottis from blocking the airway.
- **Nasopharyngeal** (trumpet): This smaller flexible airway is more commonly used in conscious patients and is inserted through one nostril, extending to the nasopharynx. It is commonly utilized in patients who need frequent suctioning.
- **Tracheostomy tubes**: Tracheostomy may be utilized for mechanical ventilation. Tubes are inserted into the opening in the trachea to provide a conduit and maintain the opening. The tube is secured with ties around the neck. Because the air entering the lungs through the tracheostomy bypasses the warming and moistening effects of the upper airway, air is humidified through a room humidifier or through the delivery of humidified air through a special mask or mechanical ventilation. If the tracheostomy is going to be long-term, eventually a stoma will form at the site, and the tube can be removed.

LARYNGEAL MASK AIRWAY

The laryngeal-mask airway (LMA) is an intermediate airway allowing ventilation but not complete respiratory control. The LMA consists of an inflatable cuff (the mask) with a connecting tube. It may be used temporarily before tracheal intubation or when tracheal intubation can't be done. It can also be a conduit for later blind insertion of an endotracheal tube. The head and neck must be in neutral position for insertion of the LMA. If the patient has a gag reflex, conscious sedation or topical anesthesia (deep oropharyngeal) is required. The LMA is inserted by sliding along the hard palate, using the finger as a guide, into the pharynx, and the ring is inflated to create a seal about the opening to the larynx, allowing ventilation with mild positive-pressure. The ProSeal LMA has a modified cuff that extends onto the back of the mask to improve seal. LMA is contraindicated in morbid obesity, obstructions or abnormalities of oropharynx, and non-fasting patients, as some aspiration is possible even with the cuff seal inflated.

ESOPHAGEAL-TRACHEAL COMBITUBE

The esophageal tracheal Combitube (ETC) is an intermediate airway that contains two lumens and can be inserted into either the trachea or the esophagus (≤91%). The twin-lumen tube has a proximal cuff providing a seal of the oropharynx and a distal cuff providing a seal about the distal tube. Prior to insertion, the Combitube cuffs should be checked for leaks (15 mL of air into distal and 85 mL of air into proximal). The patient should be non-responsive and with absent gag reflex with head in neutral position. The tube is passed along the tongue and into the pharynx, utilizing markings on the tube (black guidelines) to determine depth by aligning the ETC with the upper incisors or alveolar ridge. Once in place the distal cuff is inflated (10-15 mL) and then placement in the trachea or esophagus should be determined, so the proper lumen for ventilation can be used. The proximal cuff is inflated (usually to 50-75 mL) and ventilation begun. A capnogram should be used to confirm ventilation.

THORACENTESIS

A thoracentesis (aspiration of fluid or air from pleural space) is done to make a diagnosis, relieve pressure on the lung caused by pleural effusion, or instill medications. A chest x-ray is done prior to the procedure. A sedative may be given. The patient is in a sitting position, leaning onto a padded bedside stand, straddling a chair with head supported on the back of the chair, or lying on the opposite side with the head of the bed elevated 30-45° to ensure that fluid remains at the base. The patient should avoid coughing or moving during the procedure. The chest x-ray or ultrasound determines needle placement. After a local anesthetic is administered, a needle (with an attached 20-mL syringe and 3-way stopcock with tubing and a receptacle) is advanced intercostally into the pleural space. Fluid is drained, collected, examined, and measured. The needle is removed and a pressure dressing applied. A chest x-ray is done to ensure there is no pneumothorax. The patient is monitored for cough, dyspnea, and hypoxemia.

BRONCHOSCOPY

Bronchoscopy utilizes a thin, flexible fiberoptic bronchoscope to inspect the larynx, trachea, and bronchi for diagnostic purposes. It is also used to collect specimens, obtain biopsies, remove foreign bodies or secretions, treat atelectasis, and to excise lesions. The patient is in supine position during the procedure. The Mallampati classification may be used to determine difficulty of airway. The patient receives local anesthesia to the nares (lidocaine gel) and oropharynx (lidocaine gel, spray, or nebulizer), and usually receives a benzodiazepine (commonly midazolam or lorazepam), an opioid (fentanyl or meperidine), or propofol. Medications are usually given in small incremental doses throughout the procedure and may be combined. Over-sedation may cause physiologic depression, but undersedation may result in recall and agitation with sympathetic activation. The tube is advanced through the nares and down the trachea to the bronchi. Airway patency, respiratory rate, and oxygen saturation must be constantly monitored. Complications can include bleeding, arrhythmias, obstruction, laryngospasm, and respiratory failure.

THORACIC SURGERY

LUNG VOLUME REDUCTION

Lung volume reduction surgery (LVRS) usually involves removing about 20-35% of lung tissue that is not functioning adequately in order to reduce the lung size so that the lungs work more effectively. This procedure is most commonly used with adult emphysematous COPD patients. In adults, surgery is usually bilateral; however, some patients are not candidates for bilateral surgery because of cardiac disease or emphysema affecting only one lung. Unilateral surgery has been shown to be effective. Surgical removal of part of the lung improves ventilation and gas exchange and does not require the immunosuppressant therapy required for lung transplantation. Studies have shown that those with low risk for the surgery and with emphysematous changes in the upper lobes can benefit from the surgery, but high-risk patients with more widespread emphysematous changes have increased mortality rates. The surgery may be done through an open-chest thoracotomy or through a less invasive video-assisted thoracotomy.

PNEUMONECTOMY

Pneumonectomy is the surgical removal of one of the lungs. There are 2 surgical procedures:

- **Simple**: removal of just the lung
- **Extrapleural**: removal not only of the lung but also part of the diaphragm on the affected side and the pericardium on that same side

During the operative procedure, much care must be taken to prevent contamination of the remaining lung, including the use of bronchus blockers or prone position during surgery.

Removal of the lung is indicated for a number of conditions, including:

- Cancerous lesions (the most common reason for surgery)
- Severe bronchiectasis from chronic suppurative pneumonia, resulting in dilation of terminal bronchioles
- Severe hypoplasia
- Unilateral lung destruction with pulmonary hypertension
- Pulmonary hemorrhage
- Lobar emphysema
- Chronic pulmonary infections with destruction of lung tissue

Because the lung capacity is reduced, persistent shortness of breath may occur with exertion even many months after surgery.

LOBECTOMY AND OTHER PROCEDURES TO REMOVE PARTIAL LUNG TISSUE

Lobectomy removes one or more lobes of a lung (which has 2 on the left and 3 on the right) and is usually done for lesions or trauma that is confined to one lobe, such as tubercular lesions, abscesses or cysts, cancer (usually non-small cell in early stages), traumatic injury, or bronchiectasis. Surgery is usually done through an open thoracotomy or video-assisted thoracotomy. Complications can include hemorrhage, post-operative infection with or without abscess formation, and pneumothorax. Usually, 1-2 chest tubes are left in place in the immediate post-surgical period to remove air and/or fluid.

- **Segmental resection** removes a bronchovascular segment and is used for small lesions in the periphery, bronchiectasis or congenital cysts or blebs.
- **Wedge resection** removes a small wedged-shape portion of the lung tissue and is used for small peripheral lesions, granulomas, or blebs.
- **Bronchoplastic (sleeve) reconstruction** removes part of bronchus and lung tissue with reanastomosis of bronchus and is used for small lesions of the carina or bronchus.

Respiratory Pharmacology

PHARMACOLOGICAL AGENTS USED FOR ASTHMA

Numerous pharmacological agents are used for control of asthma, some that are long-acting to prevent attacks and others that are short-acting to provide relief for acute episodes. Listed with each are the standard med and dosage used for urgent care:

- **β-Adrenergic agonists** include both long-acting and short-acting preparations used for relaxation of smooth muscles and bronchodilation, reducing edema, and aiding clearance of mucus. Medications include salmeterol (Serevent), sustained-release albuterol (Volmax ER) and short-acting albuterol (Proventil), and levalbuterol (Xopenex). Albuterol 2.5-5.0 mg every 20 minutes, 3 doses by nebulizer.
- **Anticholinergics** aid in preventing bronchial constriction and potentiate the bronchodilating action of β-Adrenergic agonists. The most commonly used medication is ipratropium bromide (Atrovent) 500 mcg every 20 minutes, 3 doses by nebulizer.
- **Corticosteroids** provide anti-inflammatory action by inhibiting immune responses and decreasing edema, mucus, and hyper-responsiveness. Because of numerous side effects, glucocorticosteroids are usually administered orally or parenterally for ≤5 days (prednisone, prednisolone, methylprednisolone) and then switched to inhaled steroids. If a person receives glucocorticoids for more than 5 days, then dosages are tapered. Methylprednisolone 60-125 mg IV is the standard dose for respiratory failure. The Global Initiative for Asthma (GINA) recommends daily inhaled corticosteroids for all individuals with severe asthma to reduce the risk of exacerbations.
- **Methylxanthines** are used to improve pulmonary function and decrease the need for mechanical ventilation. Medications include aminophylline and theophylline.
- **Magnesium sulfate** is used to relax smooth muscles and decrease inflammation. If administered intravenously, it must be given slowly to prevent hypotension and bradycardia. When inhaled, it potentiates the action of albuterol. Standard dosage: 2 g (8 mmol), 1 dose by IV over 20 minutes.
- **Heliox** (helium-oxygen) is administered to decrease airway resistance with airway obstruction, thereby decreasing respiratory effort. Heliox improves oxygenation of those on mechanical ventilation.
- **Leukotriene inhibitors** are used to inhibit inflammation and bronchospasm for long-term management. Medications include montelukast (Singulair).

ADDITIONAL PULMONARY PHARMACOLOGY

There is a wide range of agents used for pulmonary pharmacology, depending upon the type and degree of pulmonary disease. Agents include:

- **Opioid analgesics:** Used to provide both pain relief and sedation for those on mechanical ventilation to reduce sympathetic response. Medications may include fentanyl (Sublimaze) or morphine sulfate (MS Contin).
- **Neuromuscular blockers:** Used for induced paralysis of those who have not responded adequately to sedation, especially for intubation and mechanical ventilation. Medications may include pancuronium (Pavulon) and vecuronium (Norcuron). However, there is controversy about the use of such blockers, as induced paralysis has been linked to increased mortality rates, sensory hearing loss (pancuronium), atelectasis, and ventilation-perfusion mismatch.
- **Human B-type natriuretic peptides:** Used to reduce pulmonary capillary wedge pressure. Medications include nesiritide (Natrecor).
- **Surfactants**: Reduces surface tension to prevent the collapse of alveoli. Beractant (Survanta) is derived from bovine lung tissue and calfactant (Infasurf) from calf lung tissue. They are administered as inhalants.
- **Alkalinizers**: Used to treat metabolic acidosis and reduce pulmonary vascular resistance by achieving an alkaline pH. Medications include sodium bicarbonate and tromethamine (THAM).

- **Pulmonary vasodilator (inhaled nitric oxide):** Used to relax the vascular muscles and produce pulmonary vasodilation. Some studies show it reduces the need for extracorporeal membrane oxygenation (ECMO).
- **Methylxanthines:** Used to stimulate muscle contractions of the chest and stimulate respirations. Medications include aminophylline (Aminophylline), caffeine citrate (Cafcit), and doxapram (Dopram).
- **Diuretics:** Used to reduce pulmonary edema. Medications include loop diuretics such as furosemide (Lasix) and metolazone (Mykrox).
- **Nitrates:** Used for vasodilation to reduce preload and afterload, which in turn reduces myocardial need for oxygen. Medications include nitroglycerin (Nitro-Bid) and nitroprusside sodium (Nitropress).
- **Antibiotics:** Used for treatment of respiratory infections, including pneumonia. Medications are used according to the pathogenic agent and may include macrolides such as azithromycin (Zithromax) and erythromycin (E-Mycin).
- **Antimycobacterials:** Used for treatment of TB and other mycobacterial diseases. Medications include isoniazid (Laniazid, Nydrazid), ethambutol (Myambutol), rifampin (Rifadin), streptomycin sulfate, and pyrazinamide.
- **Antivirals:** Used to inhibit replication of a virus early in a viral infection. Effectiveness decreases as time passes because the replication process has already begun. Medications include ribavirin (Virazole) and zanamivir (Relenza).

Endocrine Pathophysiology

DIABETES MELLITUS TYPES 1 AND 2

Diabetes mellitus is the most common metabolic disorder. Over 6% of adults have diabetes, but only 4% of adults are diagnosed. Insulin resistance tends to increase in older adults, so there is less ability to handle glucose. Type II is more common in older adults, with incidence increasing with age.

- **Type I:** Immune-mediated form with insufficient insulin production because of the destruction of pancreatic beta cells
  - o **Symptoms** include pronounced polyuria and polydipsia, short onset, obesity or recent weight loss, and ketoacidosis present on diagnosis.
  - o **Treatment** includes insulin as needed to control blood sugar, glucose monitoring 1–4 times daily, diet with carbohydrate control, and exercise.
- **Type II:** Insulin resistant form with defect in insulin secretion
  - o **Symptoms** include long onset, obesity with no weight loss or significant weight loss, mild or absent polyuria and polydipsia, ketoacidosis or glycosuria without ketonuria, androgen-mediated problems such as hirsutism and acne (adolescents), and hypertension.
  - o **Treatment** includes diet and exercise, glucose monitoring, and oral medications.

> **Review Video: Diabetes Mellitus: Diet, Exercise, & Medications**
> Visit mometrix.com/academy and enter code: 774388
>
> **Review Video: Diabetes: Complications**
> Visit mometrix.com/academy and enter code: 996788

DIABETIC KETOACIDOSIS

Diabetic ketoacidosis is a complication of type 1 diabetes mellitus, usually related to noncompliance with treatment, stress, illness, or lack of awareness of having diabetes (this event often being the first time that diabetes is diagnosed). Inadequate production of insulin results in glucose being unavailable for metabolism, so lipolysis (breakdown of fat) produces free fatty acids (FFAs) as an alternate fuel source. Glycerol is converted to ketone bodies which are used for cellular metabolism less efficiently than glucose. Excess ketone bodies are excreted in the urine (ketonuria) or exhalations. Acidosis of any type causes potassium in cells to shift to the serum. The ketone bodies lower serum pH, leading to ketoacidosis.

Symptoms include:

- Kussmaul respirations: "Ketone breath," or fruity smelling breath; progresses to CNS depression with loss of airway
- Fluid imbalance, including loss of potassium and other electrolytes from cellular death resulting in dehydration and diuresis with excess thirst
- Dangerous cardiac arrhythmias, related to potassium loss; hypotension, chest pain, tachycardia
- GI: Nausea/vomiting, abdominal pain, loss of appetite
- Neurological: malaise, confusion/lethargy progressing to coma

Diagnosis is based on:

- Labs: Blood glucose >250 mg/dL, lower Na and elevated K (switches after treatment), elevated beta-hydroxybutyrate (byproduct of ketones)
- ABG: pH <7.3, HCO_3 <18 mEq/L
- Urine: + glucose, ketones

TREATMENT AND POTENTIAL COMPLICATIONS

Treatment of DKA:

- **Fluids**: Priority is fluid resuscitation with 1-2 liters of isotonic fluids given in the first hour, up to 8 liters in the first 24 hours. Potassium will be added to the fluids when levels begin to fall.
- **Insulin**: Continuous drip IV, with/without loading dose. Will usually begin at 0.1 unit/kg/ hour (5-7 units an hour generally), with a goal of decreasing blood glucose 50–75 mg/dL an hour. Blood glucose is checked every hour, and when levels are < 200 mg/dL, add dextrose to IV fluids to prevent rebound hypoglycemia.
- **Potassium**: Watch carefully, as fluids and insulin will cause rapid fall in serum levels. When K <5 mEq/L, it should be added to the IV fluids (Per liter: 20 mEq for K 4-5, 40 mEq for K 3–4). If potassium falls below 3, stop insulin drip and give 10–20 an hour until >3.5.
- **Sodium and Magnesium**: Na has an inverse relationship with potassium, and will increase as potassium falls. If sodium levels rise above 150 mEq, switch fluids to 0.45 NS. Low magnesium levels prevent potassium uptake, so replace as necessary.
- **Electrolytes**: Continue to monitor electrolytes and anion gap during ICU stay. When ABG and electrolytes normalized, transition to SQ insulin.

Potential complications include:

- Sudden electrolyte shifts (potassium) leading to catastrophic arrythmias, cerebral edema, and other complications
- Vomiting and decreased LOC leading to aspiration/ARDS
- Mechanical ventilation stops respiratory alkalosis and increases acidosis

HHNK

Hyperglycemic hyperosmolar nonketotic syndrome (HHNK) occurs in people without history of diabetes or with mild type 2 diabetes, resulting in persistent hyperglycemia leading to osmotic diuresis. Fluid shifts from intracellular to extracellular spaces to maintain osmotic equilibrium, but the increased glucosuria and dehydration results in hypernatremia and increased osmolarity. This condition is most common in those 50–70 years old and often is precipitated by an acute illness, such as a stroke, medications (thiazides), or dialysis treatments. HHNK differs from ketoacidosis because, while the insulin level is not adequate, it is high enough to prevent the breakdown of fat. Onset of symptoms often occurs over a few days. Glucose levels are often higher than those in DKA due to the gradual increase over time (often greater than 600), and the body living in a state of hyperglycemia, therefore the individual is not symptomatic until the blood glucose level is at an extreme high.

Symptoms: Polyuria, dehydration, hypotension, tachycardia, changes in mental status, seizures, hemiparesis.

Diagnosis: Increased glucose, Na, osmolality (urine and serum), BUN/Creatinine.

Treatment is similar to that for ketoacidosis:

- Insulin drip with frequent (hourly) blood sugar monitoring.
- Intravenous fluids and electrolytes.
- Correct blood glucose and other labs.

ACUTE HYPOGLYCEMIA

Acute hypoglycemia (hyperinsulinism) may result from pancreatic islet tumors or hyperplasia, increasing insulin production, or from the use of insulin to control diabetes mellitus. Hyperinsulinism can cause damage to the central nervous and cardiopulmonary systems, interfering with functioning of the brain and causing neurological impairment. Other causes may include: genetic defects (chromosome 11: short arm), severe infections, and toxic ingestion of alcohol or drugs (salicylates).

Symptoms include:

- Blood glucose <50-60 mg/dL
- Central nervous system: seizures, altered consciousness, lethargy, and poor feeding with vomiting, myoclonus, respiratory distress, diaphoresis, hypothermia, and cyanosis
- Adrenergic system: diaphoresis, tremor, tachycardia, palpitation, hunger, and anxiety

Diagnosis: Blood work, patient history, presentation.

Treatment depends on underlying cause:

- Glucose/Glucagon administration to elevate blood glucose levels
- Diazoxide (Hyperstat) to inhibit release of insulin
- Somatostatin (Sandostatin) to suppress insulin production
- Careful monitoring

DIABETES INSIPIDUS

Diabetes insipidus (DI) is caused by a deficiency of the antidiuretic hormone (ADH), or vasopressin. DI may develop secondary to head trauma, primary brain tumor, meningitis, encephalitis, or surgical ablation or irradiation of the pituitary gland, or metastatic tumors. This is different from congenital nephrogenic diabetes insipidus, in which production of ADH is normal but the renal tubules do not respond.

Symptoms:

- Polydipsia—enormous quantities of fluid may be ingested (3-30 L/day)
- Polyuria—large volumes of very dilute urine is excreted (3-30 L/day); nocturia almost always occurs
- Dehydration and hypovolemia can develop quickly if urinary losses are not continuously replaced

Diagnosis: A water deprivation test is the most reliable diagnostic test, but should only be done while the patient is under constant supervision. The test measures urine production, blood electrolyte levels, and weight over about 12 hours, during which the person is not allowed to drink. At the end of the 12 hours, vasopressin is given and a diagnosis of DI is confirmed if the person's excessive urination stops, BP rises to normal, and HR is normal.

Treatment includes:

- **Hormonal drugs**—Desmopressin, a synthetic analog of vasopressin, has prolonged antidiuretic activity, lasting 12 to 24 hours in most patients, and may be given intranasally, SQ, IV, or orally. Overdosage can lead to water intoxication, so monitor neurological status.
- **Nonhormonal drugs**—Three groups of nonhormonal drugs can reduce polyuria:
  o Diuretics, primarily thiazides (hydrochlorothiazide)
  o Vasopressin-releasing drugs (chlorpropamide or carbamazepine)
  o Prostaglandin inhibitors (indomethacin)

SIADH

Syndrome of inappropriate secretion of antidiuretic hormone (SIADH) is related to hypersecretion of the posterior pituitary gland. This causes the kidneys to reabsorb fluids, resulting in fluid retention, and triggers a decrease in sodium levels (dilutional hyponatremia), resulting in production of only concentrated urine. This syndrome may result from central nervous system disorders, such as brain trauma, surgery, or tumors. It may also be triggered by other disorders, such as tumors of various organs, pneumothorax, acute pneumonia, and other lung disorders. Some medications (vincristine, phenothiazines, tricyclic antidepressants, and thiazide diuretics) may also trigger SIADH.

Symptoms: Edema, dyspnea, crackles on auscultation, anorexia with nausea and vomiting, irritability, stomach cramps, alterations of personality, stupor, and seizures (related to progressive sodium depletion).

Diagnosis: Increased urine specific gravity, decreased Na and serum osmolality.

Treatment includes: (treat underlying cause)

- Correct fluid volume excess and electrolytes.
- Monitor urine output continuously: <0.5-1 mL/kg/hour is cause for concern.
- Seizure precautions.
- With SIADH expect low serum sodium and serum osmolality with high urine osmolality.

CHRONIC ADRENAL INSUFFICIENCY (ADDISON'S DISEASE)

Adrenal/Adrenocortical insufficiency (Addison's disease) is caused by damage to the adrenal cortex related to a variety of causes, such as autoimmune disease or genetic disorders, but it may relate to destructive lesions or neoplasms. Without treatment the condition is life threatening.

Symptoms may be vague and the condition undiagnosed until 80–90% of the adrenal cortex has been destroyed:

- Chronic weakness and fatigue
- Abdominal distress with nausea and vomiting
- Salt or licorice craving as a result of aldosterone deficiency
- Pigmentary changes in skin and mucous membranes, hyperpigmentation
- Hypotension
- Hypoglycemia
- Recurrent seizures (more common in children)

Treatment includes hormone replacement therapy with glucocorticoids (cortisol) and mineralocorticoids (aldosterone), which may be taken orally or by monthly parenteral injections. Androgen replacement is sometimes recommended for women.

Note: During times of stress or illness, the demand for glucocorticoids may increase, and dosages up to 3 times the normal dosage may be needed to prevent an acute crisis.

ACUTE ADRENAL INSUFFICIENCY (ADRENAL CRISIS)

Acute adrenal insufficiency (adrenal crisis) is a sudden, life-threatening condition resulting from an exacerbation of primary chronic adrenal insufficiency (Addison's disease), often precipitated by sepsis, surgical stress, adrenal hemorrhage related to septicemia, anticoagulation complications, and cortisone withdrawal related to a decreased or inadequate dose to compensate for stress. Acute adrenal insufficiency may occur in those who do not have Addison's disease, such as those who have received cortisone for various reasons, usually a minimum of 20 mg daily for at least 5 days.

Symptoms:

- Fever
- Nausea and vomiting
- Abdominal pain
- Weakness and general fatigue
- Disorientation, confusion

- Hypotensive shock
- Dehydration
- Electrolyte imbalance with hyperkalemia, hypercalcemia, hypoglycemia, and hyponatremia

Treatment:

- IV fluids in large volume
- Glucocorticoid
- 50% dextrose if indicated (hypoglycemia)
- Mineralocorticoid may be needed after intravenous solutions
- The precipitating cause must be identified and treated as well

HYPERTHYROIDISM

Hyperthyroidism (thyrotoxicosis) usually results from excess production of thyroid hormones (Graves' disease) from immunoglobulins providing abnormal stimulation of the thyroid gland. Other causes include thyroiditis and excess thyroid medications.

Symptoms vary and may be non-specific, especially in the elderly:

- Hyperexcitability
- Tachycardia (100-160) and atrial fibrillation
- Increased systolic (but not diastolic) BP
- Poor heat tolerance, skin flushed and diaphoretic
- Dry skin and pruritis (especially in the elderly)
- Hand tremor, progressive muscular weakness
- Exophthalmos (bulging eyes)
- Increased appetite and intake but weight loss

Treatment includes:

- Radioactive iodine to destroy the thyroid gland. Propranolol may be used to prevent thyroid storm. Thyroid hormones are given for resultant hypothyroidism.
- Antithyroid medications, such as Propacil or Tapazole to block conversion of T4 to T3.
- Surgical removal of thyroid is used if patients cannot tolerate other treatments or in special circumstances, such as large goiter. Usually one-sixth of the thyroid is left in place and antithyroid medications are given before surgery.

> **Review Video: 7 Symptoms of Hyperthyroidism**
> Visit mometrix.com/academy and enter code: 923159
>
> **Review Video: Graves' Disease**
> Visit mometrix.com/academy and enter code: 516655
>
> **Review Video: Thyroid and Antithyroid**
> Visit mometrix.com/academy and enter code: 666133

THYROTOXIC STORM

Thyrotoxic storm is a severe type of hyperthyroidism with sudden onset, precipitated by stress such as injury or surgery, in those un-treated or inadequately treated for hyperthyroidism. If not promptly diagnosed and treated, it is fatal. Incidence has decreased with the use of antithyroid medications but can still occur with medical emergencies or pregnancy. Diagnostic findings are similar to hyperthyroidism and include increased T3 uptake and decreased TSH.

Symptoms:

- Increase in symptoms of hyperthyroidism
- Increased temperature >38.5 °C
- Tachycardia >130 with atrial fibrillation and heart failure
- Gastrointestinal disorders such as nausea, vomiting, diarrhea, and abdominal discomfort
- Altered mental status with delirium progressing to coma

Treatment:

- Controlling production of thyroid hormone through antithyroid medications such as propylthiouracil and methimazole
- Inhibiting release of thyroid hormone with iodine therapy (or lithium)
- Controlling peripheral activity of thyroid hormone with propranolol
- Fluid and electrolyte replacement
- Glucocorticoids, such as dexamethasone
- Cooling blankets
- Treatment of arrhythmias as needed with antiarrhythmics and anticoagulation

HYPOTHYROIDISM

Hypothyroidism occurs when the thyroid produces inadequate levels of thyroid hormones. Conditions may range from mild to severe myxedema. There are a number of **causes**:

- Chronic lymphocytic thyroiditis (Hashimoto's thyroiditis)
- Excessive treatment for hyperthyroidism
- Atrophy of thyroid
- Medications such as lithium and iodine compounds
- Radiation to the area of the thyroid
- Diseases that affect the thyroid such as scleroderma
- Iodine imbalances

Symptoms may include chronic fatigue, menstrual disturbances, hoarseness, subnormal temperature, low pulse rate, weight gain, thinning hair, thickening skin. Some dementia may occur with advanced conditions. Clinical findings may include increased cholesterol with associated atherosclerosis and coronary artery disease. Myxedema may be characterized by changes in respiration with hypoventilation and CO_2 retention resulting in coma.

Treatment involves hormone replacement with synthetic levothyroxine (Synthroid) based on TSH levels, but this increases the oxygen demand of the body, so careful monitoring of cardiac status must be done during early treatment to avoid myocardial infarction while reaching euthyroid (normal) level.

HYPERPARATHYROIDISM

Hyperparathyroidism occurs when there is **overproduction of parathyroid hormone (PTH)**. Normal range is 10-55 pg/mL. This occurs more often in women and those over 50 years old. Hypercalcemia (total Ca^{++} >10.4 mg/dL) is the most common finding in hyperparathyroidism. Patients may complain signs of hypercalcemia which can be easily remembered with *bones, stones, groans, and moans.* This includes **bone pain** due to demineralization, **kidney stones**, **abdominal groans** (nausea, vomiting, constipation, loss of appetite), and **psychiatric moans** (nervous system issues: muscle weakness, fatigue, lethargy, depression, confusion). Polyuria can occur with renal failure. Cardiac arrhythmias, hypertension, and even coma can occur. Ca^{++} levels

>12 mg/dL may be due to cancer, and therefore cancer must be ruled out, especially if Ca⁺⁺ levels rise rapidly. Hyperparathyroidism is treated with parathyroidectomy of affected glands.

HYPOPARATHYROIDISM

Hypoparathyroidism is the **deficiency of PTH**. This is more common in women and is usually due to accidental damage during thyroid/neck surgery, radioactive iodine treatment for hyperthyroidism, radiation, or due to autoimmune causes. As Ca⁺⁺ levels drop, patients may complain of paresthesia of the fingers, toes, and perioral area. Patients will show other signs of neuromuscular irritability with muscle aches, hyperreflexia, carpopedal spasm (tetany), laryngospasm, and facial grimacing. A positive Chvostek sign (unilateral spasm of the facial muscles when the facial nerve is tapped) and a positive Trousseau sign (carpal spasm when upper arm is compressed with a blood pressure cuff) may be present. Irritability, confusion, fatigue, seizures, brittle hair and nails, and personality changes may occur. Diagnose with an ionized Ca⁺⁺ level (<4.7 mg/dL), reduced PTH, and elevated phosphate. Treat with Ca⁺⁺ and vitamin D supplements. Patients with renal failure must also reduce the amount of phosphate in their diet. Patients with tetany are treated with IV calcium gluconate.

CUSHING SYNDROME AND CUSHING'S DISEASE

Cushing syndrome results when **cortisol levels** are increased. Most commonly, this is due to steroid treatment with **prednisone**. Endogenous causes include a pituitary adenoma producing excess amounts of adrenocorticotropic hormone (ACTH) which leads to elevated cortisol (termed **Cushing's disease**) or a primary tumor of the adrenal gland causing increased cortisol secretion. Forms of cancer (e.g., lung, carcinoid) can present with ectopic sources of ACTH secretion. Patients will develop proximal muscle weakness, muscular atrophy, truncal obesity with thin arms and legs, round facies, buffalo hump, and purple striae usually across the abdomen. Patients may bruise easily, have non-healing sores, and women may be affected with hirsutism and oligomenorrhea/amenorrhea. Osteoporosis can occur as can glucose intolerance. For diagnosis a patient should be screened with one of the following: 24-hour urine free cortisol x3, low dose (1 mg) dexamethasone suppression test, midnight serum or salivary cortisol. Once Cushing syndrome is established, determine the cause using an ACTH and simultaneous cortisol measurement (elevated = adrenal adenoma or carcinoma) or a high-dose (8 mg overnight, or 2-day) dexamethasone suppression test (differentiates between pituitary cause and ectopic ACTH cause). Patients should be weaned off prednisone if possible. Removal of a pituitary adenoma can decrease ACTH production. Removal of an adrenal adenoma or other ectopic source of hormone secretion can decrease cortisol levels. Complications include hypertension, CV disease, DM, osteoporosis, risk of adrenal crisis, and psychosis.

Endocrine Pharmacology

ORAL HYPOGLYCEMIC AGENTS

Oral hypoglycemic agents are **anti-diabetic treatments** generally used in the treatment of Type II Diabetes. There are five classic categories of oral hypoglycemic agents: sulfonylureas, biguanides, meglitinides, competitive inhibitors of alpha-glucosidases (located in the intestinal brush border), and thiazolidinediones. More recently, two additional novel classes of oral hypoglycemics, DPP-4 inhibitors and SGLT2 inhibitors, were introduced with proven effectiveness when used in conjunction with changes in diet and exercise. Some examples of sulfonylurea oral hypoglycemic agents include the first-generation agents tolbutamide, tolazamide, chlorpropamide, and acetohexamide; and second-generation agents glyburide, glimepiride, and glipizide. The biguanide oral hypoglycemic agent is metformin. Metformin has the distinct advantage of not causing weight gain or hypoglycemic reactions. The meglitinide agent is repaglinide. Examples of alpha-glucosidase inhibitors are acarbose and miglitol. Alpha-glucosidase inhibitors bind tightly to intestinal alpha-glucosidases and decrease the postprandial rise in glucose levels. The only available thiazolidinedione oral hypoglycemic agent is currently pioglitazone; troglitazone was removed from US market in 2000, and rosiglitazone was removed from US market in 2011. Examples of DPP-4 inhibitors include linagliptin, vildagliptin, sitagliptin, and saxagliptin. Examples of SGLT2 inhibitors include canagliflozin, dapagliflozin, and empagliflozin.

INSULIN USED TO TREAT GLYCEMIC DISORDERS

There are a number of different types of **insulin** with varying action times. Insulin is used to metabolize **glucose** for those whose pancreas does not produce insulin. People may need to take a combination of insulins (short- and long-acting) to maintain glucose control. Duration of action may vary according to the individual's metabolism, intake, and level of activity:

- **Humalog** (Lispro H) is a fast-acting, short-acting insulin with onset in 5–15 minutes, peaking at 45–90 minutes and lasting 3–4 hours.
- **Regular** (R) is a relatively fast-acting insulin with onset in 30 minutes, peaks in 2–5 hours, and lasts 5–8 hours.
- **NPH** (N) insulin is intermediate-acting with onset in 1–3 hours, peaking at 6–12 hours, and lasting for 16–24 hours.
- **Insulin Glargine** (Lantus) is a long-acting insulin with onset in 3–6 hours, no peak, and lasting for 24 hours.
- **Combined NPH/Regular** (70/30 or 50/50) has an onset of 30 minutes, peaks at 7–12 hours, and lasts 16–24 hours.

Immunologic Pathophysiology

IMMUNE DEFICIENCIES

There are multiple disorders that fall into the category of **primary immunodeficiency diseases.** These disorders are genetic or inherited disorders in which the body's immune system does not function properly. These disorders may involve low levels of antibodies, defects in the antibodies, or defects in cells that make up the immune system (T-cells, B-cells). Common variable immune deficiency is a common immune deficiency diagnosed in adulthood. This disorder is characterized by low levels of serum immunoglobins and antibodies, which substantially increases the risk of infection.

- **Signs and symptoms**: Recurrent infections are the hallmark sign of immune deficiency disorders. Recurrent infections most often involve the ears, sinuses, bronchi, and lungs. Lymphadenopathy may occur as well as splenomegaly. GI symptoms may include abdominal pain, nausea, vomiting, diarrhea, and weight loss. Some patients may experience polyarthritis. Granulomas are also common and may occur in the lungs, lymph nodes, liver, and skin.
- **Diagnosis**: A physical assessment and patient history are used to diagnose immune deficiency disorders. Since immune deficiency disorders are genetic or inherited, family history should also be evaluated. Lab tests such as serum antibodies, serum immunoglobin levels and a complete blood count may also be used to assist in the diagnosis of immune deficiency disorders.
- **Treatment**: Patients with immune deficiency disorders often receive immunoglobulin replacement. Long term antibiotics may also be administered for recurrent infections. Educate patients to frequently wash hands, cook foods thoroughly, avoid large crowds, and other infection prevention techniques.

CONGENITAL IMMUNODEFICIENCIES

Congenital immunodeficiencies include:

- **Common variable immunodeficiency** is primarily an IgG deficiency due to absent plasma cells and B cell differentiation. These patients have increased susceptibility to encapsulated organisms and are more likely to develop bronchiectasis from the recurrent damage. They are also at higher risk for B cell neoplasms, GI malignancy, and autoimmune disease. Test is with functional antibody response and treatment with IVIG.
- **Congenital Agammaglobulinemia** (Bruton's, x-linked) usually leads to a susceptibility to recurrent pyogenic infections and low IgG and no IgA, IgM, IgE, IgD, or B cells.
- **Selective IgA deficiency** is the most common Ig deficiency and leads to recurrent sinopulmonary infections. It has association with recurrent giardiasis, GI malignancy, and autoimmune disorders, including celiac sprue. One should withhold IVIG due to possible anaphylactic reaction to IgA.
- **Wiskott-Aldrich syndrome** is the combination of thrombocytopenia, eczema, and immunodeficiency. It has associated low IgM and elevated IgA and IgE. BMT treats this successfully.

COMPLEMENT DEFICIENCIES

There are deficiencies of all parts of the complement pathway, including the following:

- **Classical deficiency** may include C1 (q, r, s), C2, and C4. This leads to immune complex syndromes and pyogenic infection, such as recurrent sinopulmonary infections with encapsulated bacteria. There is an association with SLE and other rheumatoid diseases. C2 is the most common deficiency in Caucasians in the US.
- **C3 and alternative complement deficiency** may lead to immune complex syndromes and recurrent infections, such as severe pyogenic infections. It may also be associated with HUS.
- **Membrane attack complex (MAC) deficiency** is also known as terminal complement deficiency. This is associated with recurrent Neisseria infections (which can cause meningitis and sepsis) and immune complex diseases. The CH50 assay must be checked to determine the activity of the classical pathway. CH50 may also be used to follow disease activity in SLE.

Autoimmune System Disorders

Allergic interstitial/tubulointerstitial nephritis is inflammation and edema of the interstitial areas of the kidneys. Up to 92% of cases caused by allergic reaction to medications, such as antibiotics (B-lactams, fluoroquinolones, macrolides, and anti-tuberculin drugs), antivirals, NSAIDs, PPIs, antiepileptics, diuretics, chemotherapy, and allopurinol. **Symptoms** include fever, rash, and renal enlargement as well as fatigue, nausea, vomiting, and weight loss. **Diagnosis** is by renal biopsy. Urine tests may show eosinophils, blood, RBC casts and sterile pyuria. Increased protein may be seen in response to NSAIDs. **Treatment** is primarily supportive but requires stopping the triggering medication.

Eosinophilic esophagitis is the accumulation of eosinophils in the esophagus, resulting in chronic inflammation. Damage from proteins produced in esophageal tissue causes scarring and narrowing, resulting in dysphagia, vomiting, choking, GERD, upper abdominal pain, heartburn, and regurgitation. **Causes** include allergic reaction to pollens or foods. **Risk factors** include cold/dry climate, male gender, family history, allergies, and asthma. **Diagnosis** is per endoscopy with biopsy. Blood tests may help confirm allergic reactions. **Treatment** may include dietary limitations, PPIs, and topical steroids. Some may require dilation of the esophagus.

Churg-Strauss syndrome (AKA **eosinophilic granulomatosis with polyangiitis**) is an idiopathic form of pulmonary vasculitis that can affect multiple systems (skin and lungs most often) as well as affecting small- and medium-sized arteries in those with asthma. **Symptoms** include dyspnea, chest pain, skin rash, myopathy, arthropathy, rhinitis, sinusitis, abdominal pain, blood in stools, and paresthesia (from the involvement of nerves). The syndrome is characterized by eosinophilia >1500 cells/mcL or >10% of peripheral total WBC count. X-rays or CTs may show transient opacities or multiple nodules. Tissue biopsies typically show allergic granulomas. **Treatment** usually begins with corticosteroids but other immunosuppressive drugs (cyclophosphamide, methotrexate, azathioprine) may be used, especially if critical organs are involved. The goal of treatment is remission, but patients usually need to take drugs at least 2 years before they are tapered off of the drugs. Up to 50% of patients have relapses.

Neutropenia

Neutropenia is identified as a **polymorphonuclear neutrophil count** equal to or less than 500/mL. **Chronic neutropenia** is a sustained condition of minimal neutrophils lasting 3 or more months. Neutropenia may occur from a decreased production of **white blood cells** (e.g., from chemotherapy or radiation therapy). It may also occur from a loss of white blood cells from autoimmune disease processes. Neutropenia is silent but dangerous. It leaves essentially no neutrophils to fight any threat of infection. Neutrophils make up as much as 70% of the white blood cells circulating in the blood. Neutropenia can be the cause of a septic situation, which can be life-threatening. Up to 70% of patients experiencing a fever while in a neutropenic state will die within 48 hours if not treated aggressively.

Leukopenia

Leukopenia is defined as a decrease in white blood cells. Neutropenia is defined as a low number of neutrophils and is often used interchangeably with the term leukopenia. With a decrease in the number of circulating white blood cells, the patient is at an increased risk for the development of an infection. Leukopenia and neutropenia can occur from either a decrease in the production of white blood cells or an increase in their destruction. Infections, malignancy, autoimmune disorders, medications (including chemotherapy) and a history of radiation therapy may contribute to the development of leukopenia/neutropenia.

Signs and symptoms: Malaise, fever, chills, night sweats, shortness of breath, headache, cough, abdominal pain, tachycardia, and hypotension. A patient with neutropenia/leukopenia is at risk for the development of infections including pneumonia, skin infections, urinary tract infections and gastrointestinal infections. In addition, the patient is at an increased risk for sepsis.

Diagnosis: Complete blood count including an absolute neutrophil count. In addition, a bone marrow biopsy may be performed to determine the cause of the decrease in neutrophils.

Treatment: Supportive therapy is used in the treatment of leukopenia including the aggressive treatment of infections that may develop. Precautions should be taken to protect the patient from additional infections, including strict adherence to sterile technique and infection control procedures. Hematopoietic growth factors may also be given to stimulate the production of neutrophils.

LYMPHEDEMA

Lymphedema results from untreated or incurable **edema**. It is a chronic condition marked by swelling and accumulated fluids within the tissue. This accumulation is a result of lymphatic drainage failure, inadequate lymph transport capacity, an increased lymph production, or a combination of these. Primary disease is a result of **inadequately developed lymphatic pathways**, while the secondary disease process is due to **damage outside of the pathways**. The process is worsened and complicated as **macrophages** are released to control inflammation caused by the increased release of fibroblasts and keratinocytes. There is a gradual increase in adipose tissue and leakage of lymph through the skin. The skin and tissues gradually thicken and change in color, texture, tone, and temperature. It begins to blister and produce hyperkeratosis, warts, papillomatosis, and elephantiasis. There is an ever-increasing risk of infection and further complications.

HIV/AIDS

AIDS is a progression of infection with **human immunodeficiency virus** (HIV). AIDS is diagnosed when the following criteria are met:

- HIV infection
- CD4 count less than 200 cells/mm^3
- AIDS defining condition, such as opportunistic infections (cytomegalovirus, tuberculosis), wasting syndrome, neoplasms (Kaposi sarcoma), or AIDS dementia complex

Because there is such a wide range of AIDS defining conditions, the patient may present with many types of **symptoms**, depending upon the diagnosis, but more than half of AIDS patients exhibit:

- Fever
- Lymphadenopathy
- Pharyngitis
- Rash
- Myalgia/arthralgia
- It is important to review the following:
  - CD4 counts to determine immune status
  - WBC and differential for signs of infection
  - Cultures to help identify any infective agents
  - CBC to evaluate for signs of bleeding or thrombocytopenia

Treatment aims to cure or manage opportunistic conditions and control underlying HIV infection through highly active anti-retroviral therapy (HAART), 3 or more drugs used concurrently.

Immunologic Pharmacology

IMMUNOSUPPRESSANT DRUGS

Drugs	Actions	Side effects
Corticosteroids	Depress cell-mediated immune response, humoral immune response, and inflammation, reducing proliferation of T cells and B cells. Used with transplantations and to prevent GVHD disease.	Weight gain, edema, Cushing syndrome, hyperglycemia, bruising, and osteoporosis. Abruptly stopping drugs may trigger Addisonian crisis.
Ciclosporin	Inhibit activation of T cells. Used to prevent transplantation rejection and to treat autoimmune diseases and nephrotic syndrome.	Tremor, excessive facial hair, gingivitis, bone marrow suppression with increased risk of infection and cancer, especially skin cancer.
Intravenous immuno-globulin G (IVIG)	Used to combat immunosuppression by increasing antibodies to prevent infection or treat acute infection, such as Guillain-Barre. Used off-label for many different disorders and infections.	Dermatitis, headache, renal failure, and venous thrombosis. Infections can occur because IVIG is extracted from pooled plasma.

> **Review Video: <u>Immunomodulators and Immunosuppressors</u>**
> Visit mometrix.com/academy and enter code: 666131

CHEMOTHERAPY

Chemotherapy may be offered during palliative care to enhance patient comfort, wellbeing, and symptom control for **enhanced quality of life**. It is understood that the treatment is not expected to provide a cure and should not be given as a means to maintain a sense of false hope within the patient or family. It should be clear that the expectation of treatment is **prolonged survival** and **control of cancer-related symptoms**. Not all patients will benefit from palliative chemotherapy. The decision to provide chemotherapy is based on the clinical indicators and the patient's wishes. The benefit and cost ratios of treatment need to be considered. Tumor response to treatment, metastasis, and other disease specific factors will help define chemotherapy's usefulness for an individual patient. Patients also need to be aware that chemotherapy involves a commitment to repeated travel, hospitalizations, invasive procedures, and assessments in order to make an informed decision.

CHEMOTHERAPEUTIC AGENTS

The major chemotherapy agents are alkylating agents, antimetabolites, plant alkaloids, antitumor antibiotics, and steroid hormones.

- **Alkylating agents** work directly by attacking the DNA of cancers such as chronic leukemias, Hodgkin's disease, lymphomas, and lung, breast, prostate, and ovary cancers.
- **Nitrosoureas** inhibit repair in damaged DNA. They are able to cross the blood-brain barrier and are frequently used to treat brain tumors, lymphomas, multiple myeloma, and malignant melanoma.
- **Antimetabolites** block cell growth. This class of chemotherapeutic drugs is used to treat leukemias, choriocarcinoma, and gastrointestinal, breast, and ovary cancers.
- **Antitumor antibiotics** are a broad category of agents that bind to DNA and prevent RNA synthesis and are used with a wide variety of cancers.

163

- **Plant (vinca) alkaloids** are extracted from plants and block cell division. These are used to treat acute lymphoblastic leukemia, Hodgkin and non-Hodgkin lymphomas, neuroblastomas, Wilms tumor, and lung, breast, and testes cancers.
- **Steroid hormones** have an unclear action but may be useful in treating hormone-dependent cancers such as ovary and breast cancer.

ROUTES OF DELIVERY

Chemotherapy treatments may be provided orally, intramuscularly, intravenously, intra-arterially, intralesionally (directly into the tumor), intraperitoneally, intrathecally, or topically. **Oral chemotherapy** is the easiest and often used in the home. **Intravenous delivery** is the most common chemotherapy route but **intramuscular delivery** may have more lasting effects. The goal of **intra-arterial chemotherapy** is to introduce the agent directly into the blood supply feeding the tumor or affected organ. Ovarian cancer with tumors greater than 2 cm in diameter may be treated with **intraperitoneal therapy**. Acute lymphocytic leukemia is primarily treated with **intrathecal administration**. **Intralesional treatments** are used for melanoma and Kaposi sarcoma. **Topical treatment** is most common with skin cancers.

SIDE EFFECTS

Not every patient will experience every symptom, or in the same degree. **Side effects** can vary greatly; some can be easily controlled with additional medications. Many side effects are due to the effects of the chemotherapy on **cells**, such as bone marrow, hair, and gastrointestinal cells, which have a rapid mitotic rate and rapid turnover. Common side effects can include bone marrow suppression, hair loss (alopecia), mouth ulcers, sore throat and gums, heartburn, nausea, vomiting, loss of appetite, weight loss, anorexia and cachexia, anemia, nerve and muscle problems, dry or discolored skin, kidney and bladder irritation, fatigue, and increased bruising, bleeding, and infection. The patient's sexual function can also be affected, including possible infertility.

RISKS

Infection is a common concern of chemotherapy because of the decreased number of **neutrophils** in the patient's system. **Neutropenia** is silent but dangerous, leaving no neutrophils to fight the threat of infections. Neutropenia can cause a septic situation, which can be life-threatening. Severe **anemia** may result in the need for blood transfusions. **Neurological damage** may include mild alterations in taste or smell, peripheral neuropathy, mental status changes, or seizures. Some anticancer drugs can cause **heart damage** if not monitored closely. Many anticancer drugs cause **kidney damage**, as well as increasing the risk of drug toxicity from decreased renal function. Anticancer drugs can also cause **cataracts** and **retina damage**.

PALLIATIVE SEDATION

Palliative sedation is a treatment method focused on controlling and easing symptoms that have proven otherwise refractory or unendurable in nature. This process was originally named **terminal sedation**. It was changed to palliative sedation to emphasize the differences between symptom management and euthanasia. The purpose of palliative sedation is **symptom control**; it does not hasten or cause death. Through the monitored use of medications such as midazolam or propofol, relief can be provided through varying levels of unconsciousness. Among terminally ill patients, palliative sedation is most often used to calm persistent agitation and restlessness. The second most frequent need is for pain control, followed by confusion, shortness of breath, muscle twitching or seizures, and anguish.

Hematologic Pathophysiology

ANEMIA

Anemia occurs when there is an insufficient number of red blood cells to sufficiently oxygenate the body. As a result of the decreased level of oxygen being supplied to the organs, the body will attempt to compensate by increasing cardiac output and redistributing blood to the brain and heart. In return, the blood supply to the skin, abdominal organs, and kidneys is decreased. Anemia can occur from blood loss, increased destruction of red blood cells (hemolytic anemia), or as a result of a decreased production in red blood cells.

Signs and symptoms: Pallor, fatigue, hypotension, weakness, and mental status changes. As perfusion decreases and the body attempts to compensate for the lack of oxygenation, tachycardia, chest pain, and shortness of breath may occur. In hemolytic anemias, jaundice and splenomegaly may occur as the result of the breakdown of red blood cells and the excretion of bilirubin.

Diagnosis: A complete blood count, reticulocyte count, and iron studies may be used to diagnose anemia.

Treatment: The treatment of anemia is focused on treating the underlying cause. Parenteral iron may be given for patients with iron deficiency anemias caused from chronic blood loss, or inadequate iron intake or absorption. Blood transfusions are used to treat patients with active bleeding as well as those patients who are displaying significant clinical symptoms. Erythropoietin stimulating proteins may also be utilized to decrease the need for a transfusion.

SICKLE CELL DISEASE

Sickle cell disease is a recessive genetic disorder of chromosome 11, causing hemoglobin to be defective so that red blood cells (RBCs) are sickle-shaped and inflexible, resulting in their accumulating in small vessels and causing painful blockage. While normal RBCs survive 120 days, sickled cells may survive only 10-20 days, stressing the bone marrow that cannot produce fast enough and resulting in severe anemia. There are 5 variations of sickle cell disease, with sickle cell anemia the most severe. Different types of crises occur (aplastic, hemolytic, vaso-occlusive, and sequestrating), which can cause infarctions in organs, severe pain, damage to organs, and rapid enlargement of liver and spleen. Complications include anemia, acute chest syndrome, congestive heart failure, strokes, delayed growth, infections, pulmonary hypertension, liver and kidney disorders, retinopathy, seizures, and osteonecrosis. Sickle cell disease occurs almost exclusively in African Americans in the United States, with 8-10% carriers.

> **Review Video: What is Sickle Cell Disease?**
> Visit mometrix.com/academy and enter code: 603869

TREATMENT

Treatment for sickle cell disease includes:

- **Prophylactic penicillin** for children from 2 months to 5 years to prevent pneumonia
- **IV fluids** to prevent dehydration
- **Analgesics** (morphine) during painful crises
- **Folic acid** for anemia
- **Oxygen** for congestive heart failure or pulmonary disease
- **Blood transfusions** with chelation therapy to remove excess iron OR erythropheresis, in which red cells are removed and replaced with healthy cells, either autologous or from a donor
- **Hematopoietic stem cells transplantation** is the only curative treatment, but immunosuppressive drugs must be used and success rates are only about 85%, so the procedure is only used on those at high risk. It requires ablation of bone marrow, placing the patient at increased risk.
- **Partial chimerism** uses a mixture of the donor and the recipient's bone marrow stem cells and does not require ablation of bone marrow. It is showing good success.

POLYCYTHEMIA VERA

Polycythemia vera is a condition in which there is abnormal production of blood cells in the bone marrow. Erythrocytes (red blood cells) are primarily affected. The disease is more common in men older than 40 years. Polycythemia may be primary or secondary, related to conditions causing hypoxia. The blood increases in viscosity, resulting in a number of **symptoms**:

- Dizziness, headache, weakness, and fatigue
- Dyspnea, especially when supine
- Flushing of skin, blue-tinged skin discoloration, and red lesions
- Itching after warm bath
- Left upper abdominal fullness and splenomegaly
- Phlebitis from blood clots
- Vision disturbances
- Complications include stroke, hemorrhage, and heart failure

Diagnosis includes CBC with differential, chemistry panel, bone marrow biopsy, and Vitamin B_{12} level. Red cell mass will be more than 25% above normal.

Treatment includes:

- **Phlebotomy** to remove 500 mL (lesser amounts for children) of blood to decrease blood viscosity, repeated weekly until hematocrit stable (less than 45%)
- Referral for **chemotherapy** (hydroxyurea) to suppress marrow production
- **Interferon** to decrease need for phlebotomy

VON WILLEBRAND DISEASE

Von Willebrand disease is a group of congenital bleeding disorders (inherited from either parent) affecting 1-2% of the population, associated with deficiency or lack of von Willebrand factor (vWF), a glycoprotein that is synthesized, stored, and secreted by vascular endothelial cells. This protein interacts with thrombocytes to create a clot and prevent hemorrhage; however, with von Willebrand disease, this clotting mechanism is impaired. There are three types:

- **Type I**: Low levels of vWF and also sometimes factor VIII (dominant inheritance)
- **Type II**: Abnormal vWF (subtypes a, b) may increase or decrease clotting (dominant inheritance)
- **Type III**: Absence of vWF and less than 10% factor VIII (recessive inheritance)

Symptoms vary in severity and include bruising, menorrhagia, recurrent epistaxis, and hemorrhage.

Treatment includes:

- **Desmopressin acetate** parenterally or nasally to stimulate production of clotting factor (mild cases)
- **Severe bleeding**: factor VIII concentrates with vWF, such as Humate-P

HEMOPHILIA

Hemophilia is an inherited disorder in which the person lacks adequate clotting factors. There are three types:

- **Type A**: lack of clotting factor VIII (90% of cases)
- **Type B**: lack of clotting factor IX
- **Type C**: lack of clotting factor XI (affects both sexes, rarely occurs in the United States)

Both Type A and B are usually X-linked disorders, affecting only males. The severity of the disease depends on the amount of clotting factor in the blood.

Symptoms:

- Bleeding with severe trauma or stress (mild cases)
- Unexplained bruises, bleeding, swelling, joint pain
- Spontaneous hemorrhage (severe cases), often in the joints but can be anywhere in the body
- Epistaxis, mucosal bleeding
- First symptoms often occur during infancy when the child becomes active, resulting in frequent bruises

Treatment:

- Desmopressin acetate parenterally or nasally to stimulate production of clotting factor (mild cases)
- Infusions of clotting factor from donated blood or recombinant clotting factors (genetically engineered), utilizing guidelines for dosing
- Infusions of plasma (Type C)

DISSEMINATED INTRAVASCULAR COAGULATION

PATHOLOGY

Disseminated intravascular coagulation (DIC) (consumption coagulopathy) is a secondary disorder that is triggered by another disorder such as trauma, congenital heart disease, necrotizing enterocolitis, sepsis, and severe viral infections. DIC triggers both coagulation and hemorrhage through a complex series of events. Trauma causes tissue factor (transmembrane glycoprotein) to enter the circulation and bind with coagulation factors, triggering the coagulation cascade. This stimulates thrombin to convert fibrinogen to fibrin, causing aggregation and destruction of platelets and forming clots that can be disseminated throughout the intravascular system. These clots increase in size as platelets adhere to the clots, causing blockage of both the microvascular systems and larger vessels, which can result in ischemia and necrosis. Clot formation triggers fibrinolysis and plasmin to breakdown fibrin and fibrinogen, causing the destruction of clotting factors and resulting in hemorrhage. Both processes, clotting and hemorrhage, continue at the same time, placing the patient at high risk for death, even with treatment.

SYMPTOMS AND TREATMENT

The onset of symptoms of DIC may be very rapid or be a slower chronic progression from a disease. Those who develop the chronic manifestation of the disease usually have fewer acute symptoms and may slowly develop ecchymosis or bleeding wounds.

Symptoms include:

- Bleeding from surgical or venous puncture sites
- Evidence of GI bleeding with distention, bloody diarrhea
- Hypotension and acute symptoms of shock
- Petechiae and purpura with extensive bleeding into the tissues
- Laboratory abnormalities:
    - Prolonged prothrombin and partial prothrombin times
    - Decreased platelet counts and fragmented RBCs
    - Decreased fibrinogen

Treatment includes:

- Identifying and treating underlying cause
- Massive blood transfusion protocol; replacement of blood products, such as platelets and fresh frozen plasma
- Anticoagulation therapy (heparin) to increase clotting time
- Cryoprecipitate to increase fibrinogen levels
- Coagulation inhibitors and coagulation factors

THROMBOCYTOPENIA

Thrombocytopenia is a deficiency of circulating platelets in the blood. It can be caused by a decrease in the production of platelets from the bone marrow or an increase in destruction of platelets. Thrombocytopenia may also be caused from the use of heparin. Heparin induced thrombocytopenia can occur after heparin therapy (average 4-14 days post therapy) and is characterized by a decrease in platelet count to less than 50% of baseline or the occurrence of an unexplained thrombolytic event. A decreased production of platelets within the bone marrow can occur as a result of malignancy, bone marrow failure, infection, alcohol abuse, or a nutritional deficiency. An increase in the destruction of platelets may occur in disseminated intravascular coagulation, vasculitis, thrombotic thrombocytopenic purpura, sepsis, or idiopathic thrombocytopenic purpura.

Signs and symptoms: Signs and symptoms may include petechiae, ecchymosis, bleeding from the mouth or gums, epistaxis, pallor, weakness, fatigue, splenomegaly, blood in the urine or stool, and jaundice.

Diagnosis: Physical exam and lab studies including complete blood count, partial thromboplastin time and prothrombin time may be used to diagnosis thrombocytopenia. A bone marrow biopsy may be indicated to determine the cause of the decreased production of platelets.

Treatment: Treatment of thrombocytopenia involves identifying and treating the underlying cause. Medications that decrease the platelet count should be held. Platelet transfusions may be administered to patients with extremely low counts (less than 50,000) or if spontaneous bleeding occurs. Platelet transfusions are contraindicated in patients with thrombotic thrombocytopenia purpura.

ITP

The autoimmune disorder **idiopathic thrombocytopenic purpura (ITP)** causes an immune response to platelets, resulting in decreased platelet counts. ITP affects primarily children and young women although it can occur at any age. The acute form primarily occurs in children, but the chronic form affects primarily adults. Platelet counts are usually 150,000–400,000 per mcL. With ITP, platelet levels are less than 100,000. Maintaining a platelet count of at least 30,000 is necessary to prevent intracranial hemorrhage, the primary concern. The cause of ITP is unclear and may be precipitated by viral infection, sulfa drugs, and conditions, such as lupus erythematosus. ITP is usually not life threatening and can be controlled. **Symptoms** include:

- Bruising and petechiae with hematoma in some cases
- Epistaxis
- Increased menstrual flow in post-puberty females

Treatment includes:

- Corticosteroids to depress immune response and increase platelet count
- Splenectomy may be indicated for chronic conditions
- Platelet transfusions
- Avoiding aspirin, ibuprofen, or other NSAIDs

HITTS

Heparin-induced thrombocytopenia and thrombosis syndrome (HITTS) occurs in patients receiving heparin for anticoagulation. There are two types:

- **Type I** is a transient condition occurring within a few days and causing depletion of platelets ($<100,000$ mm^3), but heparin may be continued as the condition usually resolves without intervention.
- **Type II** is an autoimmune reaction to heparin that occurs in 3–5% of those receiving unfractionated heparin and also occurs with low-molecular-weight heparin. It is characterized by low platelets ($<50,000$ mm^3) that are $\geq 50\%$ below baseline. Onset is 5–14 days but can occur within hours of heparinization. Death rates are $<30\%$. Heparin-antibody complexes form and release platelet factor 4 (PF4), which attracts heparin molecules and adheres to platelets and endothelial lining, stimulating thrombin and platelet clumping. This puts the patient at risk for thrombosis and vessel occlusion rather than hemorrhage, causing stroke, myocardial infarction, and limb ischemia with symptoms associated with the site of thrombosis. Treatment includes:
  - Discontinuation of heparin
  - Direct thrombin inhibitors (lepirudin, argatroban)
  - Monitor for signs/symptoms of thrombus/embolus

Hematological Procedures and Interventions

TRANSFUSION COMPONENTS

Blood components that are commonly used for transfusions include:

- **Packed red blood cells:** RBCs (250-300 mL per unit) should be warmed >30 °C (optimal 37 °C) before administration to prevent hypothermia and may be reconstituted in 50-100 mL of normal saline to facilitate administration. RBCs are necessary if blood loss is about 30% (1,500-2,000 mL lost; Hgb ≤7). Above 30% blood loss, whole blood may be more effective. RBCs are most frequently used for transfusions.
- **Platelet concentrates:** Transfusions of platelets are used if the platelet count is <50,000 cells/mm^3. One unit increases the platelet count by 5,000-10,000 cells/mm^3. Platelet concentrates pose a risk for sensitization reactions and infectious diseases. Platelet concentrate is stored at a higher temperature (20-24 °C) than RBCs. This contributes to bacterial growth, so it is more prone to bacterial contamination than other blood products and may cause sepsis. Temperature increase within 6 hours should be considered an indication of possible sepsis. ABO compatibility should be observed but is not required.
- **Fresh frozen plasma** (FFP) (obtained from a unit of whole blood frozen ≤6 hours after collection) includes all clotting factors and plasma proteins, so each unit administered increases clotting factors by 2-3%. FFP may be used for deficiencies of isolated factors, excess warfarin therapy, and liver-disease-related coagulopathy. It may be used for patients who have received extensive blood transfusions but continue to hemorrhage. It is also helpful for those with antithrombin III deficiency. FFP should be warmed to 37 °C prior to administration to avoid hypothermia. ABO compatibility should be observed if possible, but it is not required. Some patients may become sensitized to plasma proteins.
- **Cryoprecipitate** is the precipitate that forms when FFP is thawed. It contains fibrinogen, factor VIII, von Willebrand, and factor XIII. This component may be used to treat hemophilia A and hypofibrinogenemia.

TRANSFUSION ADMINISTRATION

Prior to the transfusion of any blood component, the nurse should obtain the patient's transfusion history along with a consent form. A type and crossmatch must be completed on the patient's blood and an IV in place for administration. An 18-gauge catheter is standard, but 22-gauge can also be used at a slower rate. Baseline vital signs need to be taken prior to starting the infusion, and then the patient should be under direct observation for at least the first 15 minutes. Vital signs should be monitored at 5 minutes, 15 minutes, and then at least every 30 minutes during the transfusion and one hour post-transfusion.

TRANSFUSION-RELATED COMPLICATIONS

There are a number of transfusion-related complications, which is the reason that transfusions are given only when necessary. Complications include:

- **Infection**: Bacterial contamination of blood, especially platelets, can result in severe sepsis. A number of infective agents (viral, bacterial, and parasitic) can be transmitted, although increased testing of blood has decreased rates of infection markedly. Infective agents include HIV, hepatitis C and B, human T-cell lymphotropic virus, CMV, WNV, malaria, Chagas' disease, and variant Creutzfeldt-Jacob disease (from contact with mad cow disease).
- **Transfusion-related acute lung injury (TRALI):** This respiratory distress syndrome occurs ≤6 hours after transfusion. The cause is believed to be antileukocytic or anti-HLA antibodies in the transfusion. It is characterized by non-cardiogenic pulmonary edema (high protein level) with severe dyspnea and arterial hypoxemia. Transfusion must be stopped immediately and the blood bank notified. TRALI may result in fatality but usually resolves in 12-48 hours with supportive care.

- **Graft vs. host disease:** Lymphocytes cause an immune response in immunocompromised individuals. Lymphocytes may be inactivated by irradiation, as leukocyte filters are not reliable.
- **Post-transfusion purpura:** Platelet antibodies develop and destroy the patient's platelets, so the platelet count decreases about 1 week after transfusion.
- **Transfusion-related immunosuppression:** Cell-mediated immunity is suppressed, so the patient is at increased risk of infection, and in cancer patients, transfusions may correlate with tumor recurrence. This condition relates to transfusions that include leukocytes. RBCs cause a less pronounced immunosuppression, suggesting a causative agent is in the plasma. Leukoreduction is becoming more common to reduce transmission of leukocyte-related viruses.
- **Hypothermia**: This may occur if blood products are not heated. Oxygen utilization is halved for each 10 °C decrease in normal body temperature.

AUTOTRANSFUSION

Autotransfusion (autologous blood transfusion) is collecting of the patient's blood and re-infusing it. This is life-saving if another donor's blood is not available. Blood in trauma cases is usually collected from a body cavity, such as pleural (hemothorax with ≥1,500 mL blood) or peritoneal space (rare). **Autotransfusion** is contraindicated if malignant lesions are present in the area of blood loss, contamination of pooled blood, or wounds more than 4-6 hours old. Commercial collection/transfusion kits (Pleur-Evac, Thora-Klex) are available, but blood can be collected through the chest tube into a sterile bottle, which is then disconnected and connected to IV tubing for infusion, or the blood in the bottle may be transferred to a blood collection bag for use. Commercial kits use either a chest tube or suction tube to withdraw blood and provide specific procedures. Blood is filtered. Heparin is not routinely used, but citrate phosphate dextrose (CPD) (25-70 mL per 500 mL blood) is often added to the aspirant to prevent clotting. Complications from autotransfusion are rare.

PLASMAPHERESIS

With plasmapheresis, whole blood is removed from the body, anticoagulant is added, cellular components are separated from the plasma (which is removed), and cellular components are suspended in saline, albumin (most common), or another substitute for plasma. This is reinfused into the patient. The purpose is to remove harmful antibodies found in plasma. ACE inhibitors increase risk of hypotension and should be withheld for 24 hours before the procedure. Machine settings may vary. Typically, the patient's height and weight are entered into the automated system to aid in calculating the plasma volume. The patient must be carefully monitored during the procedure for signs of hypocalcemia (perioral/fingertip tingling, alterations in mental status, VT), which requires the administration of calcium; hypomagnesemia (confusion, headaches, dizziness, twitching), which requires administration of magnesium; and hypotension, which requires saline bolus. If the patient shows indications of transfusion reaction, the infusion must be discontinued and medications (diphenhydramine, corticosteroids) administered. The patient should be kept warm to avoid hypothermia. Post-procedure, the patient may experience thrombocytopenia and hypofibrinogenemia, so the patient must be observed for signs of bleeding.

EXCHANGE TRANSFUSION

Exchange transfusions replace a person's blood with donor blood to remove sickled blood for sickle cell anemia or to remove toxins. The exchange may be complete or partial. An automated machine is generally used, and the time on the machine ranges from 1-4 hours. (If done manually, removal and replacement are done in cycles with blood first removed followed by replacement.) A catheter is inserted (usually in the arm) to drain the blood and another, usually in the femoral area (under local or moderate sedation), to administer donor blood, plasma, or another substitute for plasma. During the exchange, the patient's VS must be carefully monitored. If the patient exhibits signs of hypocalcemia (perioral/finger tingling) then calcium is administered. Some may receive calcium routinely during administration. Blood may be taken from the femoral line for testing after the exchange. When the femoral catheter is removed, pressure must be applied to the area for at least 5 minutes and the patient instructed to lie flat for at least 30 minutes to prevent bleeding.

LEUKOCYTE DEPLETION

Red blood cell and platelet transfusions typically contain some leukocytes, which are recognized as foreign by the immune system of a patient receiving the transfusion. This can lead to adverse reactions, especially in patients who are immunocompromised. **Leukocyte depletion** is carried out by various processes, including filtration. One disadvantage to leukodepletion of RBCs is that the process results in the loss of about 10% of the RBCs, and some hemolysis may occur. Leukocyte depleted RBCs are given in volumes of 200-250 mL within a 4-hour time period.

BLOOD CONSERVATION

Blood conservation includes methods to:

- **Minimize the loss of blood during surgical procedures**: May include regional anesthesia instead of general, positioning to reduce blood loss, cell salvage, autotransfusion, non-invasive monitoring (BP, pulse oximetry), limited blood draws, normovolemic hemodilution, and medications to reduce bleeding (vitamin K, tranexamic acid, desmopressin, somatostatin, vasopressin, recombinant factor VIIa).
- **Lower the threshold for receiving transfusions**: Transfusion threshold lowered from 10 g/dL to 7 g/dL.
- **Maintain the hematocrit at acceptable levels**: Administration of oral or parenteral iron therapy to increase tolerance for blood loss. Erythropoietin alpha may also be administered perioperatively to stimulate the production of RBCs.
- **Ensure optimal oxygenation of tissue**: Hyperoxic ventilation during surgery, crystalloid/colloid volume replacement, and utilizing techniques to minimize consumption of oxygen.

Blood conservation includes a commitment to bloodless surgery as much as possible, especially through the utilization of minimally-invasive procedures.

MASSIVE TRANSFUSION PROTOCOL

A massive transfusion protocol (MTP) is a proactive standardized protocol used during an uncontrolled hemorrhage, designed to ensure effective management of massive blood loss and to improve patient outcome.

Indications for activation of **massive transfusion protocol** (MTP) include:

- Uncontrolled hemorrhage.
- Actual/anticipated use of ≥4 units of RBCs in less than 4 hours or ≥10 units in 24 hours (some may need up to 30 units in 8 hours).
- Hemodynamic instability despite initial management of bleeding and resuscitation efforts that should include avoiding hypothermia and the use of excessive crystalloid.
- Allowing permissive hypotension to 80-100 systolic BP to help control bleeding. Autotransfusion may be used when appropriate.

Protocols may vary somewhat:

- MTPs are activated by a clinician in response to massive bleeding, generally after transfusion of 4-10 units.
- Obtain baseline laboratory tests (CBC, coagulation screen, blood gases, and chemistry panel) and repeat CBC, blood gases, coagulation screen, and ionized calcium test hourly.
- MTP packs have a predetermined ratio (e.g., 1:1:1 or 2:1:1 ratio) of RBCs, FFPs, and platelet units for transfusion, prepared by the blood bank for rapid and timely delivery.
- Targets of resuscitation include:
  - Mean arterial pressure (MAP) around 60 mmHg
  - Core temperature >35 °C

- o Hemoglobin 7–9 g/dL
- o pH 7.35–7.45
- o Lactate <4 mmol/L
- o Calcium >1.1 mmol/L
- o Platelets >50,000
- o PT/aPTT <1.5 times normal
- o INR ≤1.5
- o Fibrinogen >1.5–2.0 g/L

Hematologic Pharmacology

ANTICOAGULANTS

Common anticoagulants used at home and in the hospital setting are discussed below, including possible complications and the antidotes for each:

- **Antithrombin activators**: Heparin (unfractionated) and derivatives, LWM (Dalteparin, Enoxaparin, tinzaparin), and Fondaparinux.
  - Possible complications: Thrombocytopenia, bleeding/hemorrhage, osteopenia, hypersensitivity.
  - Antidote: Protamine sulfate 1% solution—dosage varies according to drug and drug's dosage. (1 mg protamine neutralizes 100 units of heparin or 1 mg of enoxaparin.)
- **Direct thrombin inhibitors**: Hirudin analogs (bivalirudin, desirudin, lepirudin). Others: Apixaban, Argatroban, and dabigatran.
  - Possible complications: Bleeding/hemorrhage, GI upset, backpain, hypertension, headache.
  - No antidote is available.
- **Direct Xa inhibitor**: Rivaroxaban
  - Possible complications: Bleeding/hemorrhage.
  - No antidote is available.
- **Antithrombin (AT)**: Recombinant human AT, Plasma-derived AT
  - Possible complications: Bleeding/hemorrhage, hypersensitivity.
  - No antidote is available.
- **Warfarin**
  - Possible complications: Bleeding/hemorrhage. Drug interactions may cause thrombosis or increased risk of bleeding.
  - Antidote: Vitamin K_1 usually at 2.5 mg PO or 0.5–1.0 mg IV. If ineffective, FFP or fresh whole blood may be administered.

HEPARIN
PHARMACOLOGY

Heparin is an **anticoagulant** derived from the intestinal mucosa of the pig and the lung of the pig. The mechanism of action of heparin is to bind to the surface of the endothelial cell membrane. The activity of heparin depends upon plasma protease inhibitor antithrombin III. Antithrombin III inhibits thrombin and other anti-clotting proteases. In addition, heparin binding causes a change in antithrombin III inhibitor form, resulting in increased antithrombin-protease complex formation activity. After antithrombin-protease complex formation, heparin is subsequently released and is available to bind to more antithrombin molecules.

RISK FACTORS

The major risk factor of heparin use is hemorrhage. Predisposing factors for hemorrhage include advanced age and renal failure. Prolonged use of heparin can result in osteoporosis and fractures. Other risk factors of heparin use include transient thrombocytopenia, severe thrombocytopenia, paradoxical thromboembolism, and heparin-induced aggregation of platelets. These risks can be reduced by careful selection of patients who receive heparin therapy, careful control of the dosage of heparin, and meticulous monitoring of the partial thromboplastin time, or PTT. It is important to remember that thrombocytopenia or the development of a thrombus may be due to heparin itself.

CONTRAINDICATIONS

There are numerous contraindications to the use of heparin, including: hypersensitivity to heparin; diseases of the hematologic system (hemophilia, purpura, or thrombocytopenia); uncontrolled hypertension; intracranial bleed; infectious endocarditis; active tuberculosis; gastrointestinal ulcers; cancer of the gastrointestinal visceral organs; severe liver dysfunction; severe kidney dysfunction; and threatened miscarriage or abortion. Heparin is contraindicated in the following medical procedures: following brain surgery; following spinal cord surgery; following eye surgery; after a lumbar puncture; and after regional anesthesia blocks. The effects of heparin may be reversed by stopping heparin or by the use of a specific antagonist (protamine sulfate).

> **Review Video: Heparin**
> Visit mometrix.com/academy and enter code: 127426

WARFARIN

PHARMACOLOGY

Warfarin causes a deficiency in prothrombin in the plasma and is used as an **anti-thrombotic agent** and to decrease the risk of embolism in humans. This agent causes the liver to manufacture less of the proteins necessary for blood coagulation. Since it is 99% bound to albumin in the plasma, warfarin has a high bio-availability. The mechanism of action of warfarin involves prothrombin, factor VII, factor IX, factor X, and protein C. Warfarin inhibits the g-carboxylation of the glutamate residues in the aforementioned factors. The mechanism of action of warfarin also involves vitamin K. Warfarin has a slow onset of action, usually 24 hours, and a typical duration of 2 to 5 days. Using increased dosages of warfarin as loading dosages will serve to speed up the onset of anti-coagulation. Patients on warfarin must discontinue this medication five days before planned surgery due to its longer duration.

DRUG-DRUG INTERACTIONS

Warfarin has many drug-drug interactions, the most serious of which increases the risk of bleeding. Sulfinpyrazone and phenylbutazone interact with warfarin to cause enhanced decrease in prothrombin, increased inhibition of platelets, and increased risk of peptic ulcer. The following drugs can have adverse effects when co-administered with warfarin: antibiotics such as metronidazole, azithromycin, clarithromycin, dirithromycin, erythromycin, roxithromycin, and telithromycin; broad-spectrum antibiotics such as amoxicillin, imipenem, levofloxacin; antifungal agents such as fluconazole, miconazole, and ketoconazole; barbiturates; and trimethoprim-sulfamethoxazole, amiodarone, cimetidine, and disulfiram. Aspirin inhibits metabolism of the warfarin and nonsteroidal anti-inflammatory drugs (NSAIDs) inhibit the clotting of platelets. The third-generation cephalosporins increase the risk of bleeding with warfarin because these drugs destroy the intestinal bacteria that produce vitamin K. Always check on possible drug-drug interactions when administering warfarin and monitor patients who might be at risk.

> **Review Video: Warfarin**
> Visit mometrix.com/academy and enter code: 844117

THROMBOLYTICS

Thrombolytics are drugs used to dissolve clots in myocardial infarction, ischemic stroke, DVT, and pulmonary embolism. **Thrombolytics** may be given in combination with heparin or low-weight heparin to increase anticoagulation effect. Thrombolytics should be administered within 90 minutes but may be given up to 6 hours after an event. They may increase the danger of hemorrhage and are contraindicated with hemorrhagic strokes, recent surgery, or bleeding. Thrombolytics include:

- **Alteplase tissue-type plasminogen activator** (t-PA) (Activase) is an enzyme that converts plasminogen to plasmin, which is a fibrinolytic enzyme. t-PA is used for ischemic stroke, MI, and pulmonary embolism and must be given IV within 3–4.5 hours or by catheter directly to the site of occlusion within 6 hours.
- **Anistreplase** (Eminase) is used for treatment of acute MI and is given intravenously in a 30-unit dose over 2–5 minutes.
- **Reteplase** (Retavase) is a plasminogen activator used after MI to prevent CHF (contraindicated for ischemic strokes). It is given in 2 doses, a 10-unit bolus over 2 minutes and then repeated in 30 minutes.

- **Streptokinase** (Streptase) is used for pulmonary emboli, acute MI, intracoronary thrombi, DVT, and arterial thromboembolism. It should be given within 4 hours but can be given after up to 24 hours. Intravenous infusion is usually 1,500,000 units in 60 minutes. Intracoronary infusion is done with an initial 20,000-unit bolus and then 2000 units per minute for 60 minutes.
- **Tenecteplase** (TNKase) is used to treat acute MI with large ST elevation. It is administered in a one-time bolus over 5 seconds and should be administered within 30 minutes of the event.

Contraindications to thrombolytic therapy include:

- Evidence of cerebral or subarachnoid hemorrhage or other internal bleeding or history of intracranial hemorrhage, recent stroke, head trauma, or surgery (ruled out by CT scan before administration for ischemic stroke)
- Uncontrolled hypertension, seizures
- Intracranial AVM, neoplasm, or aneurysm
- Current anticoagulation therapy
- Low platelet count (<100,000 mm³)

Neurological Pathophysiology

ENCEPHALOPATHIES

HYPERTENSIVE ENCEPHALOPATHY WITH CEREBRAL EDEMA

Hypertensive encephalopathy can occur as part of a hypertensive crisis. With chronic hypertension, the brain adapts to higher pressures to regulate blood flow, but in a hypertensive crisis, autoregulation of the blood-brain barrier is overwhelmed and the capillaries leak fluid into the tissue and vasodilation takes place with resultant cerebral edema. Damage to arterioles occurs, causing increasing neurological deficits and papilledema. Hypertensive encephalopathy is relatively rare, but carries a high mortality rate and is most common in middle-aged males with long-standing hypertension. **Symptoms** usually develop over 1-2 days and include:

- Non-specific neurological deficits, such as weakness and visual abnormalities
- Alterations in mental status, including confusion
- Headache, often constant
- Nausea and vomiting
- Seizures
- Coma

TREATMENT FOR HYPERTENSIVE ENCEPHALOPATHY WITH CEREBRAL EDEMA

Hypertensive encephalopathy with cerebral edema requires prompt treatment in order to prevent neurological damage.

Treatment includes identifying and treating the underlying causes for the hypertensive crisis and taking steps to lower the blood pressure:

- **Nitroprusside sodium (Nitropress)** is usually used initially to lower BP. However, caution must be used not to lower the blood pressure too quickly, as this can lead to cerebral ischemia.
- **Positioning** of the patient to prevent obstruction of venous return from the head
- **Monitoring blood gas** and maintaining $PaCO_2$ at 33-37 mmHg to facilitate vasoconstriction of cerebral arteries
- **Preventing hyperthermia** with antipyretics and cooling devices
- **BP monitoring** and maintenance
- **Seizure control** with phenobarbital and/or phenytoin
- **Lidocaine** through endotracheal tube or intravenously prior to nasotracheal suctioning
- **Diuretics**, such as osmotic agents (mannitol) and loop diuretics (furosemide) to control fluid volume
- **Controlling metabolic demand** by measures to increase pain control and reduce stimulation
- **Barbiturates** (pentobarbital, thiopental) in high doses may be used if other treatments fail to decrease intracranial pressure

HYPOXIC ENCEPHALOPATHY

Cerebral hypoxia (hypoxic encephalopathy) occurs when the oxygen supply to the brain is decreased. If hypoxia is mild, the brain compensates by increasing cerebral blood flow, but it can only double in volume and cannot compensate for severe hypoxic conditions. Hypoxia may be the result of insufficient oxygen in the environment, inadequate exchange at the alveolar level of the lungs, or inadequate circulation to the brain. Brain cells may begin dying within 5 minutes if deprived of adequate oxygenation, so any condition or trauma that interferes with oxygenation can result in brain damage:

- Near-drowning
- Asphyxia
- Cardiac arrest

- High altitude sickness
- Carbon monoxide
- Diseases that interfere with respiration, such as myasthenia gravis and amyotrophic lateral sclerosis
- Anesthesia complications

Symptoms include increasing neurological deficits, depending upon the degree and area of damage, with changes in mentation that range from confusion to coma. Prompt identification of the cause and increase in perfusion to the brain is critical for survival.

METABOLIC ENCEPHALOPATHY

Metabolic encephalopathy (hepatic encephalopathy) is damage to the brain resulting from a disturbance in metabolism, primarily hepatic failure to remove toxins from the blood. There may be impairment in cerebral blood flow, cerebral edema, or increased intracranial pressure. It can occur as the result of the ingestion of drugs or toxins which can have a direct toxic effect on neurons, but it can also occur with liver disease, especially when stressed by co-morbidities, such as hemorrhage, hypoxemia, surgery, trauma, renal failure with dialysis, or electrolyte imbalances.

Symptoms may vary:

- Irritability and agitation
- Alterations in consciousness
- Dysphonia
- Lack of coordination, spasticity
- Seizures are common and may be the presenting symptom
- Disorientation progressing to coma

Prompt diagnosis is important because the condition may be reversible if underlying causes are identified and treated before permanent neuronal damage occurs.

Treatment varies according to the underlying cause.

INFECTIOUS ENCEPHALOPATHY

Infectious encephalopathy is an encompassing term describing encephalopathies caused by a wide range of bacteria, viruses, or prions. Common to all infections are altered brain function that results in alterations in consciousness and personality, cognitive impairment, and lethargy. A wide range of neurological symptoms may occur: myoclonus, seizures, dysphagia, and dysphonia, neuromuscular impairment with muscle atrophy and tremors or spasticity. **Treatment** depends on the underlying cause and response to treatment. Prion infections are not treatable, but bacterial infections may respond to antibiotic therapy, and viral infections may be self-limiting. HIV-related encephalopathy results from opportunistic infections as immune responses decrease, usually indicated by CD4 counts <50. Aggressive antiretroviral treatment and treatment of the infection may reverse symptoms if permanent damage has not occurred for HIV-related encephalopathy. Treatment for other infectious encephalopathies varies according to the type of infection and underlying causes.

CEREBRAL ANEURYSMS

Cerebral aneurysms, the weakening and dilation of a cerebral artery, are usually congenital (90%) while the remaining (10%) result from direct trauma or infection. Aneurysms are usually 2-7 mm in size and occur in the

Circle of Willis at the base of the brain. A rupturing aneurysm may decrease perfusion as well as increasing pressure on surrounding brain tissue. Cerebral aneurysms are classified as follows:

- **Berry/saccular:** The most common congenital type occurs at a bifurcation and grows from the base on a stem, usually at the Circle of Willis.
- **Fusiform**: Large and irregular (>2.5 cm) and rarely ruptures but causes increased intracranial pressure. Usually involves the internal carotid or vertebrobasilar artery.
- **Mycotic**: Rare type that occurs secondary to bacterial infection and aseptic emboli.
- **Dissecting**: Wall is torn apart and blood enters layers. This may occur during angiography or secondary to trauma or disease.
- **Traumatic Charcot-Bouchard (pseudoaneurysm):** Small lesion resulting from chronic hypertension.

ARTERIOVENOUS MALFORMATION

Arteriovenous malformation (AVM) is a congenital abnormality within the brain consisting of a tangle of dilated arteries and veins without a capillary bed. AVMs can occur anywhere in the brain and may cause no significant problems. Usually the AVM is "fed" by one or more cerebral arteries, which enlarge over time, shunting more blood through the AVM. The veins also enlarge in response to increased arterial blood flow because of the lack of a capillary bridge between the two. Because vein walls are thinner and lack the muscle layer of an artery, the veins tend to rupture as the AVM becomes larger, causing a subarachnoid hemorrhage. Chronic ischemia that may be related to the AVM can result in cerebral atrophy. Sometimes small leaks, usually accompanied by headache and nausea and vomiting, may occur before rupture. AVMs may cause a wide range of neurological symptoms, including changes in mentation, dizziness, sensory abnormalities, confusion, increasing ICP, and dementia.

Treatment includes:

- Supportive management of symptoms
- Surgical repair or focused irradiation (definitive treatments)

INTRACRANIAL/INTRAVENTRICULAR HEMORRHAGE
EPIDURAL AND SUBDURAL

Epidural hemorrhage is bleeding between the dura and the skull that pushes the brain downward and inward. The hemorrhage is usually caused by arterial tears, so bleeding is often rapid, leading to severe neurological deficits and respiratory arrest.

Subdural hemorrhage is bleeding between the dura and the cerebrum, usually from tears in the cortical veins of the subdural space. It tends to develop more slowly than epidural hemorrhage and can result in a subdural hematoma. If the bleeding is acute and develops within minutes or hours of injury, the prognosis is poor. Subacute hematomas that develop more slowly cause varying degrees of injury. Subdural hemorrhage is a common injury related to trauma but it can also result from coagulopathies or aneurysms. Symptoms of acute injury may occur within 24-48 hours, but subacute bleeding may not be evident for up to 2 weeks after injury. Chronic hemorrhage occurs primarily in the elderly. Symptoms vary and may include bradycardia, tachycardia, hypertension, and alterations in consciousness. Older children and adults usually require surgical evacuation of the hematoma.

SUBARACHNOID

Subarachnoid hemorrhage (SAH) may occur after trauma but is a common result of rupture of a berry aneurysm or an arteriovenous malformation (AVM). However, there are a number of disorders that may be implicated: neoplasms, sickle cell disease, infection, hemophilia, and leukemia. The first presenting symptom may be complaints of severe headache, nausea and vomiting, nuchal rigidity, palsy related to cranial nerve compression, retinal hemorrhages, and papilledema. Late complications include hyponatremia and hydrocephalus. **Symptoms** worsen as intracranial pressure rises. SAH from aneurysm is classified as follows:

- **Grade I:** No symptoms or slight headache and nuchal rigidity
- **Grade II:** Moderate to severe headache with nuchal rigidity and cranial nerve palsy
- **Grade III:** Drowsy, progressing to confusion or mild focal deficits
- **Grade IV:** Stupor, with hemiparesis (moderate to severe), early decerebrate rigidity, and vegetative disturbances
- **Grade V:** Coma state with decerebrate rigidity

Treatment includes:

- Identifying and treating underlying cause
- Observing for re-bleeding
- Anti-seizure medications (such as levetiracetam or phenytoin) to control seizures
- Antihypertensives
- Surgical repair if indicated

HYDROCEPHALUS
COMMUNICATING AND NONCOMMUNICATING

The ventricular system produces and circulates cerebrospinal fluid (CSF). The right and left lateral ventricles open into the third ventricle at the interventricular foramen (foramen of Monro). The aqueduct of Sylvius connects the third and fourth ventricles. The fourth ventricle, anterior to the cerebellum, supplies CSF to the subarachnoid space and the spinal cord (dorsal surface). The CSF circulates and then returns to the brain and is absorbed in the arachnoid villi. **Hydrocephalus** occurs when there is an imbalance between production and absorption of cerebrospinal fluid in the ventricles, resulting from impaired absorption or obstruction, which may be congenital or acquired. There are two common types of hydrocephalus:

- **Communicating:** CSF flows (communicates) between the ventricles but is not absorbed in the subarachnoid space (arachnoid villi).
- **Noncommunicating:** CSF is obstructed (non-communicating) between the ventricles, with the obstruction most often due to stenosis of the aqueduct of Sylvius.

SYMPTOMS

Symptoms of hydrocephalus depend on the age of onset. In *early infancy*, before closure of cranial sutures, head enlargement is the most common presentation, but in adults with less elasticity in the skull, neurological symptoms usually relate to increasing pressure on structures of the brain. Hydrocephalus may occur at any age, but the type that occurs in *young/middle-aged adults* is different than that common in children or those >50. Hydrocephalus in young and middle-aged adults may result from a congenital defect, hydrocephalus of infancy with shunt failure, or trauma and is characterized by:

- Headache relieved by vomiting
- Papilledema
- Lack of bladder control
- Strabismus and other visual disorders
- Ataxia
- Irritability
- Lethargy
- Confusion and impairment of cognitive abilities

With **adult-onset normal pressure hydrocephalus** (>50) cerebrospinal fluid increases and dilates the ventricles, but frequently without increasing intracranial pressure. The cause is often unclear. Symptoms include gait disturbance, bladder control issues, and mild dementia

TREATMENT

Hydrocephalus is diagnosed through CT and MRI scans, which help to determine the cause. **Treatment** may vary somewhat depending upon the underlying disorder. For example, if obstruction is caused by a tumor, surgical excision to directly remove the obstruction is required. Generally, however, most hydrocephalus is treated with shunts:

- **Ventricular-peritoneal shunt:** This procedure is the most common and consists of placing a ventricular catheter directly into the ventricles (usually lateral) at one end with the other end in the peritoneal area to drain away excess CSF. There is a one-way valve near the proximal end that prevents backflow but opens when pressure rises to drain fluid. In some cases, the distal end drains into the right atrium.
- **Third ventriculostomy:** A small opening is made in the base of the third ventricle so CSF can bypass an obstruction. This procedure is not common and is done with a small endoscope.

NEUROLOGIC INFECTIOUS DISEASE
BACTERIAL MENINGITIS

Bacterial meningitis may be caused by a wide range of bacteria, including *Streptococcus pneumoniae* and *Neisseria meningitidis.* Bacteria can enter the CNS from distant infection, surgical wounds, invasive devices, nasal colonization, or penetrating trauma. The infective process includes inflammation, exudates, WBC accumulation, and brain tissue damage with hyperemia and edema. Purulent exudate covers the brain and invades and blocks the ventricles, obstructing CSF and leading to increased intracranial pressure. **Symptoms** include abrupt onset, fever, chills, severe headache, nuchal rigidity, and alterations of consciousness with seizures, agitation, and irritability. Antibodies specific to bacteria don't cross the blood brain barrier, so immune response is poor. Some may have photophobia, hallucinations, and/or aggressive behavior or may become stuporous and lapse into coma. Nuchal rigidity may progress to opisthotonos. Reflexes are variable but Kernig and Brudzinski signs are often positive. Signs may relate to particular bacteria, such as rashes, sore joints, or a draining ear. **Diagnosis** is usually based on lumbar puncture examination of cerebrospinal fluid and symptoms. **Treatment** includes IV antibiotics and supportive care: fluids, a dark and calm environment, measures to reduce ICP, etc.

FUNGAL MENINGITIS

Fungal meningitis is the least common cause of meningitis. It occurs when a fungal organism enters into the subarachnoid space, cerebral spinal fluid, and meninges. Immune deficient patients such as those with HIV, cancer, or immunodeficiency syndromes are most at risk for the development of fungal meningitis. The most common organisms causing fungal meningitis are candida albicans and Cryptococcus neoformans. Fungal meningitis caused by candida may occur in immunosuppressed patients, in those who have had a ventricular shunt placed, or in those that have had a lumbar puncture performed. Cryptococcus is a fungus found in soil throughout the world and does not usually affect people with a healthy immune system. Cryptococcal meningitis is most commonly seen in patients with HIV/AIDS and is one of the leading causes of death in HIV/AIDS patients in certain parts of Africa.

Signs and symptoms: Headache, fever, nausea and vomiting, stiff neck, photophobia, and mental status changes.

Diagnosis: Lumbar puncture with subsequent culture of cerebral spinal fluid. In addition, blood cultures may be obtained as well as a CT of the head.

Treatment: The treatment of fungal meningitis involves a long course of anti-fungal medications, including Amphotericin B, flucytosine, and fluconazole. Anticonvulsants may be administered for seizure control.

VIRAL INFECTIONS THAT CAN IMPACT THE NEUROLOGICAL SYSTEM

Many different types of viral infections can impact the neurological system either by direct infection transmitted through the bloodstream or by spreading along the nerve pathways (such as rabies). Common viral infections affecting the neurological system include:

- **Viral encephalitis**: Arboviral infections are transmitted from an animal host to an arthropod (typically a mosquito or tick) to humans, who are typically dead-end hosts. Arboviral infections include western equine encephalitis, eastern equine encephalitis, St. Louis encephalitis, Powassan encephalitis, Colorado tick fever and La Crosse encephalitis. West Nile virus may also invade the CNS and cause encephalitis.
- **Viral meningitis**: Viral meningitis is usually self-limiting within 7 to 10 days and is less severe than bacterial meningitis.
- **Herpes virus**: Herpes simplex virus can invade the nervous system and cause herpes simplex encephalitis, which has a high mortality rate.
- **HIV**: Inflammation may affect the CNS and interfere with neuronal functions.

NEUROMUSCULAR DISORDERS
MULTIPLE SCLEROSIS

Multiple sclerosis is an autoimmune disorder of the CNS in which the myelin sheath around the nerves is damaged and replaced by scar tissue that prevents conduction of nerve impulses.

Symptoms vary widely and can include problems with balance and coordination, tremors, slurring of speech, cognitive impairment, vision impairment, nystagmus, pain, and bladder and bowel dysfunction. Symptoms may be relapsing-remitting, progressive, or a combination. Onset is usually at 20-30 years of age, with incidence higher in females. Patient may initially present with problems walking or falling or optic neuritis (30%) causing loss of central vision. Males may complain of sexual dysfunction as an early symptom. Others have dysuria with urinary retention.

Diagnosis is based on clinical and neurological examination and MRI. **Treatment** is symptomatic and includes treatment to shorten duration of episodes and slow progress.

- **Glucocorticoids**: Methylprednisolone
- **Immunomodulator**: Interferon beta, glatiramer acetate, natalizumab
- **Immunosuppressant**: Mitoxantrone
- **Hormone**: Estriol (for females)

> **Review Video: Multiple Sclerosis**
> Visit mometrix.com/academy and enter code: 417355

ALS

Amyotrophic lateral sclerosis (ALS) is a progressive degenerative disease of the upper and lower motor neurons, resulting in progressively severe symptoms such as spasticity, hyperreflexia, muscle weakness, and paralysis that can cause dysphagia, cramping, muscular atrophy, and respiratory dysfunction. ALS may be sporadic or familial (rare). Speech may become monotone; however, cognitive functioning usually remains intact. Eventually, patients become immobile and cannot breathe independently.

Diagnosis is based on history, electromyography, nerve conduction studies, and MRI. Treatment includes riluzole to delay progression of the disease. Patients in the ED usually have been diagnosed and have developed an acute complication, such as acute respiratory failure, aspiration pneumonia, or other trauma.

Treatment includes:

- Nebulizer treatments with bronchodilators and steroids
- Antibiotics for infection
- Mechanical ventilation

If **ventilatory assistance** is needed, it is important to determine if the patient has a living will expressing the wish to be ventilated or not or has assigned power of attorney for health matters to someone to make this decision.

PARKINSON'S DISEASE

Parkinson's disease (PD) is an extrapyramidal movement motor system disorder caused by loss of brain cells that produce dopamine. Typical symptoms include tremor of face and extremities, rigidity, bradykinesia, akinesia, poor posture, and a lack of balance and coordination causing increasing problems with mobility, talking, and swallowing. Some may suffer depression and mood changes. Tremors usually present unilaterally in an upper extremity.

Diagnosis includes:

- **Cogwheel rigidity test**: The extremity is put through passive range of motion, which causes increased muscle tone and ratchet-like movements.
- **Physical and neurological exam**
- **Complete history** to rule out drug-induced Parkinson akinesia

Treatment includes:

- Symptomatic support
- Dopaminergic therapy: Levodopa, amantadine, and carbidopa
- Anticholinergics: Trihexyphenidyl, benztropine
- For drug-induced Parkinson's, terminate drugs

Drug therapy tends to decrease in effectiveness over time, and patients may present with a marked increase in symptoms. Discontinuing the drugs for 1 week may exacerbate symptoms initially, but functioning may improve when drugs are reintroduced.

GUILLAIN-BARRÉ SYNDROME

Guillain-Barré syndrome (GBS) is an autoimmune disorder of the myelinated motor peripheral nervous system, causing ascending and descending paralysis. GBS is often triggered by a viral infection, but may be idiopathic in origin. Diagnosis is by history, clinical symptoms, and lumbar puncture, which often show increased protein with normal glucose and cell count although protein may not increase for a week or more.

> **Review Video: Guillain-Barre Syndrome**
> Visit mometrix.com/academy and enter code: 742900

Symptoms include:

- Numbness and tingling with increasing weakness of lower extremities that may become generalized, sometimes resulting in complete paralysis and inability to breathe without ventilatory support.
- Deep tendon reflexes are typically absent and some people experience facial weakness and ophthalmoplegia (paralysis of muscles controlling movement of eyes).

Treatment includes:

- Supportive: Fluids, physical therapy, and antibiotics for infections
- Patients should be hospitalized for observation and placed on ventilator support if forced vital capacity is reduced.
- While there is no definitive treatment, plasma exchange or IV immunoglobulin may shorten the duration of symptoms.

MUSCULAR DYSTROPHY

Muscular dystrophies are genetic disorders with gradual degeneration of muscle fibers and progressive weakness and atrophy of skeletal muscles and loss of mobility. **Pseudohypertrophic (Duchenne) muscular dystrophy** is the most common form and the most severe. It is an X-linked disorder in about 50% of the cases with the rest sporadic mutations, affecting males almost exclusively. Children typically have some delay in motor development with difficulty walking and have evidence of muscle weakness by about age 3. Pseudohypertrophic refers to enlargement of muscles by fatty infiltration associated with muscular atrophy, which causes contractures and deformities of joints. Abnormal bone development results in spinal and other skeletal deformities. The disease progresses rapidly, and most children are wheelchair bound by about 12 years of age. As the disease progresses, it involves the muscles of the diaphragm and other muscles needed for respiration. Mild to frank mental deficiency is common. Facial, oropharyngeal, and respiratory muscles weaken late in the disease. Cardiomegaly commonly occurs. Death most often relates to respiratory infection or cardiac failure by age 25. Treatment is supportive.

CEREBRAL PALSY

Cerebral palsy (CP) is a non-progressive motor dysfunction related to CNS damage associated with congenital, hypoxic, or traumatic injury before, during, or ≤2 years after birth. It may include visual defects, speech impairment, seizures, and intellectual disability. There are four **types of motor dysfunction:**

- **Spastic**: Damage to the cerebral cortex or pyramidal tract. Constant hypertonia and rigidity lead to contractures and curvature of the spine.
- **Dyskinetic**: Damage to the extrapyramidal, basal ganglia. Tremors and twisting with exaggerated posturing and impairment of voluntary muscle control.
- **Ataxic**: Damage to the extrapyramidal cerebellum. Atonic muscles in infancy with lack of balance, instability of muscles, and poor gait.
- **Mixed**: Combinations of all three types with multiple areas of damage.

Characteristics of CP include:

- Hypotonia or hypertonia with rigidity and spasticity
- Athetosis (constant writhing motions)
- Ataxia
- Hemiplegia (one-sided involvement, more severe in upper extremities)
- Diplegia (all extremities involved, but more severe in lower extremities)
- Quadriplegia (all extremities involved with arms flexed and legs extended)

MYASTHENIA GRAVIS

Myasthenia gravis is an autoimmune disorder that results in sporadic, progressive weakness of striated (skeletal) muscles because of impaired transmission of nerve impulses. Myasthenia gravis usually affects muscles controlled by the cranial nerves although any muscle group may be affected. Many patients also have thymomas.

Signs and symptoms include weakness and fatigue that worsens throughout the day. Patients often exhibit ptosis and diplopia. They may have trouble chewing and swallowing and often appear to have masklike facies.

If respiratory muscles are involved, patients may exhibit signs of respiratory failure. Myasthenic crisis occurs when patients can no longer breathe independently.

Diagnosis includes electromyography and the Tensilon test (an IV injection of edrophonium or neostigmine, which improves function if the patient has myasthenia gravis, but does not improve function if the symptoms are from a different cause). CT or MRI to diagnose thymoma.

Treatment includes anticholinesterase drugs (neostigmine, pyridostigmine) to relieve some muscle weakness, but these drugs lose effectiveness as the disease progresses. Corticosteroids may be used. Thymectomy is performed if thymoma is present. Tracheotomy and mechanical ventilation may be needed for myasthenic crisis.

SEIZURE DISORDERS
PARTIAL SEIZURES

Partial seizures are caused by electrical discharges to a localized area of the cerebral cortex, such as the frontals, temporal, or parietal lobes with seizure characteristics related to the area of involvement. They may begin in a focal area and become generalized, often preceded by an aura.

- **Simple partial:** Unilateral motor symptoms including somatosensory, psychic, and autonomic
  - Aversive: Eyes and head turned away from focal side
  - Sylvan (usually during sleep): Tonic-clonic movements of the face, salivation, and arrested speech
- **Special sensory:** Various sensations (numbness, tingling, prickling, or pain) spreading from one area. May include visual sensations, posturing or hypertonia.
- **Complex (psychomotor):** No loss of consciousness, but altered consciousness and non-responsive with amnesia. May involve complex sensorium with bad tastes, auditory or visual hallucinations, feeling of déjà vu, strong fear. May carry out repetitive activities, such as walking, running, smacking lips, chewing, or drawling. Rarely aggressive. Seizure usually followed by prolonged drowsiness and confusion. Most common ages 3 through adolescence.

GENERALIZED SEIZURES

Generalized seizures lack a focal onset and appear to involve both hemispheres, usually presenting with loss of consciousness and no preceding aura.

- **Tonic-clonic (Grand Mal):** Occurs without warning
  - Tonic period (10-30 seconds): Eyes roll upward with loss of consciousness, arms flexed; stiffen in symmetric tonic contraction of body, apneic with cyanosis and salivating
  - Clonic period (10 seconds to 30 minutes, but usually 30 seconds). Violent rhythmic jerking with contraction and relaxation. May be incontinent of urine and feces. Contractions slow and then stop.

Following seizures, there may be confusion, disorientation, and impairment of motor activity, speech, and vision for several hours. Headache, nausea, and vomiting may occur. Person often falls asleep and awakens more lucid.

- **Absence (Petit Mal):** Onset is at ages 4-12 and usually ends in puberty. Onset is abrupt with brief loss of consciousness for 5-10 seconds and slight loss of muscle tone but often appears to be daydreaming. Lip smacking or eye twitching may occur.

EPILEPSY

Epilepsy is diagnosed based on a history of seizure activity as well as supporting EEG findings. Treatment is individualized. First line treatments include antiepileptic medications for partial and generalized tonic-clonic seizures. Usually, treatment is started with one medication, but this may need to be changed, adjusted, or an additional medication added until the seizures are under control or to avoid adverse effects, which include allergic reactions, especially skin irritations and acute or chronic toxicity. Milder reactions often subside with time or adjustment in doses. Toxic reactions may vary considerably, depending upon the medication and duration of use, so close monitoring is essential. Severe rash and hepatotoxicity are common toxic reactions that occur with many of the antiepileptic drugs. Dosages of drugs may need to be adjusted to avoid breakthrough seizures during times of stress, such as during illness or surgery. Alcohol/drug abuse and sleep deprivation may also cause breakthrough seizures. Most anticonvulsant drugs are teratogenic.

STATUS EPILEPTICUS

Status epilepticus (SE) is usually generalized tonic-clonic seizures that are characterized by a series of seizures with intervening time too short for regaining of consciousness. The constant assault and periods of apnea can lead to exhaustion, respiratory failure with hypoxemia and hypercapnia, cardiac failure, and death.

Causes: Uncontrolled epilepsy or non-compliance with anticonvulsants, infections such as encephalitis, encephalopathy or stroke, drug toxicity (isoniazid), brain trauma, neoplasms, and metabolic disorders.

Treatment includes:

- Anticonvulsants usually beginning with a fast-acting benzodiazepine (lorazepam), often in steps, with administration of medication every 5 minutes until seizures subside.
- If cause is undetermined, acyclovir and ceftriaxone may be administered.
- If there is no response to the first 2 doses of anticonvulsants (refractory SE), rapid sequence intubation (RSI), which involves sedation and paralytic anesthesia, may be done while therapy continues. Combining phenobarbital and benzodiazepine can cause apnea, so intubation may be necessary.
- Antiepileptic medications are added.

BRAIN TUMORS

Any type of brain tumor can occur in adults. Brain tumors may be primary, arising within the brain, or secondary as a result of metastasis:

- **Astrocytoma**: This arises from astrocytes, which are glial cells. It is the most common type of tumor, occurring throughout the brain. There are many types of astrocytomas, and most are slow growing. Some are operable while others are not. Radiation may be given after removal. Astrocytomas include glioblastomas, aggressively malignant tumors occurring most often in adults 45-70.
- **Glioblastoma**: This is the most common and most malignant adult brain tumor/astrocytoma. Treatment includes surgery, radiation, and chemotherapy, but survival rates are very low.
- **Brain stem glioma**: This may be fast or slow growing but is generally not operable because of location, although it may be treated with radiation or chemotherapy.
- **Craniopharyngioma**: This is a congenital, slow-growing, recurrent (especially if >5 cm) and benign cystic tumor that is difficult to resect and is treated with surgery and radiation.
- **Meningioma**: Slow growing recurrent tumors are usually benign and most often occur in women, ages 40-70; however, they can cause severe impairment/death, depending on size and location. Meningiomas are surgically removed if causing symptoms.
- **Ganglioglioma**: This can occur anywhere in the brain and is usually slow growing and benign.
- **Medulloblastoma**: There are many types of medulloblastoma, most arising in the cerebellum, malignant, and fast growing. Surgical excision is often followed by radiation and chemotherapy although recent studies show using just chemotherapy controls recurrence with less neurological damage.
- **Oligodendroglioma**: This tumor most often occurs in the cerebrum, primarily the frontal or temporal lobes, involving the myelin sheath of the neurons. It is slow growing and most common in those age 40-60.

- **Optical nerve glioma**: This slow growing tumor of the optic nerve is usually a form of astrocytoma. Optic nerve glioma is often associated with neurofibromatosis type I (NF1), occurring in 15-40% of patients with NF1. Despite surgical, chemotherapy, or radiotherapy treatment, it is usually fatal.

STROKES

HEMORRHAGIC STROKES

Hemorrhagic strokes account for about 20% of all strokes and result from a ruptured cerebral artery, causing not only a lack of oxygen and nutrients but also edema that causes widespread pressure and damage:

- **Intracerebral** is bleeding into the substance of the brain from an artery in the central lobes, basal ganglia, pons, or cerebellum. Intracerebral hemorrhage usually results from atherosclerotic degenerative changes, hypertension, brain tumors, anticoagulation therapy, or use of illicit drugs, such as cocaine.
- **Intracranial aneurysm** occurs with ballooning cerebral artery ruptures, most commonly at the Circle of Willis.
- **Arteriovenous malformation**. Rupture of AVMs can cause brain attack in young adults.
- **Subarachnoid hemorrhage** is bleeding in the space between the meninges and brain, resulting from aneurysm, AVM, or trauma. This type of hemorrhage compresses brain tissue.

Treatment includes: The patient may need airway protection/artificial ventilation if neurologic compromise is severe. Blood pressure is lowered to control rate of bleeding but with caution to avoid hypotension and resulting cerebral ischemia (Goal – CPP >70). Sedation can lower ICP and blood pressure, and seizure prophylaxis will be indicated as blood irritates the cerebral cells. An intraventricular catheter may be used in ICP management; correct any clotting disorders if identified.

ISCHEMIA STROKES

Strokes (brain attacks, cerebrovascular accidents) result when there is interruption of the blood flow to an area of the brain. The two basic types are ischemic and hemorrhagic. About 80% are **ischemic**, resulting from blockage of an artery supplying the brain:

- **Thrombosis** in a large artery, usually resulting from atherosclerosis, may block circulation to a large area of the brain. It is most common in the elderly and may occur suddenly or after episodes of transient ischemic attacks.
- **Lacunar infarct** (a penetrating thrombosis in a small artery) is most common in those with diabetes mellitus and/or hypertension.
- **Embolism** travels through the arterial system and lodges in the brain, most commonly in the left middle cerebral artery. An embolism may be cardiogenic, resulting from cardiac arrhythmia or surgery. An embolism usually occurs rapidly with no warning signs.
- **Cryptogenic** has no identifiable cause.

Medical management of ischemic strokes with tissue plasminogen activator (tPA) (Activase), the primary treatment, should be initiated within 3 hours (or up to 4.5 hours if inclusion criteria are met):

- **Thrombolytic,** such as tPA, which is produced by recombinant DNA and is used to dissolve fibrin clots. It is given intravenously (0.9 mg/kg up to 90 mg) with 10% injected as an initial bolus and the rest over the next hour.
- **Antihypertensives** if MAP >130 mmHg or systolic BP >220
- **Cooling** to reduce hyperthermia
- **Osmotic diuretics** (mannitol), hypertonic saline, loop diuretics (Lasix), and/or corticosteroids (dexamethasone) to decrease cerebral edema and intracranial pressure
- **Aspirin/anticoagulation** may be used with embolism

- Monitor and treat hyperglycemia
- **Surgical Intervention:** Used when other treatment fails, may go in through artery and manually remove the clot

SYMPTOMS OF BRAIN ATTACKS IN RELATION TO AREA OF BRAIN AFFECTED

Brain attacks most commonly occur in the right or left hemisphere, but the exact location and the extent of brain damage from a brain attack affects the type of presenting symptoms. If the frontal area of either side is involved, there tends to be memory and learning deficits. Some symptoms are common to specific areas and help to identify the area involved:

- **Right hemisphere**: This results in left paralysis or paresis and a left visual field deficit that may cause spatial and perceptual disturbances, so people may have difficulty judging distance. Fine motor skills may be impacted, resulting in trouble dressing or handling tools. People may become impulsive and exhibit poor judgment, often denying impairment. Left-sided neglect (lack of perception of things on the left side) may occur. Difficulty following directions, short-term memory loss, and depression are also common. Language skills usually remain intact.
- **Left hemisphere**: Results in right paralysis or paresis and a right visual field defect. Depression is common and people often exhibit slow, cautious behavior, requiring repeated instruction and reinforcement for simple tasks. Short-term memory loss and difficulty learning new material or understanding generalizations is common. Difficulty with mathematics, reading, writing, and reasoning may occur. Aphasia (expressive, receptive, or global) is common.
- **Brain stem**: Because the brain stem controls respiration and cardiac function, a brain attack in the brain stem frequently causes death, but those who survive may have a number of problems, including respiratory and cardiac abnormalities. Strokes may involve motor or sensory impairment or both.
- **Cerebellum**: This area controls balance and coordination. Brain attacks in the cerebellum are rare but may result in ataxia, nausea and vomiting, and headaches and dizziness or vertigo.

TIA

Transient ischemic attacks (TIAs) from small clots cause similar but short-lived (minutes to hours) symptoms. Emergent treatment includes placing patient in semi-Fowlers or Fowler's position and administering oxygen. The patient may require oral suctioning if secretions pool. The patient's circulation, airway, and breathing should be assessed and IV access line placed. Thrombolytic therapy to dissolve blood clots should be administered within 1 to 3 hours. While a patient can recover fully from a TIA, they should be educated, because having a TIA increases an individual's risk for a stroke.

ACUTE SPINAL CORD INJURY

Spinal cord injuries may result from blunt trauma (such as automobile accidents), falls from a significant height, sports injuries, and penetrating trauma (such as gunshot or knife wounds). Damage results from mechanical injury and secondary responses resulting from hemorrhage, edema, and ischemia. The type of symptoms relates to the area and degree of injury. About 50% of spinal cord injuries involve the cervical spine between C4 and C7 with a 20% mortality rate, and 50% of injuries result in quadriplegia. Neurogenic shock may occur with injury above T6, with bradycardia, hypotension, and autonomic instability. Patients may develop hypoxia because of respiratory dysfunction. With high injuries, up to 70% of patients will require a tracheostomy (especially at or above C3). Patients with paralysis are at high risk for pressure sores, urinary tract infections (from catheterization), and constipation and impaction. Management varies according to the level of injury but may include mobilization, mechanical ventilation, support surfaces, ROM, assisted mobility, rehabilitation therapy, analgesia, psychological counseling, bowel training, and skin care.

BRAIN DEATH

While each state has its own laws that describe the legal definition of **brain death,** most include some variation of this description:

- Brain death has occurred if the person has "sustained irreversible cessation of circulatory and respiratory functions; or has sustained irreversible cessation of all functions of the entire brain, including the brain stem."

Some states specify the number of physicians that must make the determination and others simply say the decision must be made in accordance with accepted medical practice. Criteria for determination of brain death include coma or lack of responsiveness, apnea (without ventilation), and absence of brainstem reflexes. In many states, findings must be confirmed by at least 2 physicians. **Tests used to confirm brain death** include:

- Cerebral angiograms: Delayed intracerebral filling or obstruction
- EEG: Lack of response to auditory, visual, or somatic stimuli
- Ultrasound (transcranial): Abnormal/lack of flow
- Cerebral scintigrams: Static images at preset time intervals
- Absence of oculocephalic reflex ("Doll's eyes"): patients eyes stay fixed when head is turned side to side
- Absence of oculovestibular reflex ("cold caloric"): When ice cold water is injected into the ear, the patient's eyes exhibit no response. The patient's HOB must be at least 20° for this test to be accurate

Neurological Procedures and Interventions

CLIPPING FOR TREATMENT OF ANEURYSM

Surgical clipping of a ruptured or large, unstable **aneurysm** is necessary because of the danger of rebleeding, 4% in the first 24 hours and 1-2% each day for the next month. Mortality rates with rebleeding are about 70%. Surgical repair is usually done within 48 hours. Clipping may be done prophylactically to prevent rupture. Clipping is done to secure the aneurysm without impairing circulation. Typically, a craniotomy is done and an incision is made into the brain to access the site of the aneurysm. When bleeding is controlled, a small spring-like clip (or sometimes multiple clips) is placed about the neck of the aneurysm. The bulging part of the aneurysm is drained with a needle to make sure that it does not refill and angiography may be done to ensure patency of the artery that feeds the aneurysm. It is possible during surgery for a clot to break away from the aneurysm with resultant extensive hemorrhage. Neurological damage may occur related to surgical manipulation, especially if access is difficult. Post-op monitoring includes frequent neurological checks—sometimes every hour, checking for signs and symptoms of stroke, hemorrhage or cerebral edema/increased ICP. An angiogram may be performed after surgery to confirm placement of clips and ensure there are no leaks.

EMBOLIZATION FOR TREATMENT OF ANEURYSM OR AVM

Embolization is a minimally-invasive method that is an alternative to clipping for some aneurysms and is also used for AVMs. There are different types of embolization, but all use percutaneous transfemoral catheterization and fluoroscopy. The catheter is fed through the femoral and carotid artery to the area requiring repair:

- AVM repair by introducing small silastic beads or glue into the feeder vessels, allowing blood flow to carry the material to the site. This may also be done prior to surgical repair.
- AVM or aneurysm repair by placing one or more detachable balloons into the aneurysm or an AVM and inflating it with a liquid polymerizing agent that solidifies.
- Aneurysm repair with endovascular coiling involves feeding very small platinum coils through the catheter to fill the aneurysm.

Results of endovascular coiling have been very positive, with risk of death or disability at one year over 22% lower than those treated with clipping, although distal ischemia related to emboli is a possible complication.

SURGICAL EXCISION OF AVM

Surgical excision of AVM is the definitive treatment for AVMs as both embolization and radiotherapy treatment pose the risk that the abnormal vessels will recur. Sometimes, 2-3 different surgeries may be required for large AVMs. Usually, nonfunctioning brain tissue surrounds the AVM, so it is possible to remove the AVM without damaging brain tissue. However, reperfusion bleeding may occur as blood is diverted to surrounding arterials that had dilated because of chronic ischemia. The sudden increase in blood flow and pressure may cause leakage of blood from the vessels. There may be extensive blood loss during surgery, so constant monitoring of arterial pressure and multiple IV cannulas are important. Embolization may be done prior to surgery to reduce bleeding. Hyperventilation and mannitol are often used, and β-blockers may be used to prevent hypertension and cerebral edema. Postoperatively, blood pressure is kept low to prevent reperfusion bleeding.

EVACUATION OF HEMATOMAS

Evacuation of hematomas can be done in a number of different ways, including burr holes, needle aspiration, direct surgical craniotomy, or endoscopic craniotomy, but evacuation can pose considerable risks:

- **Epidural hematomas** are usually arterial but may be venous (20%) and are always medical emergencies and require craniotomy with evacuation before compression damage to the brain occurs. Prognosis is good if corrected early because underlying brain damage is rarely severe.

- **Subdural hematomas**, often from acceleration-deceleration accidents or abuse, involve damage to the brain tissue. Evacuation may be done if the hematoma is large and causing compression, but the brain tissue beneath hematomas is often extremely swollen. If the dura is opened, suddenly relieving the pressure may cause the brain to herniate through the opening, so aggressive therapy to reduce swelling preoperatively and careful surgical planning are necessary.

CRANIOTOMIES

Craniotomies for tumors or other surgical repair (AVMs, aneurysms) are increasingly done with micro-endoscopic equipment, but the surgical opening must be large enough to allow access and the use of necessary instruments. Procedures vary widely according to the reason for craniotomy, the type of tumor, and the age and condition of the patient. Direct craniotomies through the skull are needed in some instances, but newer approaches, including transnasal and transsphenoidal endoscopy are used when possible. Some areas of the brain are not accessible with craniotomy, but may be accessible through stereotactic radiosurgery with Gamma Knife or CyberKnife. Stereotactic radiosurgery is often used as a secondary treatment after primary removal of tumor for regrowth or residual tumor. Radiosurgery may be fractionated and given in a series of treatments. These non-invasive treatments are usually done while adults are awake.

POSTOPERATIVE CARE FOR CRANIOTOMY PATIENTS

In the post-operative period immediately following a craniotomy, the patient must be observed carefully for any **complications** or changes in condition:

- Monitor intracranial pressure
- Position the head in a midline, neutral position. HOB is elevated 30-45° for supratentorial surgery and is flat or only slightly elevated for infratentorial surgery
- Initiate anti-thromboembolism measures: Compression stockings or intermittent pneumatic compression device
- Monitor fluid balance (intake and output)
- Observe surgical wound for swelling and drainage; empty and measure drainage devices (usually bulb drains)
- Monitor oxygen saturation and ABGs to ensure proper oxygenation
- Monitor thermoregulation and prevent hyperthermia
- Administer analgesics and antiemetics routinely to maintain comfort and prevent stress or increased ICP from vomiting
- Administer corticosteroids to reduce postoperative swelling
- Administer anticoagulants (heparin) to prevent clotting
- Monitor laboratory status:
  - Complete blood count to observe for blood loss/infection
  - Electrolyte levels, especially observing for hyponatremia and/or hyperkalemia
  - Blood glucose level (may elevate with corticosteroids)

BURR HOLES

Burr holes are small holes drilled through the skull, often as an emergent procedure to relieve increased intracranial pressure (such as from subdural, epidural hematoma, or hydrocephalus), to drain blood, or to remove foreign objects. Burr holes may also be used as access points for minimally-invasive surgeries on the brain, such as to remove a brain tumor. The burr holes are generally drilled with the patient under general anesthesia, and the opening may be closed or left open with a drain in place. The patient must be monitored for indications of bleeding or other surgical complications. Perioperative complications may include increased intracranial pressure from cerebral edema, seizures, intracranial bleeding, and coma. The patient's vital signs and neurological signs should be closely monitored. If a drain is in place, the amount and character of the drainage should be monitored. The patient may receive prophylactic antibiotics to reduce the risk of infection.

NEURO-ENDOVASCULAR INTERVENTIONS

COILING

Coiling is a minimally-invasive procedure used to treat cerebral aneurysm. A catheter is inserted in the femoral area and advanced to the aneurysm. Then a microcatheter with coil attached is fed through the catheter into the aneurysm until the coil fills the aneurysm. The coil is separated with an electrical current and the catheter is removed. In some cases, more than one coil may be needed. The coil is spring like and very thin. Blood enters the aneurysm about the coils and clots so that no further blood can enter, effectively sealing the aneurysm.

THROMBECTOMY

Thrombectomy is a procedure by which an endovascular clot is removed. Various techniques may be used, but a catheter is generally inserted into the femoral vein and advanced to the clot and then the clot may be suctioned, broken up mechanically and the pieces removed, or a helical thrombectomy device wrapped around the clot so that it can be removed. Thrombectomy is used as treatment for stroke to restore blood flow as well as for removal of clots in the arms or legs.

Neurological Pharmacology

ANTICONVULSANTS

Carbamazepine (Tegretol)

Use: Partial, tonic-clonic, and absence seizures; analgesia for trigeminal neuralgia

Side effects: Dizziness, drowsiness, nausea, and vomiting. Toxic reactions include severe skin rash, agranulocytosis, aplastic anemia, and hepatitis

Clonazepam (Klonopin)

Use: Akinetic, absence, and myoclonic seizures; Lennox-Gastaut syndrome

Side effects: Behavioral changes, hirsutism or alopecia, headaches, and drowsiness. Toxic reactions include hepatotoxicity, thrombocytopenia, ataxia, and bone marrow failure.

Ethosuximide (Zarontin)

Use: Absence seizures

Side effects: Headaches and gastrointestinal disorders. Toxic reactions include skin rash, blood dyscrasias (sometimes fatal), hepatitis, and lupus erythematosus.

Felbamate (Felbatol)

Use: Lennox-Gastaut syndrome

Side effects: Headache, fatigue, insomnia, and cognitive impairment. Toxic reactions include aplastic anemia and hepatic failure. It is recommended only if other medications have failed.

Fosphenytoin (Cerebyx)

Use: Status epilepticus prevention and treatment during neurosurgery

Side effects: CNS depression, hypotension, cardiovascular collapse, dizziness, nystagmus, and pruritus.

Gabapentin (Neurontin)

Use: Partial seizures; post-herpetic neuralgia

Side effects: Dizziness, somnolence, drowsiness, ataxia, weight gain, and nausea. Toxic reactions include hepatotoxicity and leukopenia.

Lamotrigine (Lamictal)

Use: Partial and primary generalized tonic-clonic seizures; Lennox-Gastaut syndrome

Side effects: Tremor, ataxia, weight gain, dizziness, headache, and drowsiness. Toxic reactions include severe rash, which may require hospitalization.

Levetiracetam (Keppra)

Use: Partial onset, myoclonic, and generalized tonic-clonic seizures

Side effects: Idiopathic generalized epilepsy, dizziness, somnolence, irritability, alopecia, double vision, sore throat, and fatigue. Toxic reactions include bone marrow suppression and liver failure.

Oxcarbazepine (Trileptal)

Use: Partial seizures

Side effects: Double or abnormal vision, tremor, abnormal gait, GI disorders, dizziness, and fatigue. A toxic reaction is hepatotoxicity.

Phenobarbital (Luminal)

Use: Tonic-clonic and cortical local seizures; acute convulsive episodes; insomnia

Side effects: Sedation, double vision, agitation, and ataxia. Toxic reactions include anemia and skin rash.

Phenytoin (Dilantin)

Use: Tonic-clonic and complex partial seizures

Side effects: Nystagmus, vision disorders, gingival hyperplasia, hirsutism, dysrhythmias, and dysarthria. Toxic reactions include collapse of cardiovascular system and CNS depression.

Primidone (Mysoline)

Use: Grand mal, psychomotor, and focal seizures

Side effects: Double vision, ataxia, impotence, lethargy, and irritability. Toxic reactions include skin rash.

Tiagabine (Gabitril)

Use: Partial seizures

Side effects: Concentration problems, weak knees, dysarthria, abdominal pain, tremor, dizziness, fatigue, and agitation.

Topiramate (Topamax)

Use: Partial and tonic-clonic seizures; migraines

Side effects: Anorexia, weight loss, somnolence, confusion, ataxia, and confusion. Toxic reactions include kidney stones.

Valproate/Valproic acid (Depakote, Depakene)

Use: Complex partial, simple, and complex absence seizures; bipolar disorder

Side effects: Weight gain, alopecia, tremor, menstrual disorders, nausea, and vomiting. Toxic reactions include hepatotoxicity, severe pancreatitis, rash, blood dyscrasias, and nephritis.

Zonisamide (Zonegran, Excegran)

Use: Partial seizures

Side effects: Anorexia, nausea, agitation, rash, headache, dizziness, and somnolence. Toxic reactions include leukopenia and hepatotoxicity.

HYPERTONIC SALINE SOLUTION

Hypertonic saline solution (HSS) has a sodium concentration higher than 0.9% (NS) and is used to reduce intracranial pressure/cerebral edema and treat traumatic brain injury. Concentrations usually range from 2% to 23.4%. The hypertonic solution draws fluid from the tissue through osmosis. As edema decreases, circulation improves. HSS also expands plasma, increasing CPP, and counteracts hyponatremia that occurs in the brain after injury.

Administration:

- Peripheral lines: HSS <3% only
- Central lines: HSS ≥3%

HSS can be administered continuously at rates varying from 30-150 mL/hr. Rate must be carefully controlled. Fluid status must be monitored to prevent hypovolemia, which increases risk of renal failure. Boluses (typically 30 mL of 23.4%) may be administered over 15 minutes for acute increased ICP or transtentorial herniation.

Laboratory monitoring includes:

- Sodium (every 6 hours): Maintain at 145-155 mmol/L. Higher levels can cause heart/respiratory/renal failure.
- Serum osmolality (every 12 hours): Maintain at 320 mOsm/L. Higher levels can cause renal failure.

MANNITOL

Mannitol is an osmotic diuretic that increases excretion of both sodium and water and reduces intracranial pressure and brain mass, especially after traumatic brain injury. Mannitol may also be used to shrink the cells of the blood-brain barrier in order to help other medications breach this barrier. Mannitol is administered per intravenous infusion:

- 2 g/kg in a 15-25% solution over 30-60 minutes

Cerebral spinal fluid pressure should show decrease within 15 minutes. Fluid and electrolyte balances must be carefully monitored as well as intake and output and body weight. Concentrations of 20-25% require a filter. Crystals may form if the mannitol solution is too cold and the mannitol container may require heating (in 80 °C water) and shaking to dissolve crystals, but the solution should be cooled to below body temperature prior to administration. Mannitol cannot be administered in polyvinylchloride bags as precipitates form. Side effects include fluid and electrolyte imbalance, nausea, vomiting, hypotension, tachycardia, fever, and urticaria.

Gastrointestinal Pathophysiology

PERITONITIS

Peritonitis (inflammation of the peritoneum) may be primary (from infection of blood or lymph) or, more commonly, secondary, related to perforation or trauma of the gastrointestinal tract. Common causes include perforated bowel, ruptured appendix, abdominal trauma, abdominal surgery, peritoneal dialysis or chemotherapy, or leakage of sterile fluids, such as blood, into the peritoneum.

Symptoms: Diffuse abdominal pain with rebound tenderness (Blumberg's sign), abdominal rigidity, paralytic ileus, fever (with infection), nausea and vomiting, and sinus tachycardia.

Diagnosis: Increased WBC (>15,000), abdominal x-ray/CT, paracentesis, blood and peritoneal fluid culture.

Treatment includes:

- Intravenous fluids and electrolytes
- Broad-spectrum antibiotics
- Laparoscopy as indicated to determine cause of peritonitis and effect repair

APPENDICITIS

Appendicitis is inflammation of the appendix often caused by luminal obstruction and pressure within the lumen; secretions build up and can eventually perforate the appendix. Diagnosis can be made difficult by the fact that there is some variation in the exact location of the appendix in some patients. Appendicitis can occur in all ages, but children younger than 2 years usually present with peritonitis or sepsis because of difficulty in early diagnosis. **Symptoms** include:

- Acute abdominal pain, which may be epigastric, periumbilical, right lower quadrant, or right flank with rebound tenderness
- Anorexia
- Nausea and vomiting
- Positive psoas and obturator signs
- Fever may develop after 24 hours
- Malaise
- Bowel irregularity and flatulence

Diagnosis is based on clinical presentation, CBC (although leukocytosis may not be present), urinalysis, and imaging studies (usually an abdominal CT with contrast).

CHOLECYSTITIS

Cholecystitis can result in obstruction of the bile duct related to calculi as well as pancreatitis from obstruction of the pancreatic duct. In acute cholecystitis, there is fever, leukocytosis, right upper quadrant abdominal pain, and inflammation of the gallbladder. The disease is most common in overweight women 20-40 years of age, but can occur in pregnant women and people of all ages, especially those who are diabetic or elderly. Cholecystitis may develop secondary to cystic fibrosis, obesity, or total parenteral nutrition. Many times, cholecystitis may resolve in about 7-10 days on its own, but acute cholecystitis may need surgical intervention to prevent complications such as gangrene in the gallbladder or perforation. Diagnosis is confirmed by ultrasound of gallbladder showing thickening of gallbladder walls or positive Murphy's sign, or a HIDA scan showing failure to fill.

Symptoms:

- Severe right upper quadrant or epigastric pain (ranging from 2-6 hours per episode)
- Nausea and vomiting

- Jaundice
- Altered mental status
- Positive Murphy's sign

Treatment:

- Antibiotics for sepsis/ascending cholangitis
- Antispasmodic agents (glycopyrrolate) for biliary colic and vomiting
- Analgesics (note that opioids result in increased sphincter of Oddi pressure)
- Antiemetics
- Surgical consultation for possible laparoscopic or open cholecystectomy

EROSIVE VS. NONEROSIVE GASTRITIS

Gastritis is inflammation of the epithelium or endothelium of the stomach. Types include:

- **Erosive**: Typically caused by alcohol, NSAIDs, illness, portal hypertension, and/or stress. Risk factors include severe illness, mechanical ventilation, trauma, sepsis, organ failure, and burns. Patients may be essentially asymptomatic but may have hematemesis or "coffee ground" emesis. Treatment depends on cause and severity but often includes a proton pump inhibitor (such as omeprazole 20-40 mg per day). Some may receive an H2-rceptor (such as famotidine). Those with portal hypertension may respond to propranolol or nadolol or portal decompression.
- **Nonerosive**: Typically caused by Helicobacter pylori infection or pernicious anemia. H. pylori infection can lead to gastric and duodenal ulcers. Treatment for H. pylori is per antibiotics and proton pump inhibitors with standard triple or standard quadruple therapy. Pernicious anemia is treated with vitamin B-12. Gastritis may also be caused by a wide range of pathogens, including parasites, so treatment depends on the causative agent.

GASTROENTERITIS

VIRAL GASTROENTERITIS

Viral gastroenteritis (commonly referred to as stomach flu) is characterized by nausea, vomiting, abdominal cramping, watery (may become bloody) diarrhea, headache, muscle aches, and fever. Viral gastroenteritis is spread through the fecal-oral route. Common **causes** include:

- **Norovirus**: Symptoms generally include diarrhea and vomiting with symptoms persisting for 1-3 days. Most people do not require treatment, but if diarrhea or vomiting is severe, an antiemetic or antidiarrheal may be prescribed if the patient is younger than 65. If severe dehydration occurs, the patient may require intravenous fluids until she is able to resume adequate oral intake.
- **Rotavirus**: Symptoms include watery diarrhea, nausea, vomiting, abdominal pain and cramping, lack of appetite and fever. Patients may become easily dehydrated and require rehydration with Pedialyte or Rice-Lyte or IV fluids. Medications are usually not needed but the rotavirus vaccine prevents severe rotavirus-related diarrhea and is given in 3 doses (2 months, 4 months, and 6 months).

BACTERIAL GASTROENTERITIS

Bacterial gastroenteritis generally results in cramping, nausea, and severe diarrhea. Some bacteria cause gastroenteritis because of enterotoxins that adhere to the mucosa of the intestines and others because of exotoxins that remain in contaminated food. Some bacteria directly invade the intestinal mucosa. Bacterial gastroenteritis is commonly **caused** by:

- *Salmonella*: Sudden onset of bloody diarrhea, abdominal cramping, nausea, and vomiting, leading to dehydration. Infection may become systemic and life-threatening. Treatment is supportive although antibiotics may be administered to those at risk.

- *Campylobacter*: Bloody diarrhea, cramping, fever, for up to 7 days that usually resolves but may become systemic in those who are immunocompromised. Treatment is primarily supportive with antibiotics only for those at risk.
- *Shigella* **spp.**: Most common in children <5 and presents with fever, abdominal cramping, and bloody diarrhea, persisting 5-7 days. Treatment is primarily supportive (rehydration) although those at risk (very young, old, immunocompromised) may receive antibiotics because the disease may become systemic.
- *Escherichia coli*: Different strains are associated with traveler's diarrhea and food-borne illnesses, and severity varies. Most result in diarrhea, nausea, vomiting, and cramping, but some strains (O157) may develop into life-threatening hemolytic uremic syndrome (HUS). Treatment is supportive. Antibiotics increase risk of developing HUS.

PARASITIC GASTROENTERITIS

Parasitic gastroenteritis is generally caused by infection with protozoa (one-celled pathogens):

- *Giardia intestinalis*: Common cause of waterborne (drinking and recreational) disease and non-bacterial diarrhea, resulting from fecal contamination. Symptoms include diarrhea, abdominal cramping, flatulence, greasy floating stools, nausea and vomiting as well as weight loss. Symptoms usually persist for up to 3 weeks although some develop chronic disease. Metronidazole is the drug of choice: Adults, 250 mg TID for 5-7 days. Pediatrics, 15 mg/kg/day in 3 doses for 5-7 days.
- *Cryptosporidium parvum*: About 10,000 cases occur in the US each year, usually from contact with fecal-contaminated water. Symptoms include watery diarrhea, abdominal pain, nausea, vomiting, weight loss, and fever and persist for up to 2 weeks although a severe chronic infection may occur in those who are immunocompromised. Treatment for non-HIV-infected patients (medications ineffective for HIV patients): Adults and children >11, Nitazoxanide 500 mg BID for 3 days. Pediatrics, 1-3 years 100 mg BID for 3 days; 4-11 years 200 mg BID for 3 days.

CONSTIPATION AND IMPACTION

Constipation is a condition with bowel movements less frequent than normal for a person, or hard, small stool that is evacuated fewer than 3 times weekly. Food moves through the GI from the small intestine to the colon in semi-liquid form. Constipation results from the colon, where fluid is absorbed. If too much fluid is absorbed, the stool can become too dry. People may have Abdominal distension and cramps and need to strain for defecation.

Fecal impaction occurs when the hard stool moves into the rectum and becomes a large, dense, immovable mass that cannot be evacuated even with straining, usually as a result of chronic constipation. In addition to abdominal cramps and distention, the person may feel intense rectal pressure and pain accompanied by a sense of urgency to defecate. Nausea and vomiting may also occur. Hemorrhoids will often become engorged. Fecal incontinence, with liquid stool leaking about the impaction, is common.

MEDICAL PROCEDURES TO EVALUATE CAUSES OF CONSTIPATION

Medical procedures to evaluate causes of constipation should be preceded by a careful history as this may help to define the type and guide the choice of diagnostic procedures. Most tests are necessary only for severe constipation that does not respond to treatment. Medical **diagnostic procedures** may include the following:

- **Physical exam** should include rectal exam and abdominal palpation to assess for obvious hard stool or impaction.
- **Blood tests** can identify hypothyroidism and excess parathyroid hormone.
- **Abdominal x-ray** may show large amounts of stool in the colon.
- **Barium enema** can indicate tumors or strictures causing obstruction.
- **Colonic transit studies** can show defects of the neuromuscular system.
- **Defecography** shows the defecation process and abnormalities of anatomy.

- **Anorectal manometry studies** show malfunction of anorectal muscles.
- **Colonic motility studies** measure the pattern of colonic pressure.
- **Colonoscope** allows direct visualization of the lumen of the rectum and colon.

BOWEL OBSTRUCTIONS

Bowel obstruction occurs when there is a mechanical obstruction of the passage of intestinal contents because of constriction of the lumen, occlusion of the lumen, adhesion formation, or lack of muscular contractions (paralytic ileus). **Symptoms** include abdominal pain, rigidity, and distention, n/v, dehydration, constipation, respiratory distress from the diaphragm pushing against the pleural cavity, sepsis, and shock. **Treatment** includes strict NPO, insertion of naso/orogastric tube, IV fluids and careful monitoring; may correct spontaneously, severe obstruction requires surgery.

BOWEL INFARCTIONS

Bowel infarction is ischemia of the intestines related to severely restricted blood supply. It can be the result of a number of different conditions, such as strangulated bowel or occlusion of arteries of the mesentery, and may follow untreated bowel obstruction. Patients present with acute abdomen and shock, and mortality rates are very high even with resection of infarcted bowel. **Treatment** includes replacing volume, correcting the underlying issue, improving blood flow to the mesentery, insertion of NGT, and/or surgery.

INTESTINAL PERFORATION

Intestinal perforation is a partial or complete tear in the intestinal wall, leaking intestinal contents into the peritoneum. Causes include trauma, NSAIDs (elderly, patients with diverticulitis), acute appendicitis, PUD, iatrogenic (laparoscopy, endoscopy, colonoscopy, radiotherapy), bacterial infections, IBS, and ingestion of toxic substances (acids) or foreign bodies (toothpicks). The danger posed by infection after perforation varies depending upon the site. The stomach and proximal portions of the small intestine have little bacteria, but the distal portion of the small intestine contains aerobic bacteria, such as *E. coli,* as well as anaerobic bacteria.

Signs/Symptoms: (appear within 24-48 hours): Abdominal pain and distention and rigidity, fever, guarding and rebound tenderness, tachycardia, dyspnea, absent bowel sounds/paralytic ileus with nausea and vomiting; Sepsis and abscess or fistula formation can occur.

Diagnosis: Labs: elevated WBC; lactic acid and pH change as late signs. X-ray and CT will show free air in abdominal cavity.

Treatment includes:

- Prompt antibiotic therapy and surgical repair with peritoneal lavage
- The abdominal wound may be left open to heal by secondary intention and to prevent compartment syndrome

GASTROESOPHAGEAL REFLUX

Gastroesophageal reflux (GER) occurs when the lower esophageal sphincter fails to remain closed, allowing the contents of the stomach to back into the esophagus. This reflux of the acid containing contents of the stomach may cause irritation of the lining of the esophagus. Over time, damage to the lining of the esophagus can occur. In some patients, this may lead to the formation of Barrett's esophagus. In Barrett's esophagus, the lining of the esophagus begins to resemble the tissue lining the intestine. Patients with Barrett's esophagus have an increased risk of developing esophageal adenocarcinoma.

Signs and symptoms: Heartburn, dysphagia, belching, water brash, sore throat, hoarseness, and chest pain.

Diagnosis: Clinical signs/symptoms, ambulatory esophageal reflux monitoring (this test uses a thin pH probe that is placed in the esophagus). Data is collected on the amount of acid entering the esophagus along with the presence of clinical symptoms. Endoscopy may be used in the diagnosis of GERD in patients with persistent or progressive symptoms.

Treatment: GER is often treated with proton pump inhibitors (inhibit gastric acid secretion). Surgical therapy may be utilized if medical management is unsuccessful. Patients are taught to eliminate foods that trigger symptoms (chocolate, caffeine, alcohol, and highly acidic foods). In addition, patients with GERD should avoid meals 2-3 hours before bed and may find it helpful to sleep with the head of the bed elevated to alleviate symptoms.

Peptic Ulcer Disease

Peptic ulcer disease (PUD) includes both ulcerations of the duodenum and stomach. They may be primary (usually duodenal) or secondary (usually gastric). Gastric ulcers are commonly associated with **H. pylori** infections (80%) but may be caused by aspirin and NSAIDs. *H. pylori* are spread in the fecal-oral route from person to person or contaminated water and cause a chronic inflammation and ulcerations of the gastric mucosa. PUD is 2 to 3 times more common in males and is associated with poor economic status that results in a crowded, unhygienic environment, although it can occur in others. Usually, other family members have a history of ulcers as well.

Symptoms include abdominal pain, nausea, vomiting, and GI bleeding in children younger than 6 years with epigastric and postprandial pain and indigestion in older children and adults.

Treatment includes:

- Antibiotics for *H. pylori*: amoxicillin, clarithromycin, metronidazole
- Proton pump inhibitors: lansoprazole or omeprazole
- Bismuth
- Histamine-receptor antagonists: cimetidine or famotidine

> **Review Video: Peptic Ulcers and GERD**
> Visit mometrix.com/academy and enter code: 184332

Inflammatory Bowel Disease
Ulcerative Colitis

Ulcerative colitis is superficial inflammation of the mucosa of the colon and rectum, causing ulcerations in the areas where inflammation has destroyed cells. These ulcerations, ranging from pinpoint to extensive, may bleed and produce purulent material. The mucosa of the bowel becomes swollen, erythematous, and granular. Patients may present emergently with **severe ulcerative colitis** (having >6 blood stools a day, fever, tachycardia, anemia) or with **fulminant colitis** (>10 blood stools per day, severe bleeding, and toxic symptoms) These patients are at high risk for megacolon and perforation. For patients with severe and fulminant ulcerative colitis:

Symptoms:

- Abdominal pain
- Anemia
- F&E depletion
- Bloody diarrhea/rectal bleeding
- Diarrhea
- Fecal urgency
- Tenesmus
- Anorexia
- Weight loss

- Fatigue
- Systemic disorders: Eye inflammation, arthritis, liver disease, and osteoporosis as immune system triggers generalized inflammation

Treatment:

- Glucocorticoids
- Aminosalicylates
- Antibiotics if signs/symptoms of toxicity
- D/C anticholinergics, NSAIDS, and antidiarrheals
- If fulminant: Admitted & monitored for deterioration. Kept NPO, and given IV F&E replacement. NGT for decompression if intestinal dilation is present. Knee-elbow position to reposition gas in bowel. Colectomy for those with megacolon or who are unresponsive to therapy.

> **Review Video: Ulcerative Colitis**
> Visit mometrix.com/academy and enter code: 584881

CROHN'S DISEASE

Crohn's disease manifests with inflammation of the GI system. Inflammation is transmural (often leading to intestinal stenosis and fistulas), focal, and discontinuous with aphthous ulcerations progressing to linear and irregular-shaped ulcerations. Granulomas may be present. Common sites of inflammation are the terminal ileum and cecum. The condition is chronic, but patients with severe or fulminant disease (fevers, persistent vomiting, abscess, obstruction) often present emergently for treatment.

Symptoms:

- Perirectal abscess/fistula in advanced disease
- Diarrhea
- Watery stools
- Rectal hemorrhage
- Anemia
- Abdominal pain (commonly RLQ)
- Cramping
- Weight loss
- Nausea and vomiting
- Fever
- Night sweats

Treatment:

- Triamcinolone for oral lesions, aminosalicylates, glucocorticoids, antidiarrheals, probiotics, avoid lactose, and identify and eliminate food triggers.
- For patients who present with toxic symptoms: hospitalization for careful monitoring, IV glucocorticoids, aminosalicylates, antibiotics, and bowel rest. Parenteral nutrition for the malnourished.
- For repeated relapses (refractory):
  - Immunomodulatory agents (azathioprine, mercaptopurine, methotrexate) or Biologic therapies (infliximab). Bowel resection if unresponsive to all treatment or with ischemic bowel.

DIVERTICULAR DISEASE

Diverticular disease is a condition in which diverticula (saclike pouchings of the bowel lining that extend through a defect in the muscle layer) occur anywhere within the GI tract. About 20% of patients with diverticular disease will develop acute diverticulitis, which occurs as diverticula become inflamed when food or bacteria are retained within the diverticula. This may result in abscess, obstruction, perforation, bleeding, or fistula. Diagnosis is best confirmed by abdominal CT with contrast (showing a localized thickening of the bowel wall, increased density of soft tissue, and diverticula in the colon). Many patients have normal lab studies, but some present with leukocytosis, elevated serum amylase, and pyuria on urinalysis.

Symptoms (similar to appendicitis):

- Steady pain in left lower quadrant
- Change in bowel habits
- Tenesmus
- Dysuria from irritation
- Recurrent urinary infections from fistula
- Paralytic ileus from peritonitis or intra-abdominal irritation
- Toxic reactions: fever, severe pain, leukocytosis

Treatment:

- Rehydration and electrolytes per IV fluids
- Nothing by mouth initially
- Antibiotics, broad spectrum (IV if toxic reactions)
- NG suction if necessary, for obstruction
- Careful observation for signs of perforation or obstruction

ACUTE GASTROINTESTINAL HEMORRHAGE

Gastrointestinal (GI) hemorrhage may occur in the upper or lower gastrointestinal track. The primary cause (50-70%) of GI hemorrhage is gastric and duodenal ulcers, generally caused by stress, NSAIDs or infection with *Helicobacter pylori*.

Symptoms: Abdominal pain and distention, coffee-ground emesis/hematemesis, bloody or tarry stools, hypotension with tachycardia.

Diagnosis: Stool occult blood (Guaiac test), EGD, colonoscopy, GI Bleed scan.

Treatment includes:

- Medications: Fluid replacement with blood transfusions if necessary, antibiotic therapy for *Helicobacter pylori,* continuous pantoprazole IV to prevent further irritation
- Endoscopic thermal therapy to cauterize or injection therapy (hypertonic saline, epinephrine, ethanol) to cause vasoconstriction
- Arteriography with intra-arterial infusion of vasopressin and/or embolizing agents, such as stainless-steel coils, platinum microcoils, or Gelfoam pledgets
- Vagotomy and pyloroplasty if bleeding persists

Prevention: Prophylactic medications (pantoprazole [Protonix] IV is common).

HEPATIC CIRRHOSIS

COMPENSATED

Cirrhosis is a chronic hepatic disease in which normal liver tissue is replaced by the fibrotic tissue that impairs liver function. There are three **types**:

- **Alcoholic** (from chronic alcoholism) is the most common type and results in fibrosis about the portal areas. The liver cells become necrotic, replaced by fibrotic tissue, with areas of normal tissue projecting in between, giving the liver a hobnail appearance.
- **Post-necrotic** with broad bands of fibrotic tissue is the result of acute viral hepatitis.
- **Biliary**, the least common type, is caused by chronic biliary obstruction and cholangitis, with resulting fibrotic tissue about the bile ducts.

Cirrhosis may be either compensated or decompensated. **Compensated** cirrhosis usually involves non-specific symptoms, such as intermittent fever, epistaxis, ankle edema, indigestion, abdominal pain, and palmar erythema. Hepatomegaly and splenomegaly may also be present.

DECOMPENSATED

Decompensated cirrhosis occurs when the liver can no longer adequately synthesize proteins, clotting factors, and other substances so that portal hypertension occurs.

Symptoms:

- Hepatomegaly
- Chronic elevated temperature
- Clubbing of fingers
- Purpura resulting from thrombocytopenia, with bruising and epistaxis
- Portal obstruction resulting in jaundice and ascites
- Bacterial peritonitis with ascites
- Esophageal varices
- Edema of extremities and presacral area resulting from reduced albumin in the plasma. Vitamin deficiency from interference with formation, use, and storage of vitamins, such as A, C, and K
- Anemia from chronic gastritis and decreased dietary intake
- Hepatic encephalopathy with alterations in mentation
- Hypotension
- Atrophy of gonads

Treatment varies according to the symptoms and is supportive rather than curative as the fibrotic changes in the liver cannot be reversed:

- Dietary supplements and vitamins
- Diuretics (potassium sparing), such as Aldactone and Dyrenium, to decrease ascites
- Colchicine to reduce fibrotic changes
- Liver transplant (the definitive treatment)

FULMINANT HEPATITIS

Fulminant hepatitis is a severe acute infection of the liver that can result in hepatic necrosis, encephalopathy, and death within 1 to 2 weeks. Most hepatitis is caused by infection with hepatitis viruses A, B, C, D, or E, but it can also be caused by numerous viruses, toxic chemicals (carbon tetrachloride), metabolic diseases (Wilson disease), and drugs, such as acetaminophen. Fulminant hepatitis can result from any of these factors.

Fulminant hepatitis can be divided into three stages according to the duration from jaundice to encephalopathy:

$$0 \text{ to } 7 \text{ days} = \text{Hyperacute liver failure}$$
$$7 \text{ to } 28 \text{ days} = \text{Acute liver failure}$$
$$28 \text{ to } 72 \text{ days} = \text{Subacute liver failure}$$

Symptoms:

- Poor feeding/anorexia
- Increased intracranial pressure with cerebral edema and encephalopathy
- Coagulopathies
- Renal failure
- Electrolyte imbalances

Treatment:

- Identify and treat underlying cause
- Intracranial pressure monitoring and treatment
- Diuresis; liver transplantation may be necessary
- Survival rates vary from 50-85%

PORTAL HYPERTENSION

Portal hypertension occurs when obstructed blood flow increases blood pressure throughout the portal venous system, preventing the liver from filtering blood and causing the development of collateral blood vessels that return unfiltered blood to the systemic circulation. Increasing serum aldosterone levels cause sodium and fluid retention in the kidneys, resulting in hypervolemia, ascites and esophageal varices. Portal hypertension can be caused by any liver disease, especially cirrhosis and inherited or acquired coagulopathies that cause thrombosis of the portal vein.

Symptoms: Ascites with distended abdomen, esophageal varices with bleeding, dyspnea, abdominal discomfort, fluid/electrolyte imbalances.

Diagnosis: Labs (CBC, BMP, liver panel, Hep B &C), abdominal ultrasound or CT/MRI, EGD, Hemodynamic measurement of the hepatic venous pressure gradient (HVPG)

Treatment includes:

- Restricted sodium intake & use diuretics as needed
- Endoscopic treatment of obstruction
- Portal vein shunting redirecting blood from the portal vein to the vena cava
- Liver transplant in severe cases
- These patients are at high risk for esophageal varices, which, if they rupture, can cause instantaneous hemorrhage and death

ESOPHAGEAL VARICES

Esophageal varices are torturous, dilated veins in the submucosa of the esophagus (usually the distal portion). They are a complication of cirrhosis of the liver, in which obstruction of the portal vein causes an increase in collateral vessels and resulting decrease in circulation to the liver, increasing the pressure in the collateral vessels. This causes the vessels to dilate. Because they tend to be fragile and inelastic, they tear easily, causing sudden, massive esophageal hemorrhage.

Signs/Symptoms: Usually asymptomatic until rupture; projectile vomiting bright red blood, dark stools, and shock.

Diagnosis: EGD, capsule endoscopy, CT, and MRI.

Treatment (in the case of rupture) includes:

- Emergent fluid and blood replacement
- IV vasopressin, somatostatin, and octreotide to decrease venous pressure and provide vasoconstriction/clotting
- Endoscopic injection with sclerosing agents and band ligation
- Esophagogastric balloon tamponade using Sengstaken-Blakemore and Minnesota tubes (Note: always inflate gastric balloon first, keep scissors nearby in case of balloon migration, do not use longer than 24 hrs as there is increased risk of ulceration from pressure.)
- Transjugular intrahepatic portosystemic shunting (TIPS) creates a channel between systemic and portal venous systems to reduce portal hypertension

Hepatic Coma

Hepatic coma or hepatic encephalopathy occurs when the liver's inability to remove ammonia and other toxins from the bloodstream causes a decrease in neurologic function. Hepatic encephalopathy often occurs in patients with severe liver disease, most commonly in patients diagnosed with cirrhosis of the liver. The fibrous tissue that forms in cirrhosis affects the liver structure and impedes the blood flow to the liver, ultimately causing the liver to fail. There are four stages of hepatic encephalopathy ranging from grade 0 to grade 4. Grade 4 encephalopathy is defined as hepatic coma. Neurologic alterations may progress slowly and if left untreated may result in irreversible neurologic damage.

Signs and symptoms: Altered mental status, personality or mood changes, poor judgment, and poor concentration. As symptoms progress, patients may experience agitation, disorientation, drowsiness, increasing confusion, lethargy, slurred speech, tremors, and seizures. In grade 4 encephalopathy, patients become unresponsive and ultimately comatose.

Diagnosis: Physical assessment, lab tests including a complete blood count, liver function tests, serum ammonia levels, BUN, creatinine and electrolyte levels, CT or MRI of the brain, and electroencephalogram may be used to diagnose hepatic encephalopathy.

Treatment: Address precipitating factors such as infection, gastrointestinal bleeding, dehydration, hypotension, or alcohol use. Other treatment options may include limiting protein intake, administration of lactulose to prevent the absorption of ammonia, and the administration of an antibiotic such as neomycin, rifaximin, or Flagyl to reduce the serum ammonia level.

Acute Pancreatitis

Acute pancreatitis is related to chronic alcoholism or cholelithiasis in 90% of patients, but may have unknown etiology. It may also be triggered by a variety of drugs (tetracycline, thiazides, acetaminophen, and oral contraceptives). Complications may include shock, acute respiratory distress syndrome, and MODs.

Signs/Symptoms: acute pain (mid-epigastric, LUQ, or generalized), nausea and vomiting, Abdominal distension.

Diagnosis: Serum lipase (>2x normal), amylase (less accurate), CT with contrast, abdominal U/S, MRI cholangiopancreatography, ERCP.

Treatment (supportive) includes:

- **Medications**: IV fluids, antiemetics, antibiotics (if necrosis is secondary to infection), and analgesia. NOTE: do not give morphine, can cause spasms in sphincter of Oddi, making pain worse.
- **TPN, NPO, or restricted to clear liquids** may help manage vomiting, ileus, and aspiration.
- **Surgical**: may remove gallbladder and biliary duct obstructions if cause of recurrent pancreatitis.

Prevention: Avoid smoking and alcohol consumption; limit fat intake and increase fresh fruits/vegetables and water.

HERNIAS

Hernias are protrusions into or through the abdominal wall and may occur in children and adults. Hernias may contain fat, tissue, or bowel. There are a number of **types**:

- **Direct inguinal hernias** occur primarily in adults and rarely incarcerate.
- **Indirect inguinal hernias** related to congenital defect is most common on the right in males and can incarcerate, especially during the first year and in females.
- **Femoral hernias** occur primarily in women and may incarcerate.
- **Umbilical hernias** occur in children, especially those of African-American descent, and rarely incarcerate. They may also occur in adults, primarily women, and may incarcerate.
- **Incisional hernias** are usually related to obesity or wound infections, and may incarcerate.

Hernias are evident on clinical examination.

Symptoms of incarceration include:

- Severe pain
- Nausea and vomiting
- Soft mass at hernia site
- Tachycardia
- Temperature

Treatment for hernias includes:

- Reduction if incarceration is very recent with patient in Trendelenburg position and gentle compression
- Surgical excision and fixation
- Broad-spectrum antibiotics

BILIARY ATRESIA

Biliary atresia is a rare life-threatening condition that occurs in infancy of unknown cause. Bile ducts are tubes that transport bile from the liver to the gallbladder (where it is stored) and the small intestine (where it aids in digestion). Biliary atresia occurs when the bile ducts (either inside or outside of the liver) become inflamed, causing damage to the ducts and an impedance of bile flow. Without treatment, the trapped bile causes damage to the liver eventually causing it to fail. The life expectancy for infants with untreated biliary atresia is approximately 2 years.

Signs and symptoms: Early identification is key in successfully treating biliary atresia. Signs and symptoms include dark urine, gray or white stools, slow weight gain and delayed growth, jaundice, abdominal swelling, and itching.

Diagnosis: Physical assessment, abdominal films, ultrasound, lab tests including bilirubin levels, and liver biopsy.

Treatment: The only treatment options for biliary atresia are liver transplant or the Kasai procedure. Named after the surgeon who invented it, the Kasai procedure involves using a loop of intestine to act as a new bile duct and removing the damaged ducts. Flow of bile is then restored to the small intestine. The Kasai procedure is most successful when performed on younger infants (less than 3 months old).

Gastrointestinal Procedures and Interventions

NG Tubes, Sump Tubes, and Levin Tubes

Nasogastric **(NG) tubes** are plastic or vinyl tubes inserted through the nose, down the esophagus, and into the stomach. **Sump tubes** are radiopaque with a vent lumen to prevent a vacuum from forming with high suction. **Levin tubes** have no vent lumen and are used only with low suction. NG tubes drain gastric secretions, allow sampling of secretions, or provide access to the stomach and upper GI tract. They are used for lavage after medication overdose, for decompression, and for instillation of medications or fluids. NG tubes are contraindicated with obstruction proximal to the stomach or gastric pathology, such as hemorrhage.

Tube-insertion length is estimated: earlobe to xiphoid + earlobe to nose tip + 15 cm.

The tube is inserted through the naris with the patient upright, if possible, and swallowing sips of water. Vasoconstrictors and topical anesthetic reduce gag reflex. Placement is checked with insufflation of air or aspiration of stomach contents and verified by x-ray. The NG is secured and drainage bag provided. Tubes attached to continuous low or intermittent high suction must be monitored frequently.

Levin Tube

Marking to indicate tube placement

Single Lumen for suction

PEG Tube

Percutaneous endoscopic gastrostomy (PEG), used for tube feedings, involves intubation of the esophagus with the endoscope and insertion of a sheathed needle with a guidewire through the abdomen and stomach wall so that a catheter can be fed down the esophagus, snared, and pulled out through the opening where the needle was inserted and secured. The PEG tube should not be secured to the abdomen until the PEG is fully healed, which usually takes 2 to 4 weeks, because tension caused by taping the tube against the abdomen may cause the tract to change shape and direction. The tract should be straight to facilitate insertion and removal of catheters. Once the tract has healed, the original PEG tube can generally be replaced with a balloon gastrostomy tube. External stabilizing devices can be applied to the skin to hold the tube in place but should be placed 1 to 2 cm above the skin surface to prevent excessive tension that may result in buried bumper syndrome (BBS) in which the internal fixation device becomes lodged in the mucosal lining of the gastric wall, resulting in ulceration.

DRAINS

The following are different types of drains a patient may have, including pertinent nursing considerations:

- **Simple drains** are latex or vinyl tubes of varying sizes/lengths. They are usually placed through a stab wound near the area of involvement.
- **Penrose drains** are flat, soft rubber/latex tubes placed in surgical wounds to drain fluid by gravity and capillary action.

Latex or silicone tubing

Safety pin is attached to the end of the tubing leaving the wound to prevent the tube from slipping inside of the wound

- **Sump drains** are double-lumen or tri-lumen tubes (with a third lumen for infusions). The multiple lumens produce venting when air enters the inflow lumen and forces drainage out of the large lumen.
- **A percutaneous drainage catheter** is inserted into the wound to provide continuous drainage for infection/fluid collection. Irrigation of the catheter may be required to maintain patency. Skin barriers and pouching systems may also be necessary.

SAFE PERCUTANEOUS DRAINAGE KIT

Multi Drain

Standard Drain

Forty Drain

- **Closed drainage systems** use low-pressure suction to provide continuous gravity drainage of wounds. Drains are attached to collapsible suction reservoirs that provide negative pressure. The nurse must remember to always re-establish negative pressure after emptying these drains. There are two types in frequent use:
  - *Jackson-Pratt is* a bulb-type drain that is about the size of a lemon. A thin plastic drain from the wound extends to a squeeze bulb that can hold about 100 mL of drainage.

JACKSON PRATT DRAIN

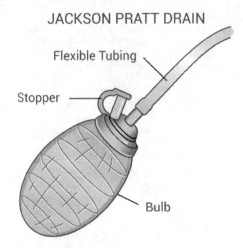

Flexible Tubing

Stopper

Bulb

  - *Hemovac* is a round drain with coiled springs inside that are compressed after emptying to create suction. The device can hold up to 500 mL of drainage.

ENTERAL SUPPORT AND PARENTERAL SUPPORT

Enteral nutrition is a method of providing nutrition to a patient through a tube; the tube may be placed in either the nose (a nasogastric tube), the stomach (a percutaneous endoscopic gastrostomy [PEG] tube), or the small bowel (a percutaneous endoscopic jejunal [J] tube). When the tube has been placed, nutrition can be administered through the tube and absorbed by the patient's digestive system. Various **enteric formulas** exist, and the choice is dependent on the nutritional requirements of the patient.

Parenteral nutrition (also called total parenteral nutrition [**TPN**]) is a method of providing nutrition that completely bypasses the digestive system by administering nutrition through an intravenous line. Enteral support is the preferred method of providing nutrition, although in patients suffering from some compromise of the gastrointestinal tract, parenteral nutrition is the only option.

TROUBLE-SHOOTING PROBLEMS RELATED TO ENTERAL FEEDINGS

Feeding tubes are commonly found in the critical care setting, as many patients are intubated and unable to take oral nutrition or medication. General maintenance involves checking placement before flushing anything into the tube (prevents aspiration), flushing the tubes with at least 30 mL of water before and after use, and every 4 hours. Never crush enteric-coated medications, and keep the HOB inclined at least 30° at all times during feeding. **Complications** include:

- **Vomiting/aspiration:** Caused by incorrect placement, gastric emptying, and/or formula intolerance.
  - Treatment: Confirm placement by checking pH (preferred to air bolus); delay feeding one hour and check residual volume before resuming. Refrigerate formula, check expiration, and use only for 24 hours.
- **Diarrhea:** Caused by rapid feeding, antibiotics/medications, intolerance of formula or hypertonic formula, and/or tube migration.
  - Treatment: Reduce rate of feeding, evaluate medications, avoid hanging feedings longer than 8 hours, and add fiber or decrease sodium in the feed.

- **Displacement of tube:**
  - Treatment: For NG tube, replace using the other nostril, only if not surgically placed. For G-tube or J-tube, cover the site and notify the physician.
  - Prevention: secure all tubes with the appropriate device and mark placement to identify migration.
- **Tube occlusion:**
  - Treatment: Check for kinks and obvious problems. Aspirate fluid, instill warm water, and aspirate to loosen occlusion. The physician may order an enzyme or sodium bicarb solution.

GASTROINTESTINAL SURGERY
WHIPPLE

The Whipple (pancreaticoduodenectomy) procedure is used to surgically remove the head of the pancreas, the gallbladder, part of the bile duct, the duodenum, and sometimes the distal portion of the stomach. After excision, the remaining pancreas, bile duct, and intestinal stump are sutured to the intestine so that secretions empty into the intestine. The Whipple procedure may be done as an open procedure or laparoscopically. This procedure is used primarily for malignant or benign tumors of the head of the pancreas but can also be used for chronic pancreatitis, duodenal cancer, cancer of the ampulla, and cholangiocarcinoma. Whipple is recommended only if the cancer has not spread beyond the pancreas and has not invaded major vessels. Usually, the pancreas is still able to produce adequate insulin, but the production of pancreatic enzymes may be impaired. A pylorus-preserving variation preserves the stomach and part of the pylorus to decrease nutritional deficiencies and weight loss associated with the standard Whipple.

Post-op treatment includes monitoring fluid/electrolyte balance and monitoring drains. These patients have a very high risk of developing numerous complications, including peritonitis, bowel obstruction, sepsis, and acute abdomen, along with others.

ESOPHAGECTOMY AND ESOPHAGOGASTRECTOMY

Esophageal cancer starts in the inner layer of the esophagus and spreads. It may develop after long-term reflux because of cell changes brought about by gastric acid. Symptoms include throat or epigastric discomfort, increasing dysphagia and inability to swallow solids, unexplained weight loss, hoarseness, hiccups, hematemesis, and the feeling of something in the throat. *Treatment* for esophageal cancer involves surgical removal of the affected portion of the esophagus. Two common procedures include:

- **Esophagectomy** is the removal of all or part of the esophagus with the distal end resutured to the stomach or an intestinal graft used to replace the excised portion of the esophagus.
- **Esophagogastrectomy** is the removal of the distal portion of the esophagus, lymph nodes, and the upper portion of the stomach, after which the remaining esophagus and stomach are reattached.

POSTOPERATIVE MANAGEMENT
Postoperative management for esophagectomy/gastrectomy includes the following:

- Monitor intubation and ventilation (increased risk for ARDS), encourage pulmonary hygiene, and monitor chest tubes (change in color or sudden increase in drainage could indicate leak; notify physician).
- Subcutaneous emphysema in the chest/neck could indicate a leak in the anastomosis and should be reported immediately.
- Manage pain, which is often severe; a PCA or epidural may be used initially.
- Hemodynamics: IV fluids, 100-200 mL/hr, bolus PRN; however, be cautious as there is an increased risk of pulmonary edema.
- Monitor the NG tube; **NEVER replace or irrigate the NG tube**, as it could damage the anastomosis. Notify MD if complications arise.
- Maintain NPO for 5-7 days; nutrition should be provided via J-tube or TPN.

- Drains: Penrose, Jackson-Pratt, possible drainage collection bag at the base of the cervical incision for saliva if >250 mL in 8 hr.
  NOTE: Patients often have history of alcohol abuse; observe for signs of DTs/withdrawal.
- Prior to initiating oral intake, a fluoroscopic examination with water-soluble contrast will be done to check for leaks. If no leaks, patients begin with clear liquids and progress to 6 to 8 small meals per day.

BARIATRIC GASTROINTESTINAL SURGERY

Bariatric surgery is used to promote weight loss in the morbidly obese (100 pounds over normal weight or BMI of 35-40). Surgery is done to restrict intake and/or prevent the absorption of calories. Procedures are open surgical or laparoscopic and include:

- **Banding** places a band around the upper portion of the stomach, creating a small pouch with a small distal opening to slow gastric emptying.
- **Sleeve gastrectomy** removes about 2/3 of the stomach, and a distal part of the small intestine is attached, bypassing part of the small intestine, reducing absorption.
- **Roux-en-Y** uses staples and a vertical band to decrease the size of the stomach, creating a small pouch. Then, a section of the small intestine is attached to the pouch, bypassing the first and second segments of the intestine to reduce absorption.
- **Gastric ballooning** places a balloon in the stomach and fills it with liquid to decrease stomach capacity; this is used primarily in Europe.

Nursing considerations: Use extreme caution with post-bariatric NG/PEG tubes – generally do not check placement/irrigate with normal amounts (risk of rupturing stomach); ensure patient maintains strict NPO. There is an increased risk of respiratory complications post-surgery.

INDWELLING FECAL MANAGEMENT SYSTEMS

Indwelling fecal management systems are used for incontinent clients with loose or watery stools in order to prevent skin breakdown, discomfort, odor, and contamination of wounds, and to control the spread of organisms, such as *Clostridium difficile,* in bedridden or immobile clients. A number of different devices, such as the Flexi-Seal FMS, are available and work similarly. A typical management system includes:

- A silicone catheter
- A silicone retention balloon at end of the catheter
- A 45-mL syringe
- Charcoal filter collection bags

The application of the fecal management system is relatively simple: The catheter is inserted into the rectum and the balloon is inflated with water or saline (using the 45-mL syringe) to hold it in place and to block fecal leakage. Some systems, such as Flexi-Seal FMS, have a pop-up button to indicate when the balloon is adequately filled for the size of the rectum. The catheter contains an irrigation port so that irrigating fluid can be instilled if necessary. The charcoal filter collection bag is attached to the end of the silicone catheter to contain fecal material.

Gastrointestinal Pharmacology

HISTAMINE RECEPTOR ANTAGONISTS

Histamine (H) receptor antagonists (actually reverse agonists) are used to treat conditions in which excessive stomach acid causes heartburn and GERD. They block histamine 2 (H_2) (parietal) cell receptors in the stomach, thereby decreasing acid production. These drugs are used less commonly now than proton-pump inhibitors. **Common H_2 antagonists** include:

- **Cimetidine (Tagamet)**: The first H_2 antagonist, it is used less frequently than others because of inhibition of enzymes that results in drug interactions, especially with contraceptive agents and estrogen.
- **Famotidine (Pepcid)**: This may be combined with an antacid to increase the speed of effects as it has a slow onset. It may be used pre-surgically to reduce post-operative nausea.
- **Nizatidine**: The last H_2 antagonist developed, it is used to treat ulcers and GERD. It is about equal in potency and action to ranitidine, which was discontinued due to the presence of NDMA, a cancer-causing contaminant, when stored in high temperatures.

ANTACIDS

Antacids are medications used to reduce stomach acids by raising the pH and neutralizing the acids present. They are commonly used to treat heartburn or indigestion. Adverse reactions are relatively rare unless taken to excess or with renal impairment. Drugs include:

- **Aluminum hydroxide** (Amphojel) may cause constipation and with renal impairment, hypophosphatemia and osteomalacia.
- **Magnesium hydroxide** (Milk of Magnesia) may cause diarrhea and with renal impairment can cause hypermagnesemia.
- **Aluminum hydroxide with magnesium hydroxide** (Maalox, Mylanta) may cause nausea, vomiting and diarrhea, yeast infection (thrush), or hypophosphatemia.
- **Calcium carbonate** (TUMS, Rolaids, Titralac) may cause gastric distention. Excess calcium intake may cause toxic reactions, including kidney stones and renal failure, so excess intake should be avoided.
- **Alka-Seltzer** combines sodium bicarbonate with aspirin and citric acid so this compound may cause gastric irritation, nausea and vomiting, and tarry stools.
- **Bismuth subsalicylate** (Pepto-Bismol). Pepto-Bismol may react with sulfur in the body to create a black tongue and black stools, but this is temporary. Pepto-Bismol has been associated with Reye's syndrome in children with influenza or chickenpox.

PROTON PUMP INHIBITORS

Proton pump inhibitors (PPIs) are now used more frequently than histamine receptor antagonists. PPIs interfere with an acid-producing enzyme in the stomach wall, reducing stomach acid. PPIs are used to treat GERD, stomach ulcers, and *H. pylori* (with antibiotics). PPIs are similar in action and include:

- Esomeprazole (Nexium)
- Lansoprazole (Prevacid)
- Omeprazole (Prilosec)
- Pantoprazole (Protonix)
- Rabeprazole (Aciphex)
- Omeprazole/sodium bicarbonate (Zegerid) (Long-acting form of omeprazole)

Common side effects include gastrointestinal upset (nausea, diarrhea, and constipation), headache, and rash. In rare instances, PPIs may cause severe muscle pain; however, they are usually well-tolerated with few adverse effects. PPIs may interfere with the absorption of some drugs, such as those that are affected by stomach acid. Absorption of ketoconazole is impaired, and absorption of digoxin is increased, sometimes leading to toxicity.

Omeprazole impacts the hepatic breakdown of drugs more than other PPIs and may cause increased levels of diazepam, phenytoin, and warfarin.

ANTI-LIPIDS

Anti-lipid medications are frequently used to **lower cholesterol levels** if dietary modifications are unsuccessful in order to decrease coronary artery disease. Four primary **types** of medications include the following:

- **Statins** (3-hydroxy-3-methylglutaryl coenzyme A reductase inhibitors), such as atorvastatin (Lipitor), rosuvastatin (Crestor), fluvastatin (Lescol), lovastatin (Altoprev), pravastatin (Pravachol), and simvastatin (Zocor), inhibit the liver enzyme that produces cholesterol, but different statins vary in the ability to reduce cholesterol and in drug/other interactions (protease inhibitors, erythromycin, grapefruit juice, niacin, and fibric acids). Adverse effects include rhabdomyolysis (which causes severe muscle pain and weakness), headache, rash, weakness, and gastrointestinal disorders.
- **Nicotinic acid** (Niacor, Niaspan) decreases synthesis of lipoprotein, lowers low-density lipoprotein (LDL) and triglycerides, and increases high-density lipoprotein (HDL). It is used for low elevations of cholesterol and may be combined with statins. Adverse effects include flushing, hyperglycemia, gout, upper gastrointestinal disorders, and hepatotoxicity. Liver function must be monitored.
- **Bile acid sequestrants,** such as cholestyramine (Questran, Prevalite), colesevelam (WelChol), and colestipol HCL (Colestid), decrease LDL, increase HDL, and do not affect triglyceride levels. They bind to bile acids in the intestines so that more are excreted in the stool rather than returned to the liver, so the liver has to produce bile acids by converting cholesterol. Adverse effects include gastrointestinal disorders and decrease in absorption of other drugs.

SEROTONIN ANTAGONISTS

Serotonin antagonists block 5-HT$_2$ receptors of serotonin in the central and peripheral nervous systems and gastrointestinal system. An open channel can result in agitation, nausea, and vomiting, but antagonists close the channel and reduce these symptoms. Serotonin antagonists are frequently used to prevent and treat nausea associated with chemotherapy and anesthesia. Medications include:

- **Metoclopramide** (Reglan) is used to reduce nausea and vomiting from a wide range of causes. It is also a prokinetic drug that increases gastrointestinal contractions and promotes faster gastric emptying, so it is used for heartburn, GERD, and diabetic gastroparesis.
- **Ondansetron** (Zofran) reduces vagal stimulation of the medulla oblongata (vomiting center) and is used for nausea related to chemotherapy.
- **Granisetron** (Sancuso) is used to reduce nausea related to chemotherapy, surgery, and radiation.

Serotonin antagonists have fewer side effects than other antiemetics, but they may cause muscle cramping, agitation, diarrhea/constipation, dizziness, and headache.

LAXATIVES

The following are different types of laxatives:

- **Bulk formers** have high fiber content and both soften stool and create more formed stools. These include products such as Metamucil, Citrucel, and FiberCon, which are usually added to liquids because without adequate fluids, they can increase constipation.
- **Lubricants** include both oral mineral oil and glycerin suppositories. They coat the stool, preventing fluid absorption and keeping the stool soft. Mineral oil absorbs fat soluble vitamins and should be used only temporarily

- **Saline**, such as Milk of Magnesia and Epsom Salt, contain ions, such as magnesium phosphate, magnesium hydroxide, and citrate, which are not absorbed through the intestines and draw more fluid into the stool. The magnesium in the preparations also stimulates the bowel. People with impairment of kidney function should avoid magnesium products, and saline laxatives should be used infrequently to avoid dependence. Epsom Salt often has a purging effect and is rarely used.
- **Stool softeners** (emollients, such as Colace, and Philip's Liqui-Gels) use wetting agents, such as docusate sodium, to increase liquid in the stool, thereby softening it. They should not be used with mineral oil because of increased absorption of the oil through the intestines.
- **Hyperosmotics** (available by prescription) contain materials that are not digestible and serve to retain fluid in the stool. Products, such as Kristalose and MiraLAX soften the stool but may result in increased Abdominal distension and flatus, especially initially. There are three types of hyperosmolar laxatives: lactulose, polymer, and saline. Lactulose types use a form of sugar and work similarly to saline laxatives, but more slowly, and may be used for long-term treatment. The salines empty the bowels quickly and are used short-term. The polymers contain polyethylene glycol, which retains fluid in the stool and is used short-term.
- **Combinations** use two or more types, such as stool softener with stimulant, and should be used only short-term.

STIMULANTS

Stimulants increase intestinal motility, moving the stool through the bowel faster and reducing the absorption of fluids so that the stool remains softer. Common ingredients include cascara in Castor oil and senna in Senokot. Stimulants work quickly and are effective but can result in electrolyte imbalance, Abdominal distension, and cramping. Chronic use may cause a cycle of constipation and diarrhea. Stimulant suppositories, such as Dulcolax, are also available.

> **Review Video: Gastroenterological Drugs**
> Visit mometrix.com/academy and enter code: 455152

Genitourinary Pathophysiology

URINARY INCONTINENCE

Urinary incontinence occurs more commonly in women than men and can range from an intermittent leaking of urine to a full loss of bladder control. Causes of urinary incontinence may include neurologic injury (including cerebral vascular accidents), infections, weakness of the muscles of the bladder, and certain medications, including diuretics, antihistamines, and antidepressants. **Stress incontinence** is defined as an involuntary leakage of urine with sneezing, coughing, laughing, lifting, or exercising. **Urge incontinence** is defined as an uncontrollable need to urinate on a frequent basis. **Total incontinence** is the full loss of bladder control.

Signs and symptoms: Urinary frequency and urgency may accompany the inability to control urine. If urinary incontinence is severe, incontinence-associated dermatitis may occur, predisposing the patient to skin breakdown and the development of pressure ulcers.

Diagnosis: Physical assessment and presence of symptoms. Ultrasound, urinalysis, urodynamic testing, and cystoscopy may be used to determine the underlying cause.

Treatment: Treatment options are dependent on the type of urinary incontinence and the severity. Bladder training and pelvic muscle exercises may be utilized to strengthen muscles to control leakage of urine. In female patients with stress incontinence, a vaginal pessary may be inserted into the vagina to help support the bladder. Suburethral slings may also be surgically implanted to support the urethra. Anticholinergics, antispasmodics, and tricyclic antidepressants may also be used in the treatment of urinary incontinence.

HYDRONEPHROSIS

Hydronephrosis is a symptom of a disease involving swelling of the kidney pelvises and calyces because of an obstruction that causes urine to be retained in the kidney. In chronic conditions, symptoms may be delayed until severe kidney damage has occurred. Over time, the kidney begins to atrophy. The primary conditions that predispose to hydronephrosis include:

- Vesicoureteral reflux
- Obstruction at the ureteropelvic junction
- Renal edema (non-obstructive)
- Any condition that impairs drainage of the ureters can cause backup of the urine

Symptoms vary widely depending upon cause and whether the condition is acute or chronic.

- Acute episodes are usually characterized by flank pain, abnormal creatinine and electrolyte levels, and increased pH.
- The enlarged kidney may be palpable as a soft mass.

Treatment includes:

- Identifying the cause of obstruction and correcting it to ensure adequate drainage.
- A nephrostomy tube, ureteral stent or pyeloplasty may be done surgically in some cases.
- A urinary catheter may be inserted if there is outflow obstruction from the bladder.

ACUTE TUBULAR NECROSIS

Acute tubular necrosis (ATN) occurs when a hypoxic condition causes renal ischemia that damages tubular cells of the glomeruli so they are unable to adequately filter the urine, leading to acute renal failure. Causes include hypotension, hyperbilirubinemia, sepsis, surgery (especially cardiac or vascular), and birth complications. ATN may result from nephrotoxic injury related to obstruction or drugs, such as chemotherapy, acyclovir, and antibiotics, such as sulfonamides and streptomycin. Symptoms may be non-specific initially and can include life-threatening complications.

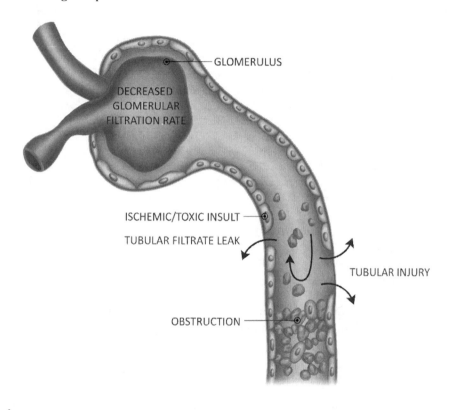

Symptoms include:

- Lethargy
- Nausea and vomiting
- Hypovolemia with low cardiac output and generalized vasodilation
- Fluid and electrolyte imbalance leading to hypertension, CNS abnormalities, metabolic acidosis, arrhythmias, edema, and congestive heart failure
- Uremia leading to destruction of platelets and bleeding, neurological deficits, and disseminated intravascular coagulopathy (DIC)
- Infections, including pericarditis and sepsis

Treatment includes:

- Identifying and treating underlying cause, discontinuing nephrotoxic agents
- Supportive care
- Loop diuretics (in some cases), such as Lasix
- Antibiotics for infection (can include pericarditis and sepsis)
- Kidney dialysis

ACUTE KIDNEY INJURY

Acute kidney injury (AKI), previously known as acute renal failure, is an acute disruption of kidney function that results in decreased renal perfusion, a decrease in glomerular filtration rate and a buildup of metabolic waste products (azotemia). Azotemia is the accumulation of urea, creatinine and other nitrogen containing end products into the bloodstream. The regulation of fluid volume, electrolyte balance and acid base balance is also affected. The causes of acute kidney injury are divided into pre-renal (caused by a decrease in perfusion), intrarenal or intrinsic (occurring within the kidney) and post-renal (caused by the inadequate drainage of urine). Acute kidney injury is common in hospitalized patients and even more common in critically ill patients, carrying a mortality rate of 50-80%. Risk factors for acute kidney injury include advanced age, the presence of co-morbid conditions, pre-existing kidney disease and a diagnosis of sepsis.

Signs and symptoms: Malaise, fatigue, lethargy, confusion, weakness, change in urine color, change in urine volume, and flank pain.

Diagnosis: Urinalysis, serum BUN and creatinine levels, renal ultrasound, CT or MRI and renal biopsy.

Treatment: The treatment of acute kidney injury is based on the underlying cause. Treatment options may include fluid and electrolyte replacement, diuretic therapy, fluid restriction, renal diet, and low dose dopamine to increase renal perfusion. Hemodialysis may also be necessary in patients with acute kidney injury.

RENAL AND URETERAL CALCULI

Renal and urinary calculi occur frequently, more commonly in males, and can relate to diseases (hyperparathyroidism, renal tubular acidosis, gout) and lifestyle factors, such as sedentary work. Calculi can form at any age, most composed of calcium, and can range in size from very tiny to larger than 6 mm. Those smaller than 4 mm can usually pass in the urine easily.

Diagnostic studies include clinical findings, UA, pregnancy test to rule out ectopic pregnancy, BUN and creatinine if indicated, ultrasound (for pregnant women and children), IV urography. Helical CT (non-contrast) is diagnostic.

Symptoms occur with obstruction and are usually of sudden onset and acute:

- Severe flank pain radiating to abdomen and ipsilateral testicle or labium majus, abdominal or pelvic pain (young children)
- Nausea and vomiting
- Diaphoresis
- Hematuria

Treatment includes:

- Instructions and equipment for straining urine
- Antibiotics if concurrent infection
- Extracorporeal shock-wave lithotripsy
- Surgical removal: percutaneous/standard nephrolithotomy
- Analgesia: opiates and NSAIDs

CHRONIC KIDNEY DISEASE

Chronic kidney disease (CKD) occurs when the kidneys are unable to filter and excrete wastes, concentrate urine, and maintain electrolyte balance because of hypoxic conditions, kidney disease, or obstruction in the urinary tract. It results first in azotemia (increase in nitrogenous waste in the blood) and then in uremia (nitrogenous wastes cause toxic symptoms). When >50% of the functional renal capacity is destroyed, the kidneys can no longer carry out necessary functions, and progressive deterioration begins over months or years. Symptoms are often non-specific in the beginning, with loss of appetite and energy.

Symptoms and complications are as follows:

- Weight loss
- Headaches, muscle cramping, general malaise
- Increased bruising and dry or itchy skin
- Increased BUN and creatinine
- Sodium and fluid retention with edema
- Hyperkalemia
- Metabolic acidosis
- Calcium and phosphorus depletion, resulting in altered bone metabolism, pain, and retarded growth
- Anemia with decreased production on RBCs. Increased risk of infection
- Uremic syndrome

Treatment includes:

- Supportive/symptomatic therapy
- Dialysis and transplantation
- Diet control: low protein, salt, potassium, and phosphorus
- Fluid limitations
- Calcium and vitamin supplementation
- Phosphate binders

UREMIC SYNDROME

Uremic syndrome is a number of disorders that can occur with end-stage renal disease and renal failure, usually after multiple metabolic failures and decrease in creatinine clearance to <10 mL/min. There is compromise of all normal functions of the kidney: fluid balance, electrolyte balance, acid-base homeostasis, hormone production, and elimination of wastes. Metabolic abnormalities related to uremia include:

- **Decreased RBC production**: The kidney is unable to produce adequate erythropoietin in the peritubular cells, resulting in anemia, which is usually normocytic and normochromic. Parathyroid hormone levels may increase, causing calcification of the bone marrow, causing hypoproliferative anemia as RBC production is suppressed.
- **Platelet abnormalities**: Decreased platelet count, increased turnover, and reduced adhesion leads to bleeding disorders.
- **Metabolic acidosis**: The tubular cells are unable to regulate acid-base metabolism, and phosphate, sulfuric, hippuric, and lactic acids increase, leading to congestive heart failure and weakness.
- **Hyperkalemia**: The nephrons cannot excrete adequate amounts of potassium. Some drugs, such as diuretics that spare potassium may aggravate the condition.
- **Renal bone disease**: Decreased calcium, elevated phosphate, elevated parathyroid hormone, decreased utilization of vitamin D lead to demineralization. In some cases, calcium and phosphate are deposited in other tissues (metastatic calcification).
- **Multiple endocrine disorders**: Thyroid hormone production is decreased and abnormalities in reproductive hormones may result in infertility/impotence. Males have decreased testosterone but elevated estrogen and LH. Females experience irregular cycles, lack of ovulation and menses. Insulin production may increase but with decreased clearance, resulting in episodes of hypoglycemia or decreased hyperglycemia in those who are diabetic.
- **Cardiovascular disorders**: Left ventricular hypertrophy is most common, but fluid retention may cause congestive heart failure and electrolyte imbalances, dysrhythmias. Pericarditis, exacerbation of valvular disorders, and pericardial effusions may occur.
- **Anorexia and malnutrition**: Nausea and poor appetite contribute to hypoalbuminemia, sometimes exacerbated by restrictive diets.

PYELONEPHRITIS

Pyelonephritis is a potentially organ-damaging bacterial infection of the parenchyma of the kidney. Pyelonephritis can result in abscess formation, sepsis, and kidney failure. Pyelonephritis is especially dangerous for those who are immunocompromised, pregnant, or diabetic. Most infections are caused by *Escherichia coli*. **Diagnostic studies** include urinalysis, blood and urine cultures. Patients may require hospitalization or careful follow-up.

Symptoms vary widely but can include:

- Dysuria and frequency, hematuria, flank and/or low back pain
- Fever and chills
- Costovertebral angle tenderness
- Change in feeding habits (infants)
- Change in mental status (geriatric)
- Young women often exhibit symptoms more associated with lower urinary infection, so the condition may be overlooked.

Treatment includes:

- Analgesia
- Antipyretics
- Intravenous fluids
- Antibiotics: started but may be changed based on cultures
    - IV ceftriaxone with fluoroquinolone orally for 14 days
    - Monitor BUN. Normal 7-8 mg/dL (8-20 mg/dL >age 60). Increase indicates impaired renal function, as urea is end product of protein metabolism.

CYSTITIS

Cystitis is a common and often-chronic low-grade kidney infection that develops over time, so observing for symptoms of urinary infections and treating promptly are very important.

Changes in **character of urine**:

- **Appearance**: The urine may become cloudy from mucus or purulent material. Hematuria may be present.
- **Color**: Urine usually becomes concentrated and may be dark yellow/orange or brownish in color.
- **Odor**: Urine may have a very strong or foul odor.
- **Output**: Urinary output may decrease markedly.

Pain: There may be lower back or flank pain from inflammation of the kidneys.

Systemic: Fever, chills, headache, and general malaise often accompany urine infections. Some people suffer a lack of appetite as well as nausea and vomiting. Fever usually indicates that the infection has affected the kidneys. Children may develop incontinence or loose stools and cry excessively.

Treatment:

- Increased fluid intake
- Antibiotics

NEPHROTOXIC AGENTS

Medications are a common cause of renal damage, especially among older patients. The **nephrotoxic effects** may be reversible if the drug is discontinued before permanent damage occurs. Those at increased risk include patients who are older than 60, have a history of renal insufficiency, suffer from volume depletion, or have diabetes mellitus, sepsis, or heart failure. Initial signs may be quite subtle. Preventive measures include baseline renal function tests and monitoring of renal function and vital signs during treatment. The following are some common effects, and the drugs that may cause them:

- **Chronic interstitial nephritis**: Acetaminophen, lithium, carmustine, cisplatin, cyclosporine.
- **Acute interstitial nephritis**: NSAIDs, acyclovir, beta-lactams, rifampin, quinolones, sulfonamides, vancomycin, indinavir, loop/thiazide diuretics, lansoprazole, allopurinol, phenytoin.
- **Rhabdomyolysis**: Amitriptyline, diphenhydramine, doxylamine, benzodiazepines, haloperidol, lithium, ketamine, methadone, methamphetamine, statins.
- **Crystal nephropathy**: Acyclovir, foscarnet, ganciclovir, quinolones, sulfonamides, indinavir, methotrexate, triamterene.
- **Tubular cell toxicity**: Aminoglycosides, amphotericin B, pentamidine, adefovir, tenofovir, contrast dye, zoledronate.
- **Thrombotic microangiopathy**: Cyclosporine, clopidogrel, mitomycin-C, quinine.
- **Impaired intraglomerular hemodynamics**: NSAIDs, cyclosporine, tacrolimus, ACE inhibitors.
- **Glomerulonephritis**: NSAIDs, lithium, beta-lactams, interferon-alpha, gold therapy, pamidronate.

PHIMOSIS AND PARAPHIMOSIS

Phimosis and paraphimosis are both restrictive disorders of the penis that occur in males who are uncircumcised or incorrectly circumcised. **Phimosis** is the inability to retract the foreskin proximal to the glans penis, sometimes resulting in urinary retention or hematuria. **Treatments** include:

- Dilating the foreskin with a hemostat (temporary solution)
- Circumcision
- Application of topical steroids (triamcinolone 0.025% twice daily) from end of foreskin to glans corona for 4-6 weeks

Paraphimosis occurs when the foreskin tightens above the glans penis and cannot be extended to normal positioning. This results in edema of the foreskin and circulatory impairment of the glans penis, sometimes progressing to gangrene, so immediate treatment is critical. Symptoms include pain, swelling, and inability to urinate. **Treatments** include:

- Compression of the glans to reduce edema (wrapping tightly with 2-inch elastic bandage for 5 minutes)
- Reducing edema by making several puncture wounds with 22- to 25-gauge needle
- Local anesthetic and dorsal incision to relieve pressure

TESTICULAR TORSION

Testicular torsion is a twisting of the spermatic cord within or below the inguinal canal, causing constriction of blood supply to the testis. Testicular torsion is most common at puberty but can occur at any age, sometimes precipitated by strenuous athletic participation or trauma, but it can also occur during sleep.

Symptoms include acute onset of severe testicular pain and edema, although children may present with nonspecific abdominal discomfort initially.

Diagnosis is based on clinical examination that demonstrates a firm scrotal mass. Color-flow duplex Doppler ultrasound may be helpful if diagnosis is not clear.

Treatment includes:

- **Manual detorsion** (usually 1.5 rotations) with elective surgical repair. Right testicle is usually rotated counterclockwise and left, clockwise. Reduction of pain should occur. If pain increases with rotation, then rotation should be done in the opposite direction.
- **Emergency surgical repair** (if manual detorsion not successful)

EPIDIDYMITIS AND ORCHITIS

Epididymitis, infection of the epididymis, is often associated with infection in a testis (epididymo-orchitis). In children, infection may be related to congenital anomalies that allow reflux of urine. In sexually active males 35 years or younger, it is usually related to STDs. In men older than 40, it is often related to urinary infections or benign prostatic hypertrophy with urethral obstruction.

Symptoms include progressive pain in lower abdomen, scrotum, and/or testicle. Late symptoms include large tender scrotal mass.

Diagnosis includes: Clinical examination. Pyuria. Urethral culture for STDs. Sonography.

Orchitis alone is rare but occurs with mumps, other viral infections, and epididymitis. Ultrasound may be needed to rule out testicular torsion.

Treatment for both conditions depends upon the cause, but epididymitis usually resolves with antibiotics:

- Younger than 40, associated with STDs:
  - Ceftriaxone 250 mg IM and doxycycline 100 mg twice daily for 10 days
- Older than 35, associated with other bacteria:
  - Ciprofloxacin 500 mg twice daily for 10-14 days
  - Levofloxacin 250 mg daily for 10-14 days
  - TMP/SMS DS twice daily for 10-14 days

PROSTATITIS

Prostatitis is an acute infection of the prostate gland, commonly caused by *Escherichia coli*, *Pseudomonas aeruginosa*, *Staphylococcus aureus*, or other bacteria. *Symptoms* include fever, chills, lower back pain, urinary frequency, dysuria, painful ejaculation, and perineal discomfort. PSA will often be elevated in this patient population, unrelated to prostate cancer. *Diagnosis* is based on clinical findings of perineal tenderness and spasm of rectal sphincter. *Treatments* include Ciprofloxacin 500 mg orally twice daily for 1 month **or** TMP/SMX DS twice daily for 1 month. Most patients also have a urethral culture to check for STDs. Patients with suspected bacteremia should be admitted for monitoring.

BENIGN PROSTATIC HYPERTROPHY

Benign prostatic hypertrophy/hyperplasia usually develops after age 40. The prostate may slowly enlarge, but the surrounding tissue restrains outward growth, so the gland compresses the urethra. The bladder wall also goes through changes, becoming thicker and irritated, so that it begins to spasm, causing frequent urinations. The bladder muscle eventually weakens and the bladder fails to empty completely.

Symptoms include urgency, dribbling, frequency, nocturia, incontinence, retention, and bladder distention.

Diagnosis may include IVP, cystogram, and PSA.

Treatment includes: Catheterization for urinary retention/bladder distention. Surgical excision. Avoid fluids close to bedtime, double void, avoid caffeine and alcohol, alpha-adrenergic antagonists, and 5-alpha-reductase inhibitors.

PID

Pelvic inflammatory disease (PID) comprises infections of the upper reproductive system, often ascending from vagina and cervix, and includes salpingitis, endometritis, tubo-ovarian abscess, peritonitis, and perihepatitis. *Neisseria gonorrhoeae* and *Chlamydia trachomatis* are implicated in most cases but some infections are polymicrobial. Complications include increase in ectopic pregnancy and tubal factor infertility. *Symptoms* include lower abdominal pain, vaginal pain, discharge, or bleeding, dyspareunia, dysuria, fever, and nausea and vomiting.

Diagnostic studies include:

- Pregnancy test
- Vaginal secretion testing, endocervical culture
- CBC
- Syphilis, HIV, and hepatitis testing
- Transvaginal pelvic ultrasound
- Endometrial biopsy
- Laparoscopy for definitive diagnosis

Treatments include:

- Broad spectrum antibiotics:
    - (Inpatient) Cefotetan 2 g IV every 12 hours or every 6 hours with doxycycline 100 mg every 12 hours
    - (Outpatient) Ceftriaxone 250 mg IM x 1 dose with doxycycline 100 mg orally every 12 hours for 14 days with metronidazole 500 mg twice daily for 2 weeks for patients who had gynecological procedures recently
- Laparoscopy to drain abscesses if symptoms do not improve in 72 hours or less
- Treatment specific to associated disorders (such as HIV or hepatitis)

VULVOVAGINITIS

Vulvovaginitis is inflammation of vulvar and vaginal tissues:

- **Bacterial vaginosis** (Gardnerella vaginalis or other bacteria)
- **Fungal infections** (usually Candida albicans)
- **Parasitic infections** (Trichomonas vaginalis)
- **Allergic contact vaginitis** (from soaps or other irritants)
- **Atrophic vaginitis** (postmenopause)

Symptoms include vaginal odor, swelling, discharge, or bleeding, pain and discomfort, or severe itching (common with *C. albicans*).

Diagnostic studies include:

- Physical exam and culture of discharge, pH testing with nitrazine paper: Greater than 4.5 is typical of bacterial and trichomonas infections. Less than 4.5 is typical of fungal infections.

Treatment includes:

- **Bacterial infections**: Metronidazole 500 mg orally twice daily for 7 days AND Metronidazole 0.75% gel intravaginally twice daily for 5 days AND Clindamycin 2% cream intravaginally at bedtime for 7 days

- **Fungal infections**: Fluconazole 150 mg tablet in 1 dose OR vaginal creams, tablets, or suppositories, such as butoconazole 2% cream for 3 days or tioconazole 6.5% ointment for 1 dose
- **Parasitic (trichomonas)**: Metronidazole 2 g orally in 1 dose

OVARIAN CYSTS

Ovarian cysts can grow within or on the ovaries. When a normal monthly follicle continues to grow, this is known as a functional cyst, of which there are two types:

- A follicular cyst begins when the follicle doesn't rupture or release its egg, but continues to grow.
- A corpus luteum cyst develops when fluid accumulates inside the follicle after it releases its egg.

Functional cysts are usually harmless, rarely cause pain, and often resolve on their own within 2-3 months. Other types of ovarian cyst include the following:

- **Cystadenomas** form on the exterior of an ovary and may enlarge and cause pain.
- **Endometriomas** develop as a result of endometriosis, where some of the tissue attaches to the ovary and causes pain during menses and sexual activity.
- **Dermoid cysts**, also called teratomas, can contain tissue, such as skin or teeth, because they from embryonic cells. They may enlarge and cause pain but are rarely cancerous.

Polycystic ovaries have multiple cysts. Ovarian cysts may cause problems if they rupture or hemorrhage and if they twist or become infected. Presenting symptoms include **hypotension** and **hypovolemia** if hemorrhage occurs, pain (often acute) and tenderness in the lower abdomen on the affected side, lower back pain, dysuria, and weight gain.

Diagnostic studies include a pregnancy test to rule out ectopic pregnancy, ultrasound with Doppler flow.

Treatment depends upon the type of cyst and complications:

- Emergency surgery for torsion
- Antibiotics for infection
- Hormone therapy may be useful for endometrioma

BARTHOLIN CYSTS

The Bartholin glands are small glands located on both sides of the vagina in the lips of the *labia minora*. The glands help to lubricate the vulvar area. A Bartholin cyst occurs when a duct to one gland becomes obstructed, usually because of infection or trauma, resulting in swelling and formation of a cyst (usually 1-3 cm but may be much larger with infection). Bartholin cyst is most common in women in their 20s. Blockage may result from tumors as well, but usually in women older than 40.

Symptoms of a Bartholin cyst include:

- Palpable mass on one side of the vagina (usually painless)
- Pain and tenderness and increasing size of lesion if infection and abscess occurs

Treatment includes:

- Warm, moist compresses or sitz baths
- Antibiotics for infection
- Surgical incision and drainage may be necessary in some cases

Genitourinary Procedures and Interventions

PROCEDURES FOR INSERTION AND REMOVAL OF URINARY CATHETER

Procedure for inserting and removing a urinary catheter:

1. Gather supplies (included in a urinary catheter insertion kit), perform hand hygiene, place a waterproof pad under the patient, and ensure that the light source is adequate to view the urinary meatus.
2. Place females in supine position with knees flexed and males in supine position.
3. Apply gloves and wash the perineal area with facility provided cleanser (sometimes included in the outside of the urinary catheter kit) and allow to dry.
4. Remove gloves and wash hands.
5. Using aseptic technique, place the catheter kit between the patient's legs, open the kit touching only the corners of the drape that wraps around the kit.
6. Apply sterile gloves.
7. Apply sterile drapes to the patient.
8. Following the steps provided with the kit, place the lubricant into the appropriate section of tray, remove the catheter from its plastic and place the tip into the lubricant, and pour iodine over the three cleansing swabs (if they do not come impregnated with iodine already). Attach the 10-cc syringe (filled with sterile water) to the appropriate port of the catheter.
9. Cleanse the urethral meatus with the iodine impregnated swabs.
10. Using the nondominant hand, hold the penis or open the labia to observe the urethral meatus. This hand now becomes "dirty" and cannot be used to touch the catheter.
11. Using the dominant hand, insert catheter with the drainage end attached to the collection bag. Insert until urine flows freely, advancing a little further after that point.
12. Inflate the balloon using the 10-cc sterile water syringe, and ensure the catheter is secure.
13. Secure the catheter to the patient's leg and hang the collection bag below the level of the patient. Secure any tubing to the bed and ensure no kinking is present.

Removal: Straight catheter—remove by pulling out slowly. To remove indwelling catheter, deflate the balloon using the appropriate port and gently pull the catheter out.

REDUCING INFECTION RISKS ASSOCIATED WITH URINARY CATHETERS

Strategies for reducing infection risks associated with urinary catheters include:

- Using **aseptic technique** for both the straight and indwelling catheter insertion
- **Limiting catheter use** by establishing protocols for use, duration, and removal; training staff; issuing reminders to physicians; using straight catheterizations rather than indwelling; using ultrasound to scan the bladder; and using condom catheters
- Utilizing **closed-drainage systems** for indwelling catheters
- **Avoiding irrigation** unless required for diagnosis or treatment
- Using **sampling port** for specimens rather than disconnecting catheter and tubing
- Maintaining **proper urinary flow** by proper positioning, securing of tubing and drainage bag, and keeping the drainage bag below the level of the bladder
- **Changing catheters** only when medically needed
- **Cleansing external meatal area** gently each day, manipulating the catheter as little as possible
- Avoiding placing catheterized patients adjacent to those infected or colonized with antibiotic-resistant bacteria to reduce **cross-contamination**

RENAL DIALYSIS

PERITONEAL DIALYSIS

Renal dialysis is used primarily for those who have progressed from renal insufficiency to uremia with end-stage renal disease (ESRD). It may also be temporarily for acute conditions. People can be maintained on dialysis, but there are many complications associated with dialysis, so many people are considered for renal transplantation. There are a number of different approaches to **peritoneal dialysis:**

- **Peritoneal dialysis:** An indwelling catheter is inserted surgically into the peritoneal cavity with a subcutaneous tunnel and a Dacron cuff to prevent infection. Sterile dialysate solution is slowly instilled through gravity, remains for a prescribed length of time, and is then drained and discarded.
- **Continuous ambulatory peritoneal dialysis:** a series of exchange cycles is repeated 24 hours a day.
- **Continuous cyclic peritoneal dialysis:** a prolonged period of retaining fluid occurs during the day with drainage at night.

Peritoneal dialysis may be used for those who want to be more independent, don't live near a dialysis center, or want fewer dietary restrictions.

HEMODIALYSIS

Hemodialysis, the most common type of dialysis, is used for both short-term dialysis and long-term for those with ESRD. Treatments are usually done three times weekly for 3-4 hours or daily dialysis with treatment either during the night or in short daily periods. **Hemodialysis** is often done for those who can't manage peritoneal dialysis or who live near a dialysis center, but it does interfere with work or school attendance and requires strict dietary and fluid restrictions between treatments. Short daily dialysis allows more independence, and increased costs may be offset by lower morbidity. A vascular access device, such as a catheter, fistula, or graft, must be established for hemodialysis, and heparin is used to prevent clotting. With hemodialysis, blood is circulated outside of the body through a dialyzer (a synthetic semipermeable membrane), which filters the blood. There are many different types of dialyzers. High flux dialyzers use a highly permeable membrane that shortens the duration of treatment and decreases the need for heparin.

DIALYSIS COMPLICATIONS

There are many complications associated with dialysis, especially when used for long-term treatment:

- **Hemodialysis:** Long-term use promotes atherosclerosis and cardiovascular disease. Anemia and fatigue are common, as are infections related to access devices or contamination of equipment. Some experience hypotension and muscle cramping during treatment. Dysrhythmias may occur. Some may exhibit dialysis disequilibrium from cerebral fluid shifts, causing headaches, nausea and vomiting, and alterations of consciousness.
- **Peritoneal dialysis:** Most complications are minor, but it can lead to peritonitis, which requires removal of the catheter if antibiotic therapy is not successful in clearing the infection within 4 days. There may be leakage of the dialysate around the catheter. Bleeding may occur, especially in females who are menstruating as blood is pulled from the uterus through the fallopian tubes. Abdominal hernias may occur with long use. Some may have anorexia from the feeling of fullness or a sweet taste in the mouth from the absorption of glucose.

CONTINUOUS RENAL REPLACEMENT THERAPY

Continuous renal replacement therapy (CRRT) circulates the blood by hydrostatic pressure through a semipermeable membrane. It is used in critical care and can be instituted quickly:

- **Continuous arteriovenous hemofiltration** (CAVH) circulates blood from an artery (usually the femoral) to a hemofilter using only arterial pressure and not a blood pump. The filtered blood is then returned to the patient's venous system, often with added fluids to offset those lost. Only the fluid is filtered.

- **Continuous arteriovenous hemodialysis** (CAVHD) is similar to CAVH except that dialysate circulates on one side of the semipermeable membrane to increase the clearance of urea.
- **Continuous venovenous hemofiltration** (CVVH) pumps blood through a double-lumen venous catheter to a hemofilter, which returns the blood to the patient in the same catheter. It provides continuous slow removal of fluid, is better tolerated with unstable patients, and doesn't require arterial access.
- **Continuous venovenous hemodialysis** is similar to CVVH but uses a dialysate to increase the clearance of uremic toxins.

BLADDER TRAINING

Bladder training usually requires the person to keep a toileting diary for at least three days so patterns can be assessed. There are a number of different approaches:

- **Scheduled toileting** is toileting on a regular schedule, usually every 2-4 hours during the daytime.
- **Habit training** involves an attempt to match the scheduled toileting to a person's individual voiding habits, based on the toileting diary. This is useful for people who have a natural and fairly consistent voiding pattern. Toileting is done every 2-4 hours.
- **Prompted voiding** is often used in nursing homes and attempts to teach people to assess their own incontinence status and prompts them to ask for toileting.
- **Bladder retraining** is a behavioral modification program that teaches people to inhibit the urge to urinate and to urinate according to an established schedule, restoring normal bladder function as much as possible. Bladder training can improve incontinence in 80% of cases.

PROMPTED VOIDING

Prompted voiding is a communication protocol for people with mild to moderate **cognitive impairment**. It uses positive reinforcement for recognizing being wet or dry, staying dry, urinating, and drinking liquids.

- Ask patient **every two hours** (8 a.m. to 4-8 p.m.) whether they are wet or dry.
- Verify if they are correct and give **feedback**, "You are right, Mrs. Brown, you are dry."
- **Prompt** patient, whether wet or dry, to use the toilet or urinal. If yes, assist them, record results, and give positive reinforcement by praising and visiting for a short time. If no, repeat the request again once or twice. If they are wet, and decline toileting, change and tell them you will return in two hours and ask them to try to wait to urinate until then.
- Offer **liquids** and record amount.
- **Record** results of each attempt to urinate or wet check.

BLADDER RETRAINING

Bladder retraining teaches people to control the urge to urinate. It usually takes about three months to rehabilitate a bladder muscle weakened from frequent urination, causing a decreased urinary capacity. A short urination interval is gradually lengthened to every 2-4 hours during the daytime as the person suppresses bladder urges and stays dry.

- The patient keeps a **urination diary** for a week.
- An individual program is established with **scheduled voiding times and goals**. For example, if a patient is urinating every hour, the goal might be every 80 minutes with increased output.
- The patient is taught **techniques** to withhold urination, such as sitting on a hard seat or on a tightly rolled towel to put pressure on pelvic floor muscles, doing five squeezes of pelvic floor muscles, deep breathing, and counting backward from 50.
- When the patient consistently meets the goal, a **new goal** is established.

THE KNACK TO CONTROL URINARY INCONTINENCE

The **knack** is the use of precisely timed muscle contractions to prevent **stress incontinence**. It is "the knack" of squeezing up before bearing down. The knack is a preventive use of **Kegel exercises**. Women are taught to contract the pelvic floor muscles right before and during events that usually cause stress incontinence. For example, if a woman feels a cough or sneeze coming, she immediately contracts the pelvic floor muscles and holds until the stress event is over. This contraction augments support of the proximal urethra, reducing the amount of displacement that usually takes place with compromised muscle support, thereby preventing incontinence. It is particularly useful if used before and during stress events, such as coughing, sneezing, lifting, standing, swinging a golf club, or laughing. Studies have shown that women who are taught this technique for mild to moderate urinary incontinence and use it consistently are able to decrease incontinence by 73-98%.

BOWEL TRAINING

Bowel training for defecation includes keeping a bowel diary to chart progress:

- **Scheduled defecation** is usually daily, but for some people 3-4 times weekly, depending on individual bowel habits. Defecation should be at the same time, so work hours and activities must be considered. Defecation is scheduled for 20-30 minutes after a meal when there is increased motility.
- **Stimulation** is necessary. Drinking a cup of hot liquid may work, but initially many require rectal stimulation, inserting a gloved, lubricated finger into the anus and running it around the rim of the sphincters. Some people require rectal suppositories, such as glycerine. Stimulus suppositories, such as Dulcolax (bisacodyl), or even Fleet enemas are sometimes used, but the goal is to reduce use of medical or chemical stimulants.
- **Position** should be sitting upright with knees elevated slightly if possible and leaning forward during defecation.
- **Straining** includes attempting to tighten abdominal muscles and relax sphincters while defecating.
- **Exercise** increases the motility of the bowel by stimulating muscle contractions. **Walking** is one of the best exercises for this purpose, and the person should try to walk 1 or 2 miles a day. If the person is unable to walk, then other activities, such as chair exercises that involve the arms and legs and bending can be very effective. Those who are bed bound need to turn from side to side frequently and change position.
- **Kegel exercises** increase strength of the pelvic floor muscles. Kegel exercises for urinary incontinence and fecal incontinence are essentially the same, but the person tries to pull in the muscles around the anus, as though trying to prevent the release of stool or flatus. The person should feel the muscles tightening while holding for 2 seconds and then relaxing for 2 seconds, gradually building the holding time to 10 seconds or more. Exercises should be done 4 times a day.

MANAGEMENT STRATEGIES FOR CONSTIPATION AND FECAL IMPACTION

Management strategies for constipation and impaction include:

- **Enemas** and **manual removal of impaction** may be necessary initially.
- Add **fiber** with bran, fresh/dried fruits, and whole grains, to 20-35 grams per day.
- Increase **fluids** to 64 ounces each day.
- **Exercise** program should include walking if possible, and exercises on a daily basis.
- Change in **medications** causing constipation can relieve constipation. Additionally, the use of stool softeners, such as Colace (docusate), or bulk formers, such as Metamucil (psyllium), may decrease fluid absorption and move stool through the colon more quickly. Overuse of laxatives can cause constipation.
- Careful **monitoring** of diet, fluids, and medical treatment, especially for irritable bowel syndrome.
- **Pregnancy-related constipation** may be controlled through dietary and fluid modifications and regular exercise.
- **Delayed toileting** should be avoided and bowel training regimen done to promote evacuation at the same time each day. During travel, stool softeners, increased fluid, and exercise may alleviate constipation.

PURPOSE OF FIBER IN THE DIET

Most constipation is caused by insufficient **fiber** in the diet, especially if people eat a lot of processed foods. An adequate amount of fiber is 20-30 grams daily. There are both soluble and insoluble forms of fiber, and both add bulk to the stool and are not absorbed into the body. Some foods have both types:

- **Soluble fiber** dissolves in liquids to form a gel-like substance, which is why liquids are so important in conjunction with fiber in the diet. Soluble fiber slows the movement of stool through the gastrointestinal system. Food sources include bananas, potatoes, dried beans, nuts, apples, oranges, and oatmeal.
- **Insoluble fiber** changes little with the digestive process and increases the speed of stool through the colon, so too much can result in diarrhea. Food sources of insoluble fiber include wheat bran, whole grains, seeds, skins of fruits, vegetables, and nuts.

Musculoskeletal Pathophysiology

IMMOBILITY

Critical care patients are often **immobile** for extended periods of time, thereby increasing their risk of skin breakdown and the development of pressure ulcers, deep vein thrombosis, functional decline, decreased muscle mass, impaired coordination and gait, cardiovascular deconditioning, depression, and constipation. Immobility leads to impaired physical functioning in which muscle mass is lost and weakness develops. Intensive care unit acquired weakness can develop during hospitalization and is associated with an increased hospital length of stay as well as an increased mortality rate. ICU acquired weakness may last years after discharge with residual effects often affecting the patient's quality of life. Progressive mobility is defined as the gradual progression of positioning and mobility techniques and should be utilized to improve muscle strength and provide the patient a greater ability to resume activities of daily living. Patients should be assessed daily for their readiness to progress in their mobility goals in order to prevent the adverse effects of immobility.

GAIT DISORDERS

Functional movement disorders are defined as an involuntary, abnormal movement of part of the body in which pathophysiology is not fully understood. Functional tremors are the most frequent type of functional movement disorder. Dystonia, myoclonus, and Parkinsonism are other types of functional movement disorders. Functional gait disorders are another type of functional movement disorder and are common in the elderly. Gait disorders can manifest as a dragging gait, knee buckling, small slow steps or "walking on ice," swaying gait, fluctuating gait, hesitant gait, and hyperkinetic gait in which there is excessive movement of the arms, trunk, and legs when ambulating. Patients with gait disorders are at an increased risk of falling. Gait disorders are diagnosed by a thorough clinical examination (including a neurologic assessment) and health history. Treatment for functional gait disorders includes strength and balance training. Assistive devices such as walkers and canes may also be utilized.

FALLS

Falls are the most commonly occurring adverse event in the hospital setting. Confusion and agitation are factors that contribute to an increased risk for falling. In addition, impaired balance or gait, orthostatic hypotension, altered mobility, a history of falling, advanced age and the use of certain medications are additional risk factors. Approximately 30% of patient falls result in injury, some of which can significantly contribute to an increase in morbidity and mortality including fractures and subdural hematomas. Both physical and environmental factors contribute to patient falls, some of which are preventable. Fall prevention strategies include utilization of a standardized fall risk assessment to determine the patient's level of risk and subsequent care planning and interventions individualized to the patient. Fall prevention should also be balanced with progressive mobility. Many falls are related to toileting needs, and nurses often utilize scheduled rounding to address such needs.

CARPAL TUNNEL SYNDROME

Carpal tunnel syndrome is a type of entrapment neuropathy in which the median nerve is compressed by thickening of the flexor tendon sheath, skeletal encroachment, or mass in the soft tissue. Carpal tunnel syndrome is often associated with repetitive hand activities, arthritis, hypothyroidism, diabetes, and pregnancy. Patients complain of pain in wrist, radiating to forearm, and numbness and tingling in the first 2 to 3 fingers, especially during the night.

Diagnosis is based on symptoms and tests such as:

- **Positive Tinel test**: Gentle percussion over medial nerve in inner aspect of wrist elicits numbness and pain.
- **Positive Phalen test**: The backs of the hands are pressed together and the wrists sharply flexed for 1 minute to elicit pain and numbness.

Treatment includes identifying and treating the underlying cause:

- Steroid injection may relieve symptoms
- Splint during the night or during repetitive activities
- Modification of activities
- Referral for decompression surgery in recalcitrant cases or those with severe loss of sensation

INFECTIOUS ARTHRITIS

Infectious arthritis may be bacterial, viral (rubella, parvovirus, and hepatitis B), parasitic, or fungal, with bacterial arthritis causing the most rapid destruction to the joint. *Neisseria gonorrhoeae* (most common), *Staphylococcus*, *Streptococcus*, and *Escherichia coli* are the most common bacterial agents. The infection may be bloodborne or spread from an infection near the joint or from direct implantation or postoperative contamination of the wound. Usually, the infection involves just one joint.

Symptoms include acute edema, erythema, and pain in a joint. Systemic reactions, such as fever and polyarthralgia, may occur, especially with gonorrhea.

Diagnosis requires a complete history and physical examination, arthrocentesis and synovial fluid culture, and WBC.

Treatment includes:

- Antibiotics as indicated by organism
- Arthrocentesis to drain fluid accumulation in joint (may need to be repeated)
- Analgesia

BURSITIS AND TENDINITIS

Bursitis is inflammation of the bursa, fluid-filled spaces or sacs that form in tissues to reduce friction, causing thickening of the lining of the bursal walls. This can be the result of infection, trauma, crystal deposits, or chronic friction from trauma.

Tendinitis is inflammation of the long, tubular tendons and tendon sheaths adjacent to the bursa. Causes of tendinitis are similar to bursitis but tendinitis may also be caused by quinolone antibiotics. Frequently, both bursa and tendons are inflamed. Common types of bursitis include shoulder, olecranon (elbow), trochanteric (hip), and prepatellar (front of knee). Common types of tendinitis include wrist, Achilles, patellar, and rotator cuff.

Symptoms include pain with movement, edema, dysfunction, and decreased range of motion.

Diagnosis is by clinical examination, although x-rays may rule out fractures. The bursa may be aspirated diagnostically to aid in ruling out other diagnosis, like gout or infection.

Treatment for bursitis and tendinitis includes:

- Rest and immobilization
- NSAIDs
- Application of cold packs to affected area
- Steroid injections

JOINT EFFUSION AND ARTHROCENTESIS

Joint effusion is the accumulation of fluid (clear, bloody, or purulent) within a joint capsule. Joint effusion can cause pressure on the joint and severe pain. Arthrocentesis relieves the pressure and the fluid aspirated can be examined to aid in diagnosis. Arthrocentesis is usually contraindicated in the presence of overlying infection, prosthetic joint, and coagulopathy without referral to an orthopedic specialist.

Procedure:

1. Patient is **positioned** according to joint to be aspirated and encouraged to relax muscles.
2. **Overlying area** is cleansed with povidone-iodine solution, air-dried a few minutes, and cleansed of iodine with alcohol wipe.
3. **Local anesthetic** is given to the area (but not into the joint) with 25- to 30-gauge needle (lidocaine 1-2%) or a regional nerve block for severe pain.
4. The joint is **aspirated** with insertion in a straight line, using a 30-60 mL syringe (depending upon expected amount of fluid) and an 18- to 22-gauge needle or IV catheter.
5. The joint is completely **drained** of fluid.
6. Observe for **complications**: bleeding, infection, or allergic reaction.

LUMBOSACRAL PAIN

Lumbosacral (low back) pain may be related to strain, muscular weakness, osteoarthritis, spinal stenosis, herniated disks, vertebral fractures, bony metastasis, infection, or other musculoskeletal disorders. Disk herniation or other joint changes put pressure on nerves leaving the spinal cord, causing pain to radiate along the nerve. Pain may be acute or chronic (more than 3 months).

Symptoms include local or pain radiating down the leg (radiculopathy), impaired gait and reflexes, difference in leg lengths, decreased motor strength, and alteration of sensation, including numbness.

Diagnosis is by careful clinical examination and history as well as x-ray (fractures, scoliosis, dislocations), CT (identifies underlying problems), MRI (spinal pathology), and/or EMG and nerve conduction studies. Diagnostic studies may be deferred in many cases for 4-6 weeks as symptoms may resolve over time.
Treatments for nonspecific back pain include:

- Analgesia: acetaminophen, NSAIDS, opiates
- Encourage activity to tolerance but not bed rest
- Muscle relaxants: diazepam 5-10 mg every 6-8 hours
- Cold and heat compresses

STRAINS AND SPRAINS

A **strain** is an overstretching of a part of the musculature ("pulled muscle") that causes microscopic tears in the muscle, usually resulting from excess stress or overuse of the muscle. Onset of pain is usually sudden with local tenderness on use of the muscle. A **sprain** is damage to a joint, with a partial rupture of the supporting ligaments, usually caused by wrenching or twisting that may occur with a fall. The rupture can damage blood vessels, resulting in edema, tenderness at the joint, and pain on movement with pain increasing over 2-3 hours after injury. An avulsion fracture (bone fragment pulled away by a ligament) may occur with strain, so x-rays rule out fractures.

Treatment for both strains and sprains includes:

- **RICE protocol**: rest, ice, compression, and elevation
- **Ice compresses** (wet or dry) applied 20-30 minutes intermittently for 48 hours and then intermittent heat 15-20 minutes 3-4 times daily
- Monitor **neurovascular status** (especially for sprain)
- **Immobilization** as indicated for sprains for 1-3 weeks

HIGH ENERGY JOINT INJURIES

Low energy injuries include those that occur as a result of a fall from standing position or less than one-meter height, but **high energy injuries** include those with greater impact, such as from an automobile accident, fall from greater height, and sports accidents (downhill skiing, ice hockey) as well as gunshot wounds, stab wounds, and blast injuries. High energy injuries are likely to be more severe and may include:

- Fractures, both open and closed
- Compression fractures
- Dislocations and fracture-dislocations
- Comminution
- Strains and sprains, injury to ligaments and tendons
- Lacerations, bleeding
- Soft tissue trauma, edema, and ecchymosis
- Shock

Patients typically have severe pain, and the affected joint may be very unstable with obvious misalignment if fractures or dislocations are present. Older adults are particularly at risk for fractures because of osteoporosis, and healing may be impaired because of chronic disease. With high energy injuries, patients also have greater risk of complications, such as fat embolism, hemorrhage, pulmonary embolism, compartment syndrome, infection, neurological damage, avascular necrosis, and mal-union, delayed union, or non-union.

FRACTURES AND DISLOCATIONS

TYPES OF FRACTURES

Fractures and dislocations usually occur as the result of trauma, such as from falls and auto accidents, but *pathologic* fractures can result from minor force to diseased bones such as those with osteoporosis or metastatic lesions. *Stress* fractures are caused by repetitive trauma, such as from forced marching. *Salter* fractures involve the cartilaginous epiphyseal plate near the ends of long bones in children who are growing. Damage to this area can impair bone growth. Orthopedic injuries that are of special concern include:

- **Open fractures** with soft tissue injury overlying the fracture, including puncture wounds from external forces or bone fragments, can result in osteomyelitis.
- **Subluxation, partial dislocation of a joint, and luxation** (complete dislocation) can cause neurovascular compromise, which can be permanent if reduction is delayed. Dislocation of the hip can result in avascular necrosis of the femoral head.

DIAGNOSIS AND TREATMENT

Fractures and dislocations are commonly **diagnosed** by clinical examination, history, and radiographs. Careful inspection and observation of range of motion, palpation, and observation of abnormalities is important because pain may be referred. Neurovascular assessment should be done immediately to prevent vascular compromise. Radiographs should usually precede reduction of dislocations to ensure there are no fractures and follow reduction to ensure the dislocation is reduced.

Treatment includes:

- Analgesia and sedation as indicated
- Application of cold compresses and elevation of fractured area to reduce edema
- Reduction of fracture: steady and gradual longitudinal traction to realign bone
- Immobilization with brace, cast, sling, or splint indicated
- Reduction of dislocation: Varies according to area of dislocation
- Open fracture: Wound irrigation with NS
- Tetanus prophylaxis

- Antibiotic prophylaxis
- Referral to orthopedic specialist for open fractures, irreducible dislocations, and complications such as compartment syndrome or circulatory impairment

PELVIC FRACTURES

Pelvic fractures may be fairly benign or seriously life threatening, depending on the degree and type of fracture. They most often result from high-speed trauma related to vehicular accidents or skiing accidents:

- **Open book**: Pelvis is pulled apart, usually from frontal injury (may cause severe hemorrhage)
- **Closed book**: Lateral compression occurs from side injury
- **Vertical shear**: Injury occurs from fall

Indications of pelvic fracture include localized edema, tenderness, obvious pelvic deformity, abnormal pelvic movement, and abdominal bruising. Associated intra-abdominal injuries and complications are common, including paralytic ileus, hemorrhage, urethral, colon, or bladder laceration. Patients may develop sepsis, peritonitis, fat embolism syndrome, or DVT. Displaced fractures may require open reduction and internal fixation. Treatment usually includes bedrest (up to 6 weeks) with care in handling to prevent further injury. Patients should be turned and moved in accordance with specific physician's orders. Ambulation using walker or crutches may be allowed for non-displaced fractures.

ACETABULAR FRACTURES

Acetabular (hip-socket) fractures occur primarily in young adults with motor vehicle accidents or falls from a height, resulting in impact pressure from the head of the femur to the joint and frequently associated (up to 50% of cases) with other severe injuries, including dislocation (which can lead to avascular necrosis if not promptly reduced). Up to 20% of those with acetabular fractures also have pelvic fractures. The degree of displacement that occurs depends on the amount of force as well as the position of the femur during impact. Acetabular fracture may be classified as posterior-wall, posterior-column, anterior-column, or transverse. Acetabular fractures in children less than 12 years may result in growth arrest. Complications may include sepsis, chondrolysis, and injury to vessels and/or nerves. Post-traumatic arthritis of the joint may develop. **Diagnosis** is per examination, radiograph, and/or CT with Doppler ultrasound with suspected DVT. Treatment includes emergent closed reduction if necessary, longitudinal skeletal traction, and open reduction and internal fixation (ORIF) for displaced fractures and serious injury (usually delayed for 2-3 days because of initial bleeding).

CLOSED FRACTURES AND OPEN FRACTURES

Closed fractures are those in which the damage to the bone and tissue (bleeding, swelling) remains enclosed within intact skin and does not invade any internal cavity. The bone segments are more likely to be aligned, although some comminution may have occurred from splintering when the bone breaks. It may be difficult to differentiate a closed fracture from an open fracture if there are abrasions and lacerations over the area of the fractures, but it is closed if there is no continuity between the fracture and the external injury.

Open fractures, on the other hand, cause an external wound and may result from fragments of the fractured bone penetrating the skin or an external force penetrating the skin and bone. Open fractures may also appear closed on the surface but invade a body cavity. Open fractures carry a much higher risk of contamination and infection as well as severe bleeding. The external wounds associated with open fractures may vary in size, but even small wounds are considered emergent because of risk of infection.

FAT EMBOLISM AS COMPLICATION OF TRAUMATIC FRACTURE

In instances of **traumatic fracture**, the possibility of **fat embolism** should be considered; this is especially true in fractures involving the long bones (femur, humerus). When the bone is fractured, this allows for some of the fatty marrow contained within the bone to escape. Because the fracture and subsequent trauma to the area surrounding the fracture results in broken vessels, it is possible that the fatty marrow can be introduced into the bloodstream. When this happens, the events are similar to that of a deep venous thrombosis; the fat embolus dislodges from the lumen of the vessel and travels to the lung. When the embolus enters the pulmonary circulation, it eventually blocks blood flow as the caliber of the vessel through which it travels decreases, keeping blood from flowing to the lung tissue. The disruption in blood flow results in inflammation and necrosis of the lung, and eventually pulmonary failure ensues.

Osteomyelitis

Musculoskeletal infections encompass a variety of different disorders with differing pathologies. Osteomyelitis, cellulitis, and septic arthritis are examples of musculoskeletal infections that can be both serious and debilitating in nature.

Osteomyelitis is an infection of the bone that can occur from an open fracture or an infection that has occurred somewhere else in the body. Osteomyelitis can also be caused by wounds or soft tissue infections that have progressed and extended to the bone. Signs and symptoms of osteomyelitis include pain, swelling, erythema and possible drainage at the site. The patient may also experience fever and chills. Diagnosis includes lab work including a complete blood count, erythrocyte sedimentation rate (ESR), C-reactive protein (CRP), and blood cultures, as well as radiologic testing that may include CT, MRI, x-ray, bone scan, or a bone biopsy. Treatment includes the administration of IV antibiotics. A needle aspiration may be performed to determine the organism and drain the area. Surgical irrigation and debridement may also be indicated.

Compartment Syndrome

Compartment syndrome occurs when there is an increase in the amount of pressure within a grouping of muscles, nerves, and blood vessels resulting in compromised blood flow to muscles and nerves. This is a medical emergency. If left untreated, tissue ischemia and eventual tissue death will occur. **Compartment syndrome** most often occurs after a fracture, particularly a long bone fracture, but can also occur with crushing syndrome and rhabdomyolysis. Risk factors include lower extremity trauma, massive tissue injury, venous obstruction, the use of certain medications (anticoagulants), burns and compressive dressings or casts. Compartment syndrome can affect the hand, forearm, upper arm, abdomen, and lower extremities. It can be acute or chronic in nature with acute compartment syndrome requiring immediate intervention.

Signs and symptoms: Intense pain, decreased sensation and paresthesia, firmness at the affected site, swelling and tightness at the affected site, pallor and pulselessness (late signs).

Diagnosis: Physical assessment and the measurement of intra-compartmental pressures.

Treatment: The goal of treatment in compartment syndrome is decompression and the restoration of perfusion to the affected area. Surgical fasciotomy is often indicated to relieve pressure and prevent tissue death. Fasciotomy involves the opening of the skin and muscle fascia to release the pressure within the compartment and restore blood flow to the area.

Prevention: Leave large abdominal wounds open to drain, delay casting on affected extremities, and use flexible casts. Watch circumferential burns closely and perform frequent neurovascular checks on those at risk.

Rhabdomyolysis

Rhabdomyolysis occurs when damage of the cells of the skeletal muscles causes the release of toxins from injured cells into the bloodstream. Rhabdomyolysis may be caused by trauma, tissue ischemia, infection, certain medications (statins, selective serotonin reuptake inhibitors, lithium, and antihistamines), sepsis, immobilization, extraordinary physical exertion, myopathies and cocaine or alcohol abuse. Additionally, rhabdomyolysis may occur with exposure to certain toxins such as snake/insect venoms or mushroom poisoning. In rare circumstances, the identifiable cause cannot be determined. The most serious complication of rhabdomyolysis is renal failure. Rhabdomyolysis may be life threatening. Early recognition and treatment are critical to avoid serious complications and for patients to make a full recovery.

Signs and symptoms: Electrolyte imbalance, muscle pain and weakness, fever, tachycardia, dehydration, fatigue, lethargy, hypotension, and metabolic acidosis. Dark, reddish-brown urine may occur due to the presence of myoglobin released from the muscles and excreted into the urine.

Diagnosis: Laboratory studies such as creatinine kinase (CK) level, metabolic panel, urinalysis, and blood gases.

Treatment: The treatment of rhabdomyolysis includes fluid administration to eliminate toxins and prevent renal failure. Bicarbonate may be administered to correct metabolic acidosis. Mannitol or dopamine may be administered to increase renal perfusion. Electrolyte replacement may also be indicated. In severe cases, emergency dialysis may be necessary.

Musculoskeletal Procedures and Interventions

MONITORING DEVICES FOR EXTREMITY COMPARTMENT SYNDROME

Signs of extremity compartment syndrome include the 5 P's:

- Pain that is severe and out of proportion to injury
- Paresthesia
- Pallor
- Paresis
- Pulse deficit

Pressure is typically measured with a device specially intended for measurement although it can also be measured by attaching a manometer to a needle and syringe. The procedure with the **Stryker intercompartmental pressure monitor device** includes:

- First, the skin is cleansed with antiseptic and a local anesthetic administered.
- The pressure monitor device (or similar) contains a 3 mL syringe, a chamber and needle that connect to the syringe, and a pressure monitor into which the syringe is placed.
- Air is purged from the chamber and needle with the saline.
- The syringe is placed into the pressure monitoring device.
- The device is turned on, zeroed automatically by pressing the "zero" button.
- The needle is inserted into the compartment.
- Once the needle is inserted, about 0.3 mL of NS is injected and the device automatically records the compartment pressure. If the compartment pressure is over 30 mmHg, a fasciotomy is usually needed.

PELVIC STABILIZER

Pelvic stabilizers are used to prevent excessive bleeding associated with pelvic fractures, to maintain the bones in the correct position, and to prevent further damage. Maintaining pressure and reducing the fracture often reduces bleeding. Various methods of stabilizing the pelvis may be employed, including the sheet wrap method in which a sheet is folded, center under the patient, wrapped tightly about the pelvis, and secured. The pneumatic anti-shock garment (PASG) is indicated for hypovolemic shock, and hypotension associated with and for stabilization of pelvic and bilateral femur fractures. PASG is contraindicated with respiratory distress, pulmonary edema, pregnancy (after the first trimester), heart failure, myocardial infarction, stroke, evisceration, abdominal or leg impalement, head injuries, and uncontrolled bleeding above the garment. Another device is the SAM pelvic sling, which has a wide band that fits under and about the pelvis and lateral hips and a belt anteriorly that allows adjustment.

IMMOBILIZATION DEVICES

Immobilization devices include:

- **Cervical collar**: Support the head to prevent spinal cord injury with suspected injury to cervical vertebrae.
- **Cervical extrication splints**: Short board used to immobilize and protect the head and neck during extrication.
- **Backboards**: Used to immobilize the spine to prevent further injury to spinal cord. Both long and short spine boards are available in a number of different shapes and sizes.
- **Full-body splints** (such as vacuum mattress splint): Provide cushioned support to maintain body alignment.
- **Various types of splints for extremities**: Include rigid (should be padded), non-rigid (moldable), traction, and air (pneumatic devices) as well as the use of blankets, rolled towels, sheets, and pillows to maintain position. Traction splints are used for fractured femurs to keep bones in position.

- **Pneumatic anti-shock garment** (PASG): Provides pressure on lower extremities and abdomen and is used to control hemorrhage and shock to prevent pooling of blood in extremities and return blood to general circulation. Often used for pelvic fractures, but may increase risk of internal hemorrhage.

SPINAL IMMOBILIZATION

Spinal immobilization, once a standard for trauma patients, has been shown to have little effect and in some cases may cause harm. Because of these findings, spinal immobilization with backboard is now recommended only for patients with neurological complaints, such as numbness, tingling, weakness, paralysis, pain or tenderness in the spine, spinal deformity, blunt trauma associated with alterations of consciousness, and high energy injuries associated with drugs/alcohol, inability of the patient to communicate, and/or distracting injury. Cervical collars for cervical spine immobilization are to be utilized for trauma based on the NEXUS criteria or Canadian C-spine rules (CCR). According to **NEXUS criteria**, a patient who exhibits all of the following does not require a cervical collar:

- Alert and stable
- No intoxication
- No midline tenderness of the spine
- No distracting injury
- No neurological deficit

Spinal immobilization should be continued for the shortest time possible, so imaging, such as CT, should be carried out upon admission. Cervical collars are applied while the head is supported in neutral position, and the patient is logrolled onto a backboard and strapped in place.

IMMOBILIZATION OF FRACTURES AND DISLOCATIONS

Immobilization techniques for fractures and dislocations include:

- **Cast**: Plaster and fiberglass casts are applied after reduction to ensure that the bone is correctly aligned. Cast should be placed over several layers of padding that extends slightly beyond the cast ends. Cast material, such as plaster, should NOT be immersed in hot water but water slightly above room temperature (70 °F).
- **Splint**: Plaster splints use 12 or more layers of plaster measured to the correct length and then several layers of padding (longer and wider than splint should be measured and cut). The plaster splint is submerged in water to saturate, removed, laid on a flat surface, and massaged to fuse the layers. The padding is laid on top, and the splint is positioned and wrapped with gauze to hold it in place. While setting the splint, position can be maintained by holding it in place with the palm of the hand (not the fingers). After setting, the splint may be wrapped by elastic compression bandages.

AMPUTATION CARE

IMMEDIATE INTERVENTIONS FOR TRAUMATIC AMPUTATION

Amputations may be partial or complete. The amputated limb should be treated initially as though it could be reattached or revascularized. Single digits, except the thumb, are often not reattached. Initial treatment includes stabilizing patient and stopping bleeding by applying a proximal blood pressure cuff proximal to injury 30 mmHg above systolic for <30 minutes. Instruments, such as clamps and hemostats, should be avoided. Other treatment includes:

- Tetanus prophylaxis
- Analgesia
- Prophylactic antibiotics may be needed
- Irrigation of stump with NS (not antiseptics) if contaminated
- Splint and elevate stump, with saline-moistened sterile dressing in place
- Neurovascular examinations of stump

The Allen test should be done to determine arterial injury if digits are amputated. In the Allen test, both the radial and ulnar artery are compressed and the patient is asked to clench the hand repeatedly until it blanches, and then one artery is released, and the tissue on that side should flush. Then the test is repeated again, releasing the other artery.

CARE OF AMPUTATED PART PRIOR TO REATTACHMENT OR REVASCULARIZATION

The amputated part should be cooled to 4 °C to extend the time of viability and decrease damage from ischemia. (Single digits and lower limbs are not usually reattached, but the limbs should be treated as though they will until determination is made, especially for children.) The part should be reattached within 6 hours if possible but up to 24 hours if properly cooled. **Initial care of amputated part** includes:

- Removal of jewelry
- Irrigation with NS to remove debris or contamination
- Part stored wrapped in saline moistened dressing but NOT immersed in saline or hypotonic solution
- Minimal handling to prevent tissue damage
- Cool by placing wrapped part in sealed plastic bag and immersing the bag in ice water (1:1 ice to water), but avoid freezing the part

If the amputation is partial, treatment is similar but NS wrapped part is splinted and ice packs or commercial cold packs are applied over area that is devascularized.

TOURNIQUETS

Tourniquets are used to control hemorrhage in an extremity and should be applied immediately with arterial bleeds or if pressure does not stop bleeding. Commonly used **tourniquets** include adjustable bands that are tightened and secured and then include a windlass handle twisted until blood flow stops and the handle is secured. Another type is a wide elastic band that is stretched, wrapped about the extremity tightly a number of times and secured. Blood pressure cuffs may also be used to apply pressure if standard tourniquets are not available. Regardless of the type, the tourniquet should be placed as high on the extremity as possible (avoiding joints), and the date and time of placement should be documented (on the tourniquet if possible). Tourniquets may be contraindicated with DVT, Reynaud's disease, crushing injuries, sickle cell disease, severe peripheral arterial disease, and open lower extremity fractures. Risks include damage to muscles, nerves, and vessels as well as increased risk of amputation. However, the first priority is always to prevent exsanguination.

TEACHING PATIENTS HOW TO WALK WITH CRUTCHES

Crutches should be properly fitted before a patient attempts ambulation. Correct height is one hand-width below axillae. The handgrips should be adjusted so the patient supports the body weight comfortably with elbows slightly flexed rather than locked in place. The patient should be cautioned not to bear weight under the axillae as this can cause nerve damage but to hold the crutches tightly against the side of the chest wall. The type of gait that the patient uses depends on the type of injury. Typical gaits include:

- **Two-point** in which each crutch is advanced in tandem with the opposite side leg (i.e., the left crutch is advanced at the same time as the right leg, and the right crutch is advanced at the same time as the left leg).
- **Three-point** in which the injured extremity and both crutches are advanced together and then the well leg advances to (or past) the crutches.
- **Four-point** in which the injured side crutch is advanced, followed by the non-injured leg, followed by the non-injured side crutch, followed by the injured leg.

The patient should be advised whether there is partial or no weightbearing and a demonstration should be provided. Stair climbing should be practiced:

- **Ascending**: well foot goes first and then crutches and injured extremity.
- **Descending**: crutches go first and then the well foot.

Functional Status and Rehabilitation

ADLs

Activities of daily living (ADLs) are a group of activities that are used to evaluate a patient's return to normal function; these are activities that the patient had performed on a daily basis before hospitalization, and will be expected to perform once he or she has completed rehabilitation. The **rate** at which the patient accomplishes these activities, in addition to the **level of independence** maintained by the patient when performing the activities, can help caregivers determine the amount of rehabilitation required, and can also be used to monitor the progress of the patient during the rehabilitation process. ADLs are grouped into 3 different areas: **personal or physical**, **instrumental**, and **occupational**.

Grouping ADLs

The first group of ADLs, the **physical or personal group**, contains those daily activities that relate to the patient's ability to take care of him or herself. Included in this group are activities related to health management, nutritional needs, elimination of bladder and bowel contents, exercise, self-esteem, coping/stress management, cognitive abilities, communication, sexual health and ability, and relationship roles. The second group of ADLs, the **instrumental group**, contains activities such as shopping, answering the phone, and other activities that involve leaving home. The third group, **occupational activities**, includes activities that are required of being a parent, husband, or wife, as well as those required on the job.

Rehabilitation

Rehabilitation is an area of health care that is dedicated to helping patients improve and/or restore functions and abilities after a disease or injury. Although rehabilitation is usually thought of in relation to **physical therapy** (which is one of the many areas of rehabilitation), it also encompasses **drug and alcohol rehabilitation**, as well as **occupational therapy** for physically and mentally ill patients. The general goals of all types of rehabilitation include an improvement in overall function; the promotion of independence, satisfaction, and well-being; and the preservation of the individual's self-esteem in the face of illness or debilitating disease or injury.

Assessing Potential for Rehabilitation

There are various factors that are considered when assessing a patient to determine whether he or she will benefit from **rehabilitation**. A patient with the inability to perform any of the ADLs will automatically be considered for rehabilitation. At this point, however, other factors must be considered. First and foremost is whether or not the patient has a **desire to improve his or her functions** through rehabilitation; if the patient is not interested in improvement, the rehabilitation potential is poor. If the patient wants to improve function and increase independence, the potential for rehabilitation is greater. Another factor is whether or not the patient has **support at home**; even if the patient improves greatly during his or her rehabilitation stay, he or she will still most likely need some support at home. If the patient has no support at home, rehabilitation may eventually fail.

Diseases and Illnesses That Commonly Require Rehabilitation

There are some diseases, illnesses, and injuries that almost always require rehabilitation at some point during their course; in these cases, rehabilitation may be initiated before the patient even leaves the hospital to be transferred to a rehabilitation facility. It is important to know which diseases usually require rehabilitation, because the sooner evaluation and rehabilitation are initiated, the better the patient's chance of recovery. The following are diseases, illnesses, and injuries that **commonly require rehabilitation**: AIDS, amyotrophic lateral sclerosis (ALS), limb amputation, traumatic or ischemic brain injury, spinal cord injury, burns, Guillain-Barré syndrome, hip or knee replacement, multiple sclerosis (MS), and most types of cancer.

REHABILITATION SETTINGS

There are various kinds of rehabilitation settings, depending on the needs of the patient. Once the need for rehabilitation has been determined and the patient has been evaluated regarding specific rehabilitation needs, he or she can be placed in an appropriate rehabilitation setting. A **long-term acute care hospital** is a rehabilitation facility that is best for patients who are physically and psychologically stable but are receiving medical treatment such as dialysis or ventilation and thus require medical support. A **subacute care unit** is appropriate for patients who require more limited treatment, such as cancer patients. A **comprehensive inpatient rehabilitation facility** is just what the name suggests; it addresses the needs of a broad range of different patients, from burn victims to amputees. The comprehensive rehabilitation center has a "team" of medical specialists that includes a rehabilitation medicine physician, nurses trained in rehabilitation, occupational therapists, physical therapists, social workers, and speech-language pathologists. **Outpatient rehab** is designed for the high-functioning patient who can return home after rehab sessions.

INTERVENTIONS TO CONSIDER WHEN BEGINNING REHABILITATION PROCESS

When a patient is to be considered for rehabilitation, he or she must undergo a rather extensive **evaluation** in order to increase the likelihood that he or she will succeed during rehabilitation. This process of evaluation, which includes various interventions, should take place in the early stages of illness, when the patient is still in the hospital. The goal is to forestall any **secondary complications** that may inhibit the rehabilitation process. These **interventions** include health management, in which the patient and family are educated about his or her disease(s); nutritional status assessment and support; initiation of bowel and bladder management in order to prevent infection; exercises; assessment of cognitive function; and education involving self-esteem, relationship roles, sexual activity, and coping mechanisms.

OCCUPATIONAL THERAPY

Occupational therapy is defined as the use of creative activities in the treatment of disabled individuals, whether they are disabled physically or mentally. The purpose of occupational therapy is to provide disabled individuals with the skills that are necessary to live life as fully and independently as possible; after completion of occupational therapy, the individual should be able to perform at his or her **maximum potential**. The occupational therapist will typically provide the patient with **interventions** tailored to his or her disability. The OT will also visit the patient's home and/or place of employment in order to assess potential problems and provide **adaptive solutions**. As part of occupational therapy, the patient will receive regular **assessments** of his or her skills, as well as specific training. The occupational therapist is also responsible for educating the patient's family, caretakers, friends, and coworkers.

The philosophy of occupational therapy is based on the idea that **occupation** (meaning, loosely, either an activity or activities in which an individual engages) is a **basic human need**, one that is important to an individual's health and overall well-being in that it is in and of itself therapeutic in nature. The basic assumptions of occupational therapy are based on the idea of occupational therapy as stated by its creator, **William Rush Dunton**. Dunton states that occupational therapy is a human need because an individual's occupation has an effect on his or her health and general well-being. It creates **structure** in the individual's life and allows for him or her to manage and organize time. Another assumption is that individuals have different sets of values and, therefore, will value different occupations; for each person, however, the occupation that he or she chooses is meaningful to him or her.

AREAS IN WHICH OCCUPATIONAL THERAPY MAY BE INSTITUTED AND PRACTICED

Although occupational therapy is an important part of the overall rehabilitation process for hospitalized individuals, it is also beneficial in other areas because occupational therapy deals not only with physical disabilities but with **emotional and cognitive disabilities** as well. Occupational therapy as related to **physical disabilities** may be practiced in outpatient clinics, pediatric hospitals or units, acute care rehabilitation facilities, and long-term, or comprehensive, inpatient rehabilitation centers. Occupational therapy as related to **mental disabilities** may be practiced in mental health clinics, acute and long-term psychiatric hospitals, prisons, and gateway or halfway houses. Occupational therapists may also work at schools, childcare facilities, workplaces, or shelters, or they may even work with individuals in their own homes.

ASSISTIVE DEVICES

Crutches should be properly fitted before client attempts ambulation. Correct height is one hand-width below axillae. The handgrips should be adjusted so the client supports the body weight comfortably with elbows slightly flexed rather than locked in place. The client should be cautioned not to bear weight under the axillae as this can cause nerve damage but to hold the crutches tight against the side of the chest wall. The type of gait used depends on the type of injury.

A **cane** should be held in the opposite hand of the side of injury. When holding the cane in neutral position, the elbow should be bent at about a 15-degree angle and if holding the cane straight down to the side of the body, the top of the cane should be in line with the crease of the wrist.

The same is true of a **walker**, the elbow should be bent at 15 degrees when standing up straight and grasping the handles, and the handle grasps should be in line with to the crease of the wrists. The client should be able to move the walker forward without leaning over.

Integumentary Pathophysiology

CELLULITIS

Cellulitis occurs when an area of the skin becomes infected, usually following injury or trauma to the skin. Cellulitis is most likely to be caused by staphylococcus or streptococcus bacteria. Patients with peripheral vascular disease, diabetes mellitus, and immunosuppression are at a higher risk for the development of cellulitis. **Signs and symptoms** include pain, erythema, and warmth at the affected site that progresses rapidly. In addition, the patient may experience fever, chills, fatigue, and malaise. **Diagnosis** is made by physical exam. Labs include complete blood count, culture of the involved area and blood. **Treatment** for cellulitis is the administration of antibiotics. Surgical irrigation and debridement may be indicated in severe cases.

EXTRAVASATION

Extravasation occurs when an intravenously infused vesicant medication or fluid leaks from the vein and into the subcutaneous space. Vesicant medications are those that cause tissue injury if extravasated and that may ultimately lead to tissue necrosis. Extravasation and infiltration are similar in nature, with infiltration occurring when the infusate is a non-vesicant solution or medication. Extravasation occurs more commonly in peripheral IVs; however, it can also occur with central venous catheters. Common vesicant agents include several chemotherapeutic agents, vancomycin, electrolytes, dobutamine, norepinephrine, phenytoin, promethazine, propofol, and vasopressin.

Signs and symptoms: Pain, burning, erythema, and edema at the site of the extravasation. Oftentimes, a blood return from the peripheral IV or central venous catheter is not present. Long term complications include complex regional pain syndrome, tissue necrosis, and nerve or tendon damage.

Diagnosis: Physical assessment and review of patient symptoms and medications/infusions administered.

Treatment: Early recognition is key to the successful treatment of an extravasation. When an extravasation is suspected, the IV infusion should be immediately stopped and the infusion site assessed. For some medications, antidotes may be available to minimize the damage caused by the extravasation. Heat or cold therapy may also be utilized depending on the medication. In cases of severe damage, debridement, skin grafting, and even amputation may result.

SEPTIC ARTHRITIS

Septic arthritis is defined as an invasion of the joint space by bacteria, virus, or fungi. Elderly patients, immunosuppressed patients, and those with prosthetic joints are at an increased risk for septic arthritis. The most commonly affected joints include the knee, hip, shoulder, ankle, and wrist. **Signs and symptoms** include joint pain, fever, impaired range of motion, chills, edema, erythema, warmth, and the abnormal presence of fluid (effusion) surrounding the joint. **Diagnosis** is made by aspiration of the fluid with stain and culture, x-ray, and blood tests including CBC and cultures. **Treatment** is the administration of antibiotics. Surgical irrigation and debridement may also be indicated. The patient will likely undergo physical therapy as part of their recovery to improve and restore mobility and range of motion.

TISSUE DAMAGE RELATED TO ALLERGIC CONTACT DERMATITIS

Contact dermatitis is a localized response to contact with an allergen, resulting in a rash that may blister and itch. Common allergens include poison oak, poison ivy, latex, benzocaine, nickel, and preservatives, but there is a wide range of items, preparations, and products to which people may react.

Treatment includes:

- Identifying the causative agent through evaluating the area of the body affected, careful history, or skin patch testing to determine allergic responses
- Corticosteroids to control inflammation and itching
- Soothing oatmeal baths
- Pramoxine lotion to relieve itching
- Antihistamines to reduce allergic response
- Lesions should be gently cleansed and observed for signs of secondary infection
- Antibiotics are used only for secondary infections as indicated
- Rash is usually left open to dry
- Avoidance of allergen to prevent recurrence

PRESSURE ULCERS

Pressure ulcers occur when pressure from the weight of the body causes a decrease in perfusion, affecting arterial and capillary blood flow and resulting in ischemia. Ulcers may then develop from pressure, shearing, and friction. Common pressure points include the occiput, scapula, sacrum, buttocks, ischium, and heels. Patients with a decreased level of consciousness, brain/spinal cord injuries, peripheral neuropathies, malnutrition, dehydration, PVD, or impaired mobility are at a higher risk for pressure ulcers. Critically ill patients are at an increased risk due to prolonged immobility, sedation, and often incontinence of urine and stool. In addition, patients on vasopressors are at a higher risk due to the constriction of the peripheral circulation.

Signs and symptoms: Early stages include redness, tenderness, and firmness at the site of the ulcer. Once the ulcer progresses to severe tissue injury, bone, muscle, or tendons may be exposed, and there may be a yellow or black wound base in addition to pain and drainage at the site.

Diagnostics: Skin and wound assessment, including staging of the ulcer.

Treatment: Wet-to-Dry dressings, Wound VAC therapy, and hyperbaric oxygen may be used; a wound care consult is often advised.

Prevention: Begins with a risk assessment; the Braden scale is a commonly used scale. A score of 16 or below indicates that the patient is at risk. At-risk patients or patients with active ulcers should be placed on a turning and positioning schedule or on a specialty bed to relieve pressure. Moisture barriers and skin protectants may also be utilized.

NATIONAL PRESSURE INJURY ADVISORY PANEL STAGING

Pressure ulcers result from pressure or pressure with shear and/or friction over bony prominences. The **National Pressure Injury Advisory Panel (NPIAP) stages** include:

- **Suspected deep tissue injury**: Skin discolored, intact or blood blister
- **Stage I**: Intact skin with non-blanching reddened area
- **Stage II**: Abrasion or blistered area without slough but with partial-thickness skin loss
- **Stage III**: Deep ulcer with exposed subcutaneous tissue; tunneling or undermining may be evident with or without slough
- **Stage IV**: Deep ulcer, full thickness, with necrosis into muscle, bone, tendons, and/or joints
- **Unstageable**: Eschar and/or slough prevents staging prior to debridement

Patients should be placed on pressure-reducing support surfaces and turned at least every two hours, avoiding the area(s) with a pressure ulcer. Wound care depends on the stage of the wound and the amount of drainage but includes irrigation, debridement when necessary, antibiotics for infection, and appropriate dressing.

Patients should be encouraged to have adequate protein and iron in their diets to promote healing and to maintain adequate hydration.

INFECTIOUS WOUNDS

All types of wounds have the potential to become infected. Infectious wounds are commonly health care acquired. Wound infections increase a patient's risk of sepsis, multisystem organ failure and death. Trauma patients are at an increased risk of developing an infected wound due to exposure to various contaminants that they may have encountered during their injury (e.g., dirt from a motor vehicle accident).

Signs and symptoms: Erythema, edema, induration, drainage, increasing pain and tenderness, fever, leukocytosis, and lymphangitis.

Diagnosis: Wound infections are diagnosed by wound cultures (anaerobic and aerobic). Fluid or tissue biopsy may also be performed.

Treatment: Wound infections are treated with antibiotics and a wound care regimen that includes routine cleaning and dressing of the wound. Wound care treatment is based on the type and severity of the wound. Surgical irrigation and debridement may also be indicated. For deep, complex wounds, a wound-care consult is often indicated.

NECROTIZING FASCIITIS

Necrotizing fasciitis is an infection that develops deep within the fascia, causing a rapidly developing tissue necrosis resulting in destruction and death of the soft tissue and nerves. Complications of necrotizing fasciitis may include the loss of the affected limb, sepsis, and death. Group A *Streptococcus*, *Klebsiella*, *Clostridium*, *Escherichia coli*, *Staphylococcus aureus*, and *Aeromonas hydrophila* are organisms that have the potential to cause necrotizing fasciitis.

Signs and symptoms: Edema, erythema, and pain at the affected site. Nausea, vomiting, fatigue, malaise, fever, and chills may also occur.

Diagnosis: Diagnosis is based on physical assessment and patient history. In addition, excisional deep skin biopsy and gram staining may be performed to determine the causative organism. CT/MRI may also be utilized to assess the extent of the infection.

Treatment: Treatment options for necrotizing fasciitis include antibiotics and fasciotomy with radical debridement. Hyperbaric oxygen therapy may also be utilized.

SURGICAL WOUNDS

Surgical wounds or incisions are made during a surgical procedure in a sterile, controlled environment. The American College of Surgeons has defined four classes of surgical wound types. This classification can help to predict how the wound will heal and the risk of infection.

- **Class I** is defined as clean (e.g., laparoscopic surgeries and biopsies).
- **Class II** is defined as clean contaminated (e.g., GI and GU surgeries).
- **Class III** is defined as contaminated (e.g., traumatic wounds such as a gunshot wound).
- **Class IV** is defined as dirty (e.g., traumatic wound from a dirty source).

Surgical wounds should be assessed for signs and symptoms of infection including erythema, edema, fever, increasing pain, and drainage. Surgical drains are commonly placed near the surgical incision to promote drainage—inspect drains for patency, amount, and characteristics of drainage. Patients are often treated with antibiotics prophylactically to help prevent a surgical site infection. Wound vacuum assisted closure devices may also be utilized to remove blood or serous fluid from the surgical wound/incision site.

MANAGEMENT OF INFLAMMATION RESULTING FROM TATTOOS AND PIERCING

Tattoos and piercing have both been implicated in **MRSA infections**. Tattooing uses needles that inject dye, sometimes resulting in local infection with erythema, edema, and purulent discharge. Body piercing for insertion of jewelry carries similar risks. Piercings of concern include the upper ear cartilage, nipples, navel, tongue, lip, penis, and nose. Some people who do piercings use reusable piercing equipment that is difficult to adequately clean and sterilize. Infections resulting from piercing in cartilage are often resistant to antibiotics because of lack of blood supply.

Treatment includes:

- **Cleansing wounds**. Jewelry may need to be removed in some cases.
- **Antibiotics**: Culture should be obtained, but medications for community-acquired MRSA should be started immediately:
  - **Mupirocin** may be used topically 3 times daily for 7-10 days with or without systemic antimicrobials.
  - **Trimethoprim-sulfamethoxazole DS** (TMP 160 mg/SMX 800 mg), 1-2 tablets twice daily. Children, dose based on TMP: 8-12 mg/kg/day in 2 doses.

TISSUE DAMAGE

Abrasion is damage to superficial layers of skin, such as with road burn or ligature marks.

Contusion occurs when friction or pressure causes damage to underlying vessels, resulting in bruising. Contusions that are bright red/purple with clear margins have occurred within 48 hours and those with receding edges or yellow-brown discoloration are older than 48 hours.

Laceration is a tear in the skin resulting from blunt force, often from falls on protuberances, such as elbows, or other blunt trauma. Lacerations may be partial to full-thickness.

Avulsion is tissue that is separated from its base and lost or without adequate base for attachment.

Treatments include:

- Local anesthetic if needed
- Low pressure, high volume irrigation with 35-50 mL syringe of open wound with normal saline, water, or non-antiseptic nonionic surfactants, and mechanical scrubbing of surrounding tissue with disinfectant
- Topical antibiotics as indicated
- Prophylactic antibiotics or antibiotic irrigation if wound contaminated
- Suturing/debridement as needed
- Hydrocolloids, Steri-Strips, and transparent dressings to stabilize flaps

Integumentary Procedures and Interventions

WOUND VACS

Wound vacuum-assisted closure (wound VAC) (AKA negative pressure wound therapy) uses subatmospheric (negative) pressure with a suction unit and a semi-occlusion vapor-permeable dressing. The suction reduces periwound and interstitial edema, decompressing vessels, improving circulation, stimulating production of new cells, and decreasing colonization of bacteria. Wound VAC also increases the rate of granulation and re-epithelialization to hasten healing. The wound must be debrided of necrotic tissue prior to treatment. Wound VAC is used for a variety of difficult-to-heal wounds, especially those that show less than 30% healing in 4 weeks of post-debridement treatment or those with excessive exudate, including chronic stage II and IV pressure ulcers, skin flaps, diabetic ulcer, acute wounds, burns, surgical wound, and those with dehiscence and nonresponsive arterial and venous ulcers. Contraindications include:

- Wound malignancy
- Untreated osteomyelitis
- Exposed blood vessels or organs
- Non-enteric, unexplored fistulas.

Nonadherent porous foam is cut to fit and cover the wound and is secured with occlusive transparent film with an opening cut to accommodate the drainage tube, which is attached to a suction canister in a closed system. The pressure should be set at 75-125 psi and the dressing changed 2-3 times weekly.

PRESSURE REDUCTION SURFACES

Pressure reduction surfaces redistribute pressure to prevent pressure ulcers and reduce shear and friction. There are various types of support surfaces for beds, examining tables, operating tables, and chairs. Functions of pressure reduction surfaces include temperature control, moisture control, and friction/shear control. **General use guidelines** include:

- Pressure redistribution support surfaces should be used for patients with stage II, III, and IV ulcers, as well as for those that are at risk for developing pressure ulcers.
- Chairs should have gel or air support surfaces to redistribute pressure for chair-bound patients, critically ill patients, or those who cannot move independently.
- Support surface material should provide at least an inch of support under areas to be protected when in use to prevent bottoming out. (Check by placing hand palm-up under the overlay below the pressure point.)
- Static support surfaces are appropriate for patients who can change position without increasing pressure to an ulcer.
- Dynamic support surfaces are needed for those who need assistance to move or when static pressure devices provide less than an inch of support.

Integumentary Pharmacology

PHARMACOLOGIC TREATMENT OF WOUND PAIN

TOPICAL ANESTHETICS

There are numerous different types of pain medications that may be used to control pain from wounds, including **topical anesthetics**:

- **Lidocaine 2-4%** is frequently used during debridement or dressing changes. Lidocaine is useful only superficially and may take 15-30 minutes before it is effective.
- **Eutectic Mixture of Local Anesthetics (EMLA Cream)** provides good pain control. The wound is first cleansed and then the cream is applied thickly (1/4 inch) extending about 1/2 inch past the wound to the periwound tissue. The wound is then covered with plastic wrap, which is secured and left in place for about 20 minutes. The wrapped time may be extended to 45-60 minutes if necessary, to completely numb the tissue. The tissue should remain numb for about 1 hour after the plastic wrap is removed, allowing time for the wound to be cleansed, debrided, and/or redressed.

REGIONAL ANESTHESIA

Regional anesthesia (injectable subcutaneous and perineural medications) is administered locally about the wound or as nerve blocks. Medications include lidocaine, bupivacaine, and tetracaine in solution. Epinephrine is sometimes added to increase vasoconstriction and reduce bleeding, although it is avoided in distal areas of the limbs (hands and feet) to prevent ischemia.

- **Field blockade** involves injecting the anesthetic into the periwound tissue or into the wound margins. The effect may be decreased by inflammation. The effects last for limited periods of time.
- **Regional nerve blocks** may involve single injections, the effects of which are limited in duration but can provide pain relief for treatments. Techniques that use continuous catheter infusions are longer lasting and can be controlled more precisely. Blocks may involve nerves proximal to affected areas, such as peripheral nerve blocks, or large nerve blocks near the spinal cord, such as percutaneous lumbar sympathetic blocks (LSB). Long-term blocks may use alcohol-based medications to permanently inactivate the nerves.

Ear, Nose, and Throat Pathophysiology

PERITONSILLAR ABSCESS

Peritonsillar abscess (PTA), which usually derives from tonsillitis, progresses from cellulitis to abscess between the palatine tonsil and capsule. It is often polymicrobial. It usually occurs bilaterally between the ages of 20 and 30. Complications include obstruction of airway, rupture with aspiration of purulent material, septicemia, endocarditis, and epiglottitis. The infection is often polymicrobial. Symptoms include fever, pain, hoarseness, muffling of voice, dysphagia, tonsillar edema, erythema, exudate, and edema of palate with displacement of uvula.

Diagnosis:

- Aspiration of purulent material (usually diagnostic)
- CT with contrast, ultrasound
- On exam: Displacement of the uvula, with enlarged tonsils

Treatments include:

- Needle aspirations (often multiple) with needle penetrating 1 cm or less to avoid carotid artery
- Abscess incision and drainage if aspiration not successful
- IV volume replacement
- **Antibiotics**: IV ampicillin-sulbactam or clindamycin until culture results come back and in areas with high rates of CA-MRSA vancomycin may be added. Once the patient shows signs of clinical improvement, they may switch to oral antibiotics (needing 14 days total).

DENTAL AVULSIONS

Dental avulsions are the complete displacement of a tooth from its socket. The tooth may be reimplanted if done within one to two hours after displacement, although only permanent teeth are reimplanted, not primary.

Procedure:

1. Tooth can be **transported** from accident site to the emergency department in Hank solution, saline, or milk.
2. **Cleanse** tooth with sterile NS or Hank solution, handling only the crown and avoiding any disruption of fibers.
3. If tooth has been dry for 20-60 minutes, **soak** tooth in Hank solution for 30 minutes before reimplantation.
4. If tooth has been dry for more than 60 minutes, **soak** tooth in citric acid for 5 minutes, stannous fluoride 2% for 5 minutes, and doxycycline solution for 5 minutes prior to reimplantation.
5. Remove **clot** in socket and gently irrigate with NS.
6. Place tooth into **socket** firmly, cover with gauze, and have patient bite firmly on gauze until splinting can be applied.
7. Apply **splinting material and mold packing** over implanted tooth and 2 adjacent teeth on both sides (encompasses 5 teeth).

DENTAL FRACTURES

Dental fractures, most commonly of the maxillary teeth, may occur in association with other oral injuries and may be overlooked unless a careful dental examination is carried out. Fractures are classified according to severity of fracture with treatment to prevent further damage and necrosis.

- **Ellis I**: Chipping of enamel
  - Smoothen rough edges

- **Ellis II**: Fracture of enamel and dentin with pain on pressure and air sensitivity
  - Protect dentin with glass ionomer dental cement and refer to dentist within 24 hours
- **Ellis III**: Fracture of enamel, dentin, and pulp with pain on movement; air and temperature sensitivity; blood may be evident
  - Protect dentin with ionomer dental cement or calcium hydroxide base and refer to dentist for prompt treatment
  - Administer oral analgesics
- **Alveolar/root fracture:** Loose tooth and malocclusion, sensitivity to percussion
  - Prompt referral to dentist for splinting and/or root canal

> **Review Video: Anatomical and Clinical Parts of Teeth**
> Visit mometrix.com/academy and enter code: 683627

RECURRENT EPISTAXIS

Recurrent epistaxis is common in young children (2 to 10 years), especially boys, and is often related to nose picking, dry climate, or central heating in the winter. Incidence also increases between 50 and 80 years of age, and may be caused by NSAIDs and anticoagulants. Kiesselbach plexus in the anterior nares has plentiful vessels and bleeds easily. Bleeding in the posterior nares is more dangerous and can result in considerable blood loss. Bleeding from the anterior nares is usually confined to one nostril, but from the posterior nares, blood may flow through both nostrils or backward into the throat and the person may be observed swallowing. People abusing cocaine may suffer nosebleeds because of damage to the mucosa. Hematocrit and hemoglobin should be done to determine if blood loss is significant. Bleeding should stop within 20 minutes. Treatment:

- Upright position, leaning forward so blood does not flow down throat.
- Applying pressure below the nares or by pinching the nostrils firmly for 10 minutes.
- Severe bleeding: packing and/or topical vasoconstrictors.
- Humidifiers may decrease irritation.

BELL'S PALSY

Bell's palsy is caused by inflammation of cranial nerve VII, usually from a herpes simplex I or II infection, and generally affects only one side of the paired nerves. Onset is generally sudden, and symptoms peak by 48 hours with a wide range of presentation. **Symptoms** usually subside within two to six months but may persist one year:

- Mild weakness on one side of face to complete paralysis with distortion of features
- Drooping of eyelid and mouth
- Tearing in affected eye
- Taste impairment

Diagnosis includes:

- Neurological, eye, parotid gland, and ear exam to rule out other cranial nerve involvement or conditions.

Treatment includes:

- Artificial tears during daytime with lubricating ophthalmic ointment and patch at night to protect eye
- Prednisone 60 mg daily for 5 days with tapering over 5 days.
- For severe cases use prednisone AND acyclovir 400 mg 5 times daily for 7 days.

TEMPORAL ARTERITIS

Temporal arteritis (TA), also called giant cell arteritis, is inflammation of the blood vessels of the head, especially the temporal artery, and the thoracic aorta and branches. TA is commonly associated with polymyalgia rheumatica (30% or less of patients) but can occur with other systemic disorders such as lupus erythematous, Sjögren syndrome, and rheumatoid arthritis. TA is a progressive disorder that can result in blindness and is most common in those older than 50. **Symptoms** include:

- New onset of headaches
- Vision fluctuations, including decreased visual acuity and loss of vision
- Intermittent claudicating pain in jaw, tongue, and upper extremities
- Fever

Diagnosis includes:

- Temporal artery biopsy (definitive)
- ESR greater than 50 mm/hr (may be normal in about 20%)
- CRP greater than 2.45 mg/dL

Treatment should begin immediately if the diagnosis is suspected to prevent blindness:

- Prednisone 60 mg daily

TRIGEMINAL NEURALGIA

Trigeminal neuralgia (tic douloureux) is a neurological condition in which blood vessels press on the trigeminal nerve as it leaves the brainstem causing severe pain on one side of the face or jaw. The shock-like pains may involve a small area or half the face and in rare cases both sides of the face at different times. The pain lasts from seconds to two minutes and is extremely debilitating and may be precipitated by movement, vibration, or contact with the face or mouth. Trigeminal neuralgia is most common in women older than 50. Patients may go through periods of remission and recurrences. Diagnosis is by history and neurological exam.

Treatment includes:

- **Carbamazepine** is the drug of choice and usually controls pain initially, but the effects may decrease over time.
- **Phenytoin or oxcarbazepine** may be used in place of carbamazepine.
- **Baclofen** (muscle relaxant) potentiates other drugs.
- **Surgical procedures** may be done if no response to medications.

FOREIGN BODIES

FOREIGN BODIES IN THE EAR

Foreign bodies in the ear (most often in children) can be organic or inorganic materials or insects. Careful history should be done to determine the type of foreign body before attempting removal. Children may require conscious sedation or general anesthesia for deep insertions. Irrigations should not be done if tympanic membrane is ruptured or cannot be visualized. Procedure:

1. Examine ear to determine if tympanic membrane is intact.
2. Drown insects with lidocaine 2% solution and then suction.
3. Irrigate small nonorganic particles with pulsatile flow aimed at wall of the canal.
4. Use cerumen loops, right-angle hooks, and/or alligator forceps to grasp and remove item.
5. Carefully examine the ear canal after removal of the item for lacerations or abrasions.
6. Topical antibiotic if extensive cutaneous abrasion or laceration or for organic material.

FOREIGN BODIES IN THE EYE

Foreign bodies in the eye should be assessed carefully with slit lamp with corneal examination using optical sectioning before attempting removal of the foreign body. Foreign bodies that penetrate the cornea full-thickness should not be removed in the ED, but superficial foreign bodies can safely be removed. Procedure:

1. Apply topical anesthetic to both eyes (to suppress blinking in the unaffected eye).
2. Eye held open by hand or with wire eyelid speculum.
3. Foreign body is carefully removed with small gauge needle or moistened cotton swab.
4. Rust ring from metallic objects should be removed with ophthalmic burr (if not over pupil), and patient referred to ophthalmologist for further rust ring removal within 24 hours.
5. Eyelid everted and examined carefully for further foreign bodies.
6. Abrasions treated as indicated.

FOREIGN BODIES IN THE NARES

Children may insert various organic and inorganic foreign bodies in the nose. In most cases, this is observed, but persistent unilateral obstruction of nose, foul discharge, or epistaxis is suggestive of foreign body. Small or uncooperative children may need to be restrained with conscious sedation or papoose board.

Procedure:

1. Vasoconstrictor/topical anesthetic applied: 1 mL of phenylephrine with 3 mL of lidocaine 4%.
2. Aerosolized racemic epinephrine may be used for decongestion, to loosen foreign body.
3. Examine nares with speculum.

Removal techniques:

- Positive pressure: Blowing nose on command. For small children, block opposite nares and have caregiver blow puff of air in mouth, forcing item out of nares.
- Suction with catheter.
- Use alligator or bayonet forceps to grasp item.
- Pass a curette behind item, rotate, and the use to pull item out.
- Pass Fogarty vascular catheter past item, inflate balloon, pull catheter back out.

LUDWIG ANGINA

Ludwig angina is cellulitis, usually caused by *Streptococcus* or *Staphylococcus,* of the submandibular spaces and lingual space that can result in obstruction of the airway as the swelling in the mouth floor pushes the tongue superior and posterior.

Symptoms include:

- Evidence of poor dental hygiene and odontogenic abscess (usually from lower third molars or surrounding gums) that has spread into soft tissue
- Dysphagia
- Odynophagia, trismus, edema of the upper neck (midline)
- Erythema, stridor, and cyanosis (late signs of obstruction)
- Changes in mental status

Diagnosis includes:

- Examination of the head and neck to observe for swelling of the upper neck, floor of mouth, and tongue
- CT scan
- Culture (treatment should, however, begin immediately)

Treatments include:

- Nasotracheal intubation (with fiberoptic tube if necessary) and ventilation if respiratory obstruction
- IV antibiotics, such as penicillin or clindamycin
- Referral to surgeon for incision and drainage as indicated

OTITIS EXTERNA

Otitis externa is infection of the external ear canal, either bacterial or mycotic. Common pathogens include bacteria, *Pseudomonas aeruginosa*, *Staphylococcus aureus,* and fungi, *Aspergillus* and *Candida.* OE is often caused by chlorine in swimming pools killing normal flora and allowing other bacteria to multiply. Fungal infections may be associated with immune disorders, diabetes, and steroid use.

Symptoms include:

- Pain, swelling, and exudate
- Itching (pronounced with fungal infections)
- Red pustular lesions
- Black spots over tympanic membrane (fungus)

Diagnosis: On exam, tenderness when touched on tragus or when the auricle is pulled, erythema, and history.

Treatment includes:

- Irrigate ear with Burow's solution or saline to clean and remove debris or foreign objects.
- **Bacteria**: Antibiotic ear drops, such as ciprofloxacin and ofloxacin. If impetigo, flush with hydrogen peroxide 1:1 solution and apply mupirocin twice daily for 5-7 days. Lance pointed furuncles.
- **Fungus**: Solution of boric acid 5% in ethanol; clotrimazole-miconazole solution with/without steroid for 5-7 days.
- Analgesics as needed.

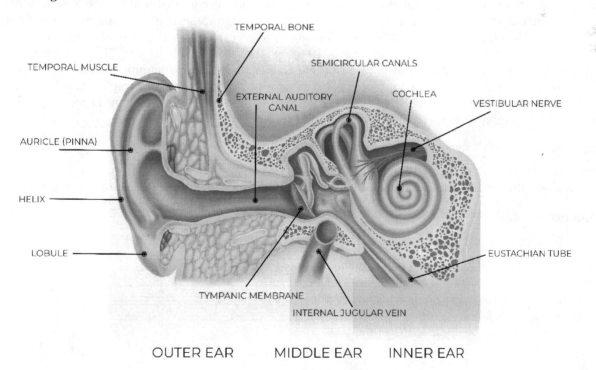

255

OTITIS MEDIA

Otitis media, inflammation of the middle ear, usually follows upper respiratory tract infections or allergic rhinitis. The eustachian tube swells and prevents the passage of air. Fluid from the mucous membrane pools in the middle ear, causing infection. Common pathogens include *Streptococcus pneumoniae, Haemophilus influenzae,* and *Moraxella catarrhalis.* Some genetic conditions, such as trisomy 21 and cleft palate, may include abnormalities of the eustachian tube, increasing risk. There are four forms:

- **Acute**: 1-3 weeks with swelling, redness, and possible rupture of the tympanic membrane, fever, pain (ear pulling), and hearing loss.
- **Recurrent**: 3 episodes in 6 six months or 4-6 in 12 months.
- **Bullous**: Acute infection with ear popping pressure in middle ear, pain, hearing loss, and bullae between layers of tympanic membrane, causing bulging.
- **Chronic**: Persists at least 3 months with thick retracted tympanic membrane, hearing loss, and drainage.

Diagnosis: Distinguishing features on assessment of acute otitis media include a bulging or perforated tympanic membrane, signs of inflammation, or purulent fluid present.

Treatment: 75-90% resolve spontaneously, so antibiotics are **withheld** for 2-3 days. Amoxicillin for 7-10 days. Referral for **tympanostomy and pressure-equalizing tubes** (PET) for severe chronic or recurrent infections.

> **Review Video: Otitis Media**
> Visit mometrix.com/academy and enter code: 328778

MASTOIDITIS

Mastoiditis usually results from extension of acute otitis media because the mucous membranes of the middle ear are continuous with the mastoid air cells in the temporal bone. All patients with otitis media should be considered at risk for mastoiditis. Patients with chronic otitis media also often develop chronic mastoiditis, which can result in formation of benign cholesteatoma. Signs and symptoms of mastoiditis include persistent fever, pain in or behind the ear (especially during the night), and hearing loss. Differential diagnoses may include Bell's palsy, otitis externa, and otitis media. **Diagnosis** is based on symptoms, CBC, audiometry, tympanocentesis or myringotomy with culture and sensitivities, and CT scan (definitive). Acute mastoiditis is treated with antibiotics, usually beginning with a 3rd generation cephalosporin or penicillin/aminoglycoside combination until culture and sensitivity results return. If spreading empyema or osteitis is present, then surgical mastoidectomy is required.

SINUSITIS

Sinusitis is inflammation of the nasal sinuses, of which there are two maxillary, two frontal, and one sphenoidal, as ethmoidal air cells. Inflammation causes obstruction of drainage with resultant discomfort.

Symptoms include:

- Frontal and maxillary presents with pain over sinuses
- Ethmoidal present with dull aching behind eye
- Tenderness to palpation and percussion of sinuses
- Mucosa of nasal cavity edematous and erythematous
- Purulent exudate

Diagnosis includes:

- Transillumination of sinus (diminished with inflammation)
- CT for those who are immunocompromised or if diagnosis is not clear
- Careful examination to rule out spreading infection, especially with signs of fever, altered mental status, or unstable vital signs

Treatment includes:

- Symptomatic relief with analgesia
- Topical decongestants and nasal irrigation
- Antimicrobial therapy if symptoms persist at least seven days or are severe (avoid routine use): Amoxicillin or TMP/SMX
- Steroid nasal spray twice daily

MENIERE'S DISEASE

Meniere's disease occurs when a blockage in the endolymphatic duct of the inner ear causes dilation of the endolymphatic space and abnormal fluid balance, which causes pressure or rupture of the inner ear membrane.

Symptoms include:

- Progressive fluctuating sensorineural hearing loss
- Tinnitus
- Pressure in the ear
- Severe vertigo that lasts minutes to hours
- Diaphoresis
- Poor balance
- Nausea and vomiting

Diagnosis includes:

- Complete physical exam and evaluation of cranial nerves
- Tuning fork sounds may lateralize to unaffected ear
- Assessment of hearing loss

Treatment:

- Low sodium diet
- Vestibular suppressant (antihistamine): Meclizine
- Benzodiazepine or SSRI for anxiety
- Antiemetics, such as promethazine suppositories
- Diuretics, such as hydrochlorothiazide
- Referral for surgical repair for persistent vertigo, but this will not correct other symptoms

LABYRINTHITIS

Labyrinthitis is a viral or bacterial inflammation of the inner ear, and it may occur secondary to bacterial otitis media. Viral labyrinthitis may be associated with mumps, rubella, rubeola, influenza, or other viral infections, such as upper respiratory tract infections. Because the labyrinth includes the vestibular system that is responsible for sensing head movement, labyrinthitis causes balance disorders. The condition often persists for 1 to 6 weeks with acute symptoms the first week and then decreasing symptoms. **Symptoms** include:

- Sudden onset of severe vertigo
- Hearing loss and sometimes tinnitus
- Nausea and vomiting
- Panic attacks from severe anxiety related to symptoms

Treatment includes:

- **Bacterial**: IV antibiotics
- **Viral**: Symptomatic as for bacterial (except for antibiotics)
- Volume replacement
- Antiemetics, such as promethazine suppositories
- Vestibular suppressant (antihistamine): Meclizine
- Benzodiazepine or SSRI for anxiety
- Referral to surgeon for I&D if necessary

TMD

Temporomandibular disorder (TMD) is jaw pain caused by dysfunction of the temporomandibular joint (TMJ) and the supporting muscles and ligaments. It may be precipitated by injury, such as whiplash, or grinding or clenching of the teeth, stress, or arthritis.

Symptoms include:

- Clicking or popping noises on jaw movement
- Limited jaw movement or "locked" jaw
- Acute pain on chewing or moving jaw
- Headaches and dizziness
- Toothaches

Diagnosis includes:

- Complete dental exam with x-rays to rule out other disorders
- MRI or CT may be needed

Treatment usually begins conservatively:

- Ice pack to jaw area for 10 minutes followed by jaw stretching exercises and warm compress for 5 minutes 3-4 times daily
- Avoidance of heavy chewing by eating soft foods and avoiding hard foods, such as raw carrots and nuts
- NSAIDs to relieve pain and inflammation
- Night mouthguard
- Referral for dental treatments to improve bite as necessary

Multisystem Pathophysiology

RANGE OF SEVERE INFECTION

There are a number of terms used to refer to severe infections which are often used interchangeably. It is important to know these terms to properly perform the continuum of care.

- **Bacteremia** is the presence of bacteria in the blood without systemic infection.
- **Septicemia** is a systemic infection caused by pathogens (usually bacteria or fungi) present in the blood.
- **Systemic inflammatory response syndrome** (SIRS) is a generalized inflammatory response affecting many organ systems. It may be caused by infectious or non-infectious agents, such as trauma, burns, adrenal insufficiency, pulmonary embolism, and drug overdose. If an infectious agent is identified or suspected, SIRS is an aspect of sepsis. Infective agents include a wide range of bacteria and fungi, including *Streptococcus pneumoniae* and *Staphylococcus aureus.* SIRS includes 2 of the following:
  o Elevated (>38 °C) or subnormal rectal temperature (<36 °C)
  o Tachypnea or $PaCO_2$ <32 mmHg
  o Tachycardia
  o Leukocytosis (>12,000) or leukopenia (<4000)
- **Sepsis** is the presence of infection either locally or systemically in which there is a generalized life-threatening inflammatory response (SIRS). It includes all the indications for SIRS as well as one of the following:
  o Changes in mental status
  o Hypoxemia without preexisting pulmonary disease
  o Elevation in plasma lactate
  o Decreased urinary output <5 mL/kg/hr for ≥1 hour
- **Severe sepsis** includes both indications of SIRS and sepsis as well as indications of increasing organ dysfunction with inadequate perfusion and/or hypotension.
- **Septic shock** is a progression from severe sepsis in which refractory hypotension occurs despite treatment. There may be indications of lactic acidosis.
- **Multi-organ dysfunction syndrome** (MODS) is the most common cause of sepsis-related death. Cardiac function becomes depressed, acute respiratory distress syndrome (ARDS) may develop, and renal failure may follow acute tubular necrosis or cortical necrosis. Thrombocytopenia appears in about 30% of those affected and may result in disseminated intravascular coagulation (DIC). Liver damage and bowel necrosis may occur.

SHOCK

There are a number of different types of shock, but there are general characteristics that they have in common. In all types of shock, there is a marked decrease in tissue perfusion related to hypotension, so that there is insufficient oxygen delivered to the tissues and inadequate removal of cellular waste products, causing injury to tissue:

- Hypotension (systolic below 90 mmHg); this may be somewhat higher (110 mmHg) in those who are initially hypertensive
- Decreased urinary output (<0.5 mL/kg/hr), especially marked in hypovolemic shock
- Metabolic acidosis
- Peripheral/cutaneous vasoconstriction/vasodilation resulting in cool, clammy skin
- Alterations in level of consciousness

Types of shock are as follows:

- **Distributive:** Preload decreased, CO increased, SVR decreased
- **Cardiogenic:** Preload increased, CO decreased, SVR increased
- **Hypovolemic:** Preload decreased, CO decreased, SVR increased

SEPTIC SHOCK

Septic shock is caused by toxins produced by bacteria and cytokines that the body produces in response to severe infection, resulting in a complex syndrome of disorders. **Symptoms** are wide-ranging:

- **Initial**: Hyper- or hypothermia, increased temperature (>38 °C) with chills, tachycardia with increased pulse pressure, tachypnea, alterations in mental status (dullness), hypotension, hyperventilation with respiratory alkalosis ($PaCO_2$ ≤30 mmHg), increased lactic acid, unstable BP, and dehydration with increased urinary output
- **Cardiovascular**: Myocardial depression and dysrhythmias
- **Respiratory**: Acute respiratory distress syndrome (ARDS)
- **Renal**: Acute kidney injury (AKI) with decreased urinary output and increased BUN
- **Hepatic**: Jaundice and liver dysfunction with an increase in transaminase, alkaline phosphatase, and bilirubin
- **Hematologic**: Mild or severe blood loss (from mucosal ulcerations), neutropenia or neutrophilia, decreased platelets, and DIC
- **Endocrine**: Hyperglycemia, hypoglycemia (rare)
- **Skin**: Cellulitis, erysipelas, and fasciitis, acrocyanotic and necrotic peripheral lesions

DIAGNOSIS AND TREATMENT

Septic shock is most common in newborns, those >50, and those who are immunocompromised. There is no specific test to confirm a diagnosis of septic shock, so **diagnosis** is based on clinical findings and tests that evaluate hematologic, infectious, and metabolic states: Lactic acid, CBC, DIC panel, electrolytes, liver function tests, BUN, creatinine, blood glucose, ABGs, urinalysis, ECG, radiographs, blood and urine cultures.

Treatment must be aggressive and includes:

- Oxygen and endotracheal intubation as necessary
- IV access with 2-large bore catheters and central venous line
- Rapid fluid administration at 0.5L NS or isotonic crystalloid every 5-10 minutes as needed (to 4-6 L)
- Monitoring urinary output to optimal >30 mL/hr (>0.5-1 mL/kg/hr)
- Inotropic or vasoconstrictive agents (dopamine, dobutamine, norepinephrine) if no response to fluids or fluid overload
- Empiric IV antibiotic therapy (usually with 2 broad spectrum antibiotics for both gram-positive and gram-negative bacteria) until cultures return and antibiotics may be changed
- Hemodynamic and laboratory monitoring
- Removing source of infection (abscess, catheter)

DISTRIBUTIVE SHOCK

Distributive shock occurs with adequate blood volume but inadequate intravascular volume because of arterial/venous dilation that results in decreased vascular tone and hypoperfusion of internal organs. Cardiac output may be normal or blood may pool, decreasing cardiac output. **Distributive shock** may result from anaphylactic shock, septic shock, neurogenic shock, and drug ingestions.

Copyright © Mometrix Media. You have been licensed one copy of this document for personal use only. Any other reproduction or redistribution is strictly prohibited. All rights reserved.
This content is provided for test preparation purposes only and does not imply an endorsement by Mometrix of any particular political, scientific, or religious point of view.

Symptoms include:

- Hypotension (systolic <90 mmHg or <40 mmHg below normal), tachypnea, tachycardia (>90) (may be lower if patient receiving β-blockers)
- Hypoxemia
- Skin initially warm, later hypoperfused
- Hyper- or hypothermia (>38 °C or <36 °C)
- Alterations in mentation
- Decreased urinary output
- Symptoms related to underlying cause

Treatment includes:

- Treating underlying cause while stabilizing hemodynamics
- Oxygen with endotracheal intubation if necessary
- Rapid fluid administration at 0.25-0.5 L NS or isotonic crystalloid every 5-10 minutes as needed to 2-3 L
- Vasoconstrictive and inotropic agents (dopamine, dobutamine, norepinephrine) if necessary, for patients with profound hypotension

NEUROGENIC SHOCK

Neurogenic shock is a type of distributive shock that occurs when injury to the CNS from trauma resulting in acute spinal cord injury (from both blunt and penetrating injuries), neurological diseases, drugs, or anesthesia, impairs the autonomic nervous system that controls the cardiovascular system. The degree of symptoms relates to the level of injury with injuries above T1 capable of causing disruption of the entire sympathetic nervous system and lower injuries causing various degrees of disruption. Even incomplete spinal cord injury can cause neurogenic shock.

Symptoms include:

- Hypotension and warm dry skin related to lack of vascular tone that results in hypothermia from loss of cutaneous heat
- Bradycardia (common but not universal)

Treatment includes:

- ABCDE (airway, breathing, circulation, disability evaluation, exposure)
- Rapid fluid administration with crystalloid to keep mean arterial pressure at 85-90 mmHg
- Placement of pulmonary artery catheter to monitor fluid overload
- Inotropic agents (dopamine, dobutamine) if fluids don't correct hypotension
- Atropine for persistent bradycardia

HYPOVOLEMIC SHOCK/VOLUME DEFICIT

Hypovolemic shock occurs when there is inadequate intravascular fluid. The loss may be *absolute* because of an internal shifting of fluid or an external loss of fluid, as occurs with massive hemorrhage, thermal injuries, severe vomiting or diarrhea, and internal injuries (such as ruptured spleen or dissecting arteries) that interfere with intravascular integrity. Hypovolemia may also be *relative* and related to vasodilation, increased capillary membrane permeability from sepsis or injuries, and decreased colloidal osmotic pressure that may occur with loss of sodium and some disorders, such as hypopituitarism and cirrhosis.

Hypovolemic shock is **classified** according to the degree of fluid loss:

- **Class I:** <750 mL or ≤15% of total circulating volume (TCV)
- **Class II:** 750-1500 mL or 15-30% of TCV
- **Class III:** 1500-2000 mL or 30-40% of TCV
- **Class IV:** >2000 mL or >40% of TCV

SYMPTOMS AND TREATMENT

Hypovolemic shock occurs when the total circulating volume of fluid decreases, leading to a fall in venous return that in turn causes a decrease in ventricular filling and preload, indicated by ↓ in right atrial pressure (RAP) and pulmonary artery occlusion pressure (PAOP). This results in a decrease in stroke volume and cardiac output. This in turn causes generalized arterial vasoconstriction, increasing afterload (↑ systemic vascular resistance), causing decreased tissue perfusion.

Symptoms: Anxiety, pallor, cool and clammy skin, delayed capillary refill, cyanosis, hypotension, increasing respirations, weak, thready pulse.

Treatment is aimed at identifying and treating the cause:

- Administration of blood, blood products, autotransfusion, colloids (such as plasma protein fraction), and/or crystalloids (such as normal saline)
- Oxygen—intubation and ventilation may be necessary
- Medications may include vasopressors, such as dopamine. **Note: Fluids must be given before starting vasopressors**!

ANAPHYLACTIC SHOCK

Anaphylactic reaction or anaphylactic shock may present with a few symptoms or a wide range of potentially lethal effects.

Symptoms may recur after the initial treatment (biphasic anaphylaxis), so careful monitoring is essential:

- Sudden onset of weakness, dizziness, confusion
- Severe generalized edema and angioedema; lips and tongue may swell
- Urticaria
- Increased permeability of vascular system and loss of vascular tone leading to severe hypotension and shock
- Laryngospasm/bronchospasm with obstruction of airway causing dyspnea and wheezing
- Nausea, vomiting, and diarrhea
- Seizures, coma, and death

Treatments:

- Establish patent airway and intubate if necessary, for ventilation
- Provide oxygen at 100% high flow
- Monitor VS
- Administer epinephrine (Epi-pen or solution)
- Albuterol per nebulizer for bronchospasm
- Intravenous fluids to provide bolus of fluids for hypotension
- Diphenhydramine if shock persists
- Methylprednisolone if no response to other drugs

HEAT-RELATED ILLNESS

Children and the elderly are particularly vulnerable to heat-related illness, especially when heat is combined with humidity. Heat-related illnesses occur when heat accumulation in the body outpaces dissipation, resulting in increased temperature and dehydration, which can then lead to thermoregulatory failure and multiple organ dysfunction syndromes. Each year in the United States, about 29 children die from heat stroke after being left in automobiles. At temperatures of 72-96 °F, the temperature in a car rises 3.2 °F every 5 minutes, with 80% of rise within 30 minutes. Temperatures can reach 117 °F even on cool days. There are three **types of heat-related illness**:

- **Heat stress**: Increased temperature causes dehydration. Patient may develop swelling of hands and feet, itching of skin, sunburn, heat syncope (pale moist skin, hypotension), heat cramps, and heat tetany (respiratory alkalosis). Treatment includes removing from heat, cooling, hydrating, and replacing sodium.
- **Heat exhaustion**: Involves water or sodium depletion, with sodium depletion common in patients who are not acclimated to heat. Heat exhaustion can result in flu-like aching, nausea and vomiting, headaches, dizziness, and hypotension with cold, clammy skin and diaphoresis. Temperature may be normal or elevated to less than 106 °F. Treatment to cool the body and replace sodium and fluids must be prompt in order to prevent heat stroke. Careful monitoring is important and reactions may be delayed.
- **Heat stroke**: Involves failure of the thermoregulatory system with temperatures that may be more than 106 °F and can result in seizures, neurological damage, multiple organ failures, and death. Exertional heat stroke often occurs in young athletes who engage in strenuous activities in high heat. Young children are susceptible to nonexertional heat stroke from exposure to high heat. Treatment includes evaporative cooling, rehydration, and supportive treatment according to organ involvement.

HYPOTHERMIA

Hypothermia occurs with exposure to low temperatures that cause the core body temperature to fall below 95 °F (35 °C). Hypothermia may be associated with immersion in cold water, exposure to cold temperature, metabolic disorders (hypothyroidism, hypoglycemia, hypoadrenalism), or CNS abnormalities (head trauma, Wernicke disease). Many patients with hypothermia are intoxicated with alcohol or drugs.

Symptoms of hypothermia include pallor, cold skin, drowsiness, alterations in mental status, confusion, and severe shivering. The patient can progress to shock, coma, dysrhythmias (T-wave inversion and prolongation of PR, QRS, and QT) including atrial fibrillation and AV block, and cardiac arrest.

Diagnosis requires low-reading thermometers to verify temperature.

Treatment includes:

- Passive rewarming if cardiac status stable
- Active rewarming (external) with immersion in warm water or heating blankets at 40 °C, radiant heat
- Active rewarming (internal) with warm humidified oxygen or air inhalation, heated IV fluids, and internal (bladder, peritoneal pleural, GI) lavage
- Warming with extracorporeal circuit, such as arteriovenous or venovenous shunt that warms the blood
- Supportive treatment as indicated

LOCALIZED COLD INJURIES

Frostnip is a superficial freeze injury that is reversible. Frostbite is damage to tissue caused by exposure to freezing temperatures, most often affecting the nose, ears, and distal extremities. As frostbite develops, the affected part feels numb and aches or throbs, becoming hard and insensate as the tissue freezes, resulting in circulatory impairment, necrosis of tissue, and gangrene. There are **three zones of injury:**

- **Coagulation** (usually distal): severe, irreversible cellular damage
- **Hyperemia** (usually proximal): minimal cellular damage
- **Stasis** (between other 2 zones): severe but sometimes reversible damage

Symptoms vary according to the degree of freezing:

- **Partial freezing** with erythema and mild edema, stinging, burning, throbbing pain
- **Full-thickness freezing** with increased edema in 3-4 hours, edema and clear blisters in 6-24 hours, desquamation with eschar formation, numbness, and then aching and throbbing pain
- Prognosis is very good for **first-degree** and good for **second-degree** frostbite
- Full-thickness and into **subdermal tissue** freezing with cyanosis, hemorrhagic blisters, skin necrosis, and "wooden" feeling, severe burning, throbbing, and shooting pains
- Freezing extends into **subcutaneous tissue**, including muscles, tendons, and bones with mottled appearance, non-blanching cyanosis, and eventual deep black eschar

Prognosis is poor for **third-degree** and **fourth-degree** freeze injuries. Determining the degree of injury can be difficult because some degree of thawing may have occurred prior to admission to the hospital.

Treatment includes:

- Rapid rewarming with warm water bath (40-42 °C [104-107.6 °F]) 10-30 minutes or until the frostbitten area is erythematous and pliable
- Treatment for generalized hypothermia

Treatment **after warming**:

- Debridement of clear blisters but not hemorrhagic blisters
- Aloe vera cream every 6 hours to blistered areas
- Dressings, separating digits
- Tetanus prophylaxis
- Ibuprofen 12 mg/kg daily in divided doses
- Antibiotic prophylaxis if indicated (penicillin G 500,000 units IV every 6 hours for 24 to 72 hours)

FEBRILE SEIZURE

Febrile seizure is a generalized seizure associated with high fever (usually more than 38°C [100.4°F]) from any type of infection (upper respiratory tract, urinary) but without intracranial infection or other cause, occurring between six months and five years of age. Careful clinical examination must be conducted to rule out more serious disorders. Laboratory tests are conducted in relation to symptoms. Lumbar puncture is not usually indicated unless intracranial infection is suspected. Seizures usually last less than 15 minutes and are without subsequent neurological deficit.

Treatment includes:

- Fever control: Acetaminophen 10-15 mg/kg every 4-6 hours OR ibuprofen 10 mg/kg every 6-8 hours. Antipyretics are NOT recommended as prophylaxis for recurrent febrile seizures.
- Tepid water bath (NOT alcohol).
- Antiepileptic drugs (AEDs) are usually not advised unless seizures are complex or continuous, child is younger than 6 months, or there is a preexisting neurological disorder: IV diazepam 0.1-0.2 mg/kg or IV lorazepam 0.05-0.1 mg/kg. (May cause lethargy.)

FIBROMYALGIA

Fibromyalgia is a complex syndrome of disorders that include fatigue, chronic generalized muscle pain, and focal areas of tenderness persisting for at least three months. The cause of fibromyalgia is not clear and has only recently been recognized as a distinct disorder. Diagnosis is by clinical exam and ruling out joint and muscle inflammation that could be cause of the pain. On clinical exam there are specific points of tenderness, usually in multiple areas of the body.

Symptoms:

- Fatigue.
- Pain and stiffness unresponsive to treatment, persisting for months.
- Sleep disorders.
- Irritable bowel syndrome.
- Stiffness in neck and shoulders associated with headache and pain in face.
- Sensitivity to odor, noises, and lights.
- Mood disorders, such as depression, anxiety.
- Dysmenorrhea.
- Paresthesia in hands and feet.

Treatment:

- **Analgesia**: Acetaminophen, tramadol, or NSAIDs.
- **Antidepressants**, such as amitriptyline, nortriptyline, or fluoxetine. Duloxetine and venlafaxine have been shown to reduce pain.
- **Antiseizure medication**: Pregabalin is the first FDA-approved treatment for the pain of fibromyalgia.
- **Referral** for physical therapy and/or cognitive therapy.

Multisystem Procedures and Interventions

TARGETED TEMPERATURE MANAGEMENT

Targeted temperature management (previously referred to as therapeutic hypothermia) is used to reduce ischemic tissue damage associated with cardiac arrest, ischemic stroke, traumatic brain/spinal cord injury, neurogenic fever, and subsequent coma (3 on Glasgow scale). Reducing the body's temperature to below normal range has a neuroprotective effect by making cell membranes less permeable, thus reducing neurologic edema and damage. Hypothermia should be initiated immediately after an ischemic event if possible, but some benefit remains up to 6 hours. Hypothermia to 33 °C may be induced by cooled saline through a femoral catheter, reducing temperature 1.5-2.0 °C/hr by an electronic control unit. Hypothermic water blankets covering ≥80% of the body's surface can also lower body temperature. In some cases, both a femoral cooling catheter and a water blanket are used for rapid reduction of temperature. Rectal probes are used to measure core temperature, but Foley temperature catheters are more common. Desflurane or meperidine is given to reduce the shivering response. Hypothermia increases risk of bleeding (decreased clotting time), infection (due to impairing leukocyte function and introducing catheters), arrhythmias, hyperglycemia, and DVT. Rewarming is done slowly at 0.5-1.0 °C/hr. through warmed intravenous fluids, warm humidified air, and/or warming blanket. The warming process is a critical time, as it causes potassium to be moved from extracellular to intracellular spaces and the patient's electrolyte levels must be monitored regularly.

CONTINUOUS TEMPERATURE MONITORING

Continuous temperature monitoring may be carried out through various means:

- Pulmonary artery catheter (most accurate but generally not recommended because of invasiveness and potential for complications)
- Rectal or Foley temperature probes
- Skin probes
- Wearable Bluetooth monitors (patch applied to the skin), which transmit information to an external monitor or the patient's electronic health record. (For external temperature monitoring, the device must be applied properly and for the correct duration of time [e.g., the TempTraQ wearable patch is applied in the underarm area and measures temperature for 72 hours].)

Indications for continuous temperature monitoring include:

- Skin flap transplantation—to assess perfusion
- Brain injury—to assess thermoregulation
- Therapeutic hypothermia—for cardiac arrest or post-cardiac surgery
- Malignant hyperthermia
- Immunocompromised patients—to assess for signs of infection
- Critically ill patients—at risk for temperature dysregulation

PERMISSIVE HYPOTENSION

Permissive hypotension procedures allow the systolic blood pressure to fall low enough to prevent or control hemorrhage while still high enough to maintain perfusion. With trauma patients, this means restricting fluid resuscitation when active bleeding is occurring. While protocols vary, permissive hypotension usually includes systolic blood pressure no higher than 80 mmHg, although this may vary. For example, permissive hypotension with systolic blood pressure maintained at 80-100 mmHg may be indicated when massive transfusion protocols are activated. Permissive hypotension helps decrease some of the adverse effects associated with rapid and high-dose fluid resuscitation (emboli, coagulopathy, and hypothermia). However, the patient does remain at risk of hypoperfusion and must be monitored carefully. Permissive hypotension is generally contraindicated with brain or spinal cord injury, although studies are ongoing (and mostly conducted with animals) and some controversy remains about the use of permissive hypotension.

SEDATION

MINIMAL SEDATION

Minimal sedation includes local/topical anesthesia, peripheral nerve blocks, administration of <50% nitrogen oxide in oxygen by itself, or administration of one sedative or analgesic medication in a dosage that does not typically require supervision. The patient should be fully aware, able to respond appropriately to verbal and tactile stimulation, and able to maintain an airway independently, as these medications should not have cardiovascular or respiratory effects. The purpose of minimal sedation is to decrease perception of pain, relax the patient, and reduce fear. The patient's level of consciousness, sedation, and pain should be monitored throughout the procedure to ensure the dosage is adequate and the patient is not excessively sedated. Medications may include benzodiazepines (diazepam, lorazepam) and opioids (fentanyl, morphine, meperidine). Reversal agents (flumazenil, naloxone) should be available. Minimal sedation is often used during labor and delivery and for minor procedures, such as skin biopsies and removal of skin lesions.

CONTINUOUS VS. INTERMITTENT SEDATION

Sedation for critically ill patients may include:

- **Intermittent sedation** is that administered through IV push, so the expected duration is relatively short. Typical agents include benzodiazepines and opioids. Intermittent sedation is most often used for endoscopic procedures but is also sometimes used for patients who are on mechanical ventilation, especially if they have regular trials of weaning. Also, intermittent sedation is less likely to result in oversedation.
- **Continuous sedation** is that administered through a steady intravenous infusion to ensure longer-lasting sedation. Typical agents include opioids, midazolam, and propofol. Continuous sedation is more commonly used for patients on mechanical ventilation because it requires less intervention and maintains a steady blood level. Daily interruptions of continuous sedation may be carried out as a trial for weaning patients on mechanical ventilation.

With both intermittent sedation and continuous sedation, the patient's vital signs, respiratory status, temperature, and oxygen saturation should be monitored. Arousal scales (Richmond or Riker Agitation/Sedation Scales) should be utilized to assess arousal and to adjust sedation dosages.

NEUROMUSCULAR BLOCKADE AGENTS

Neuromuscular blocker agents are used for induced paralysis of those who have not responded adequately to sedation, especially for intubation and mechanical ventilation. NMBAs do not produce unconsciousness, amnesia, or analgesia, therefore it is critical that they are administered *after* the patient has been adequately sedated. NMBAs include:

- **Depolarizing agents**: Succinylcholine. Risk for severe hyperkalemia after denervation injury persists for 7-10 days. Post-operative myalgia is common, and succinylcholine may trigger malignant hyperthermia and severe anaphylactic/anaphylactoid reactions.
- **Non-depolarizing agents**: Short-acting (mivacurium, rapacuronium), intermediate-acting (rocuronium, vecuronium, atracurium, cisatracurium), and long-acting (pancuronium, doxacurium, pipecuronium). Should be given for ≤2 days for those on ventilators because they may develop persistent quadriparesis. Most are not associated with malignant hyperthermia.

Eye lubricant should be applied every 2 hours and the eyes kept closed. Range of motion exercises should not extend beyond normal range because of the potential to damage joints. The patient must be repositioned frequently while paralyzed and on an adequate support surface. Pupil reactivity should be assessed every 1-4 hours to evaluate neurological status. Temperature should be monitored hourly if <36 °C or if placed under a cooling blanket because heat production is depressed. After cessation, the patient should be closely monitored to ensure that muscle function has returned to normal.

> **Review Video: Muscle Relaxants**
> Visit mometrix.com/academy and enter code: 862193

MODERATE (CONSCIOUS) SEDATION

The ASA sedation guidelines (2018) are intended for **moderate (conscious) sedation** used for procedures, such as colonoscopy. Steps include:

- **Pre-procedure evaluation**: Includes review of health records, physical examination and laboratory testing as indicated a few days or weeks prior to the procedure, and re-evaluating the patient again before the procedure.
- **Patient preparation**: Consult with a specialist if indicated, ensure the patient has informed consent and has been compliant with pre-procedure fasting, and insert intravenous line.
- **Patient monitoring**: LOC (every 5 minutes), oxygenation/ventilation (capnography, pulse oximetry), and hemodynamic with a designated person responsible for monitoring and recording.
- **Supplemental oxygen:** Use unless contraindicated by condition.
- **Emergency interventions**: Resuscitative equipment and reversal agents for opioids (naloxone) and benzodiazepines (Romazicon) must be present with a person trained in assessment and use available.
- **Sedatives**: Analgesics (opioids) and combinations of drugs as appropriate may be used (benzodiazepines and dexmedetomidine).
- **Sedative (propofol, ketamine, etomidate) and analgesics (local anesthetics, NSAIDs, and opioids) intended for general anesthesia**: Care must be consistent with that of general anesthesia and IV medications administered incrementally.
- **Recovery care**: Monitor oxygenation, ventilation, and circulation every 5-15 minutes.

SEDATION USING PROPOFOL

Sedation used for a drug-induced coma often includes **propofol**. Propofol is an IV non-opioid hypnotic anesthetic, the most common used for induction. It is also used for maintenance and postoperative sedation. Onset of action is rapid because of high lipid solubility, and propofol has a short distribution half-life and rapid clearance, so recovery is also fast. Propofol is metabolized by the liver, as well as through the lungs. Propofol decreases cerebral blood flow, metabolic rate of oxygen consumption, and ICP. Propofol causes vasodilation with resultant hypotension, but with bradycardia rather than tachycardia. Propofol is a respiratory depressant, resulting in apnea after induction and decreased tidal volume, respiratory rate, and hypoxic drive during maintenance. Propofol has antiemetic properties as well but does not produce analgesia.

DELAYED EMERGENCE

Delayed emergence (failure to emerge for 30-60 minutes after anesthesia ends) is more common in the elderly because of slowed metabolism of anesthetic agents but may have a variety of causes, such as drug overdose during surgery, overdose related to preinduction use of drugs or alcohol that potentiates intraoperative drugs. In this case, naloxone or flumazenil may be indicated if opioids or benzodiazepines are implicated. Physostigmine may also be used to reverse effects of some anesthetic agents. Hypothermia may also cause delay in emergence, especially core temperatures <33 °C, and may require forced-air warming blankets to increase the temperature. Other metabolic conditions, such as hypoglycemia or hyperglycemia, may also affect emergence. Patients suffering from delayed emergence must be evaluated for perioperative stroke, especially after neurological, cardiovascular, or cerebrovascular surgery. Metabolic disturbance may also delay emergence.

POSTANESTHETIC RESPIRATORY COMPLICATIONS

Postoperative respiratory complications are most common in the postanesthesia period, so monitoring of oxygen levels is critical to preventing hypoxemia:

- **Airway obstruction** may be partial or total. Partial obstruction is indicated by sonorous or wheezing respirations, and total by absence of breath sounds. Treatment includes supplemental oxygen, airway insertion, repositioning (jaw thrust), or succinylcholine and positive-pressure ventilation for laryngospasm. If edema of the glottis is causing obstruction, IV corticosteroids may be used.
- **Hypoventilation** ($PaCO_2$ >45 mmHg) is often mild but may cause respiratory acidosis. It is usually related to depression caused by anesthetic agents. A number of factors may slow emergence (hypothermia, overdose, metabolism) and cause hypoventilation. It may also be related to splinting because of pain, requiring additional pain management.
- **Hypoxemia** (mild is PaO_2 50-60 mmHg) is usually related to hypoventilation and/or increased right to left shunting and is usually treated with supplementary oxygen (30-60%) with or without positive airway pressure.

POSTANESTHETIC CARDIOVASCULAR COMPLICATIONS

Cardiovascular complications after surgery are sometimes related to respiratory complications, which may need to be addressed as well. Complications include:

- **Hypotension** is most often mild and requires no specific treatment. It is most commonly caused by hypovolemia and is significant if BP falls 20-30% below the normal baseline. A bolus (100-250 mL IV colloid) is used to confirm hypovolemia. If severe, then medications such as vasopressors may be indicated. Hypotension may occur with pneumothorax, so careful respiratory assessment must be done.
- **Hypertension** usually occurs ≤30 minutes after surgery and is common in those with a history of hypertension. It may be secondary to hypoxemia or metabolic acidosis. Mild increases usually don't require treatment but medications may be used for moderate (β-adrenergic blockers) or severe (nitroprusside) increases.
- **Arrhythmias** usually relate to respiratory complications or effects of anesthetic agents. Bradycardia may relate to cholinesterase inhibitors, opioids, or propranolol. Tachycardia may relate to anticholinergics, β-agonists, and vagolytic drugs. Hypokalemia and hypomagnesemia may cause premature atrial and ventricular beats.

Infectious Diseases

VIRAL INFECTIONS

HERPES SIMPLEX VIRUS INFECTIONS

There are 2 types of the herpes simplex virus (HSV), human herpesvirus 1 and 2. **HSV-1** usually causes a **gingivostomatitis** (often referred to as "cold sores" or "fever blisters") and is transmitted through **close contact**. **HSV-2** usually causes painful **genital lesions** through **sexual contact**. Either may be found in other areas of the body.

- **Incubation** period is around 2-12 days.
- The primary infection is usually more severe (causes systemic **symptoms**) than the reactivated infection, but it may be asymptomatic. After the primary infection, the virus remains dormant in the nerve ganglia, and can be reactivated especially during times of stress, illness, immunosuppression, or sun exposure. While patients are most contagious during times of active lesions, the disease may be spread while asymptomatic. The frequency of the outbreaks usually decreases over time.
- HSV **lesions** are grouped vesicles with an erythematous base. They are usually painful, and a prodrome of tingling, pain, or burning sensations may be felt hours to a couple days before the eruption. Lesions last for approximately 2-3 weeks in primary infection (up to 4 weeks with genital HSV), and 1-2 weeks in recurrent infections.
- HSV is **diagnosed** clinically and confirmed with a + culture, PCR test, or HSV antibody tests (HSV-1 or HSV-2: IgM= active or recent infection; IgG= previous infection).
- Symptomatic **treatment**, proper wound care, and antivirals (acyclovir, valacyclovir, or famciclovir) may be given.
- **Complications** include perinatal infection, keratitis, herpetic whitlow, herpes gladiatorum, secondary infections, and encephalitis.

EPSTEIN-BARR INFECTION

Epstein-Barr virus (EBV) is a **herpesvirus** (human herpesvirus 4) and is responsible for causing **infectious mononucleosis**. After the initial infection, it remains latent in B cells and epithelial cells. It has been linked to certain epithelial and lymphatic neoplasms (e.g., nasopharyngeal carcinoma, Burkitt lymphoma, Hodgkin lymphoma).

- EBV is **transmitted** through **body fluids** like saliva, so it is sometimes referred to as the kissing disease. It is most common in teenagers and college-age young adults
- **Incubation** period is typically 30-50 days.
- **Symptoms** of EBV infection range from being asymptomatic to swollen painful lymph nodes, pharyngitis (can mimic strep pharyngitis), extreme fatigue, fever, and possibly hepatosplenomegaly. The WBC count is elevated (~10,000-20,000 cells/mL) with 10-30% atypical lymphocytes in the differential.
- Confirm **diagnosis** with a Mono Spot test or EBV antibody serology tests.
- **Treatment** is supportive, and antibiotics are not helpful in treating this viral infection. Therefore, avoid unnecessary antibiotics in those with EBV, especially since administration of ampicillin or amoxicillin is often associated with a pruritic, maculopapular rash. Analgesics, warm salt water gargles, increased fluid intake, and rest will help to relieve some of the symptoms. Symptoms may last for several weeks and fatigue may last even longer. Patients should avoid contact sports for up to 2 months.
- **Complications** include hepatitis, cytopenias (e.g., thrombocytopenia), Guillain Barré syndrome, and splenic rupture.

MEASLES, MUMPS, AND RUBELLA

Measles (rubeola) virus is highly contagious, is spread through **respiratory secretions** (incubation is 7-14 days), and peaks in late winter to spring. It causes a prodrome of high fever (4-7 days), cough, congestion, conjunctivitis; then Koplik spots (pathognomonic), and finally a maculopapular rash (spreads cephalocaudally). Report suspected cases immediately to the health dept. **Diagnose** with a + IgM antibody test (collected after 3 days of rash), viral culture, or PCR. **Treatment** is supportive.

Mumps (parotitis) is a viral infection that is spread via **saliva** (incubation is 12-24 days), and often occurs during winter and spring. It causes painful swelling of the salivary glands (parotid). Report to health dept. Supportive **treatment**. Complications include orchitis (infertility), pancreatitis, and meningitis.

Rubella (German measles) is a virus that spreads via **respiratory droplets** (incubation is 2-3 weeks), and peaks in the spring. There is a mild prodrome (fever, aches, sore throat, conjunctivitis, swollen nodes [esp. suboccipital, postauricular, & posterior cervical]), then a maculopapular rash (face first, then down). Report to health dept. Confirm with rubella antibodies IgM or IgG. Symptomatic care.

INFLUENZA

Influenza is a highly contagious viral infection that affects the entire **respiratory system** from the nose to the lungs. There are 3 types of **influenza virus**: **A** (causes epidemics), **B** (only in humans), and **C**. Types A and B are seen most often and are the strains that the annual flu vaccine is most effective against; and type C is not as common and much less severe.

- Prevention is key and annual, age-appropriate influenza **vaccines** should be given to those ≥6 months; 2 vaccines are required in first-time vaccine patients if 6 mo. through 8-year-olds (separated by 28 days).
- **Incubation** period is 1-4 days and it is spread via respiratory droplets.
- Though **symptoms** can be very similar, the flu and the common cold differ in that the flu has a very sudden onset. Symptoms of influenza include a high fever (may last up to 5 days), headache, myalgias, dry cough, rhinorrhea, and fatigue. There may also be vomiting and diarrhea, although children are more prone to this.
- Clinical judgement, community patterns, and rapid influenza tests (high specificity, but lower sensitivity) aid in **diagnosis**, but RT-PCR or viral culture definitively confirm the diagnosis; pulse oximetry and CXR as needed for pulmonary issues.
- Antibiotic **treatment** is not effective unless there is a secondary bacterial infection (e.g., pneumonia). Look for signs of secondary infections (e.g., dyspnea, cyanosis, fever that goes away and returns, confusion/lethargy). Supportive treatment with rest, fluids, and analgesics. Antivirals should be considered in those who are at high risk (<5 years old, elderly, pregnant, chronic conditions). These are most effective if initiated within 24-48 hours of symptom onset. The neuraminidase inhibitors (oseltamivir, zanamivir) treat type A, type B, and avian H5N1. There is extensive resistance to the adamantanes (amantadine, rimantadine) so they are rarely used.
- **Complications** include pneumonia, ARDS, and death.

CORONAVIRUS

A coronavirus is a common virus that causes cold-like symptoms, including a cough, runny nose, sore throat, and congestion. Most cases of coronavirus are not dangerous and are often given little attention or go entirely unnoticed. However, specific coronavirus strains have led to two worldwide pandemics. The first, **severe acute respiratory syndrome (SARS)**, appeared in China in 2002 and quickly spread worldwide. Presenting symptoms of SARS were fever, cough, dyspnea, and general malaise. It was extremely virulent, spreading easily from person to person through close contact by way of contaminated droplets produced by coughing or sneezing. SARS was also very deadly, with a case fatality rate of nearly 10%. High rates of infection occurred in health care workers and others in contact with infected patients, so prompt diagnosis and proper isolation were essential. By 2004, there were no longer any documented active cases of SARS.

The most recent coronavirus outbreak was the **COVID-19** strain, which first appeared in December of 2019, in the Chinese city of Wuhan, and quickly became a global pandemic. Presentation of COVID-19 was similar to that of SARS, with the notable additional symptom of acute loss of taste/smell as a unique identifier. Much is still unknown about this strain, including exact transmission methods (though droplet transmission is suspected), effective treatment protocols, and long-term effects.

Precautions to take when treating patients with pandemic coronavirus include the following:

- Contact and droplet precautions, including eye protection and appropriate personal protection equipment.
- Airborne precautions (recommended by the CDC), especially with aerosol-producing procedures (ventilators, nebulizers, intubation).
- Immediate notification of public health authorities and institution of contact tracing.
- Activity restrictions of exposed health care workers planned in coordination with public health officials.

CYTOMEGALOVIRUS

Cytomegalovirus (CMV) is a herpes virus, occurring in most people by the time they are adults.

- **Transmission** can occur through secretions during personal contact and from mother to baby before, during or after birth.
- Most cases have no **symptoms**, although a few infants will have fetal damage, such as jaundice, hepatitis, brain damage, or growth retardation.
- **Treatment** for those with severe infections is with ganciclovir, an antiviral drug.

RESPIRATORY SYNCYTIAL VIRUS

Respiratory syncytial virus (RSV) is a virus that infects the respiratory tract, causing symptoms of nasal congestion, cough, sore throat, and headache. Severe cases can lead to high fever, breathing difficulties, severe cough, and cyanosis.

- Respiratory syncytial virus may **manifest** as a cold in adults and older children; however, there are some children who are more at risk of developing complications.
- **Transmission** is through contact with droplets from an infected person's nose or throat, generally through coughing and sneezing.
- Infants born prematurely, children with chronic lung disease, children with cystic fibrosis, and children who are in an immunocompromised state because of surgery or illness are at **high risk** of breathing difficulties, poor oxygenation, and even death from RSV.

BACTERIAL INFECTIONS

DIPHTHERIA

Diphtheria, caused by ***Corynebacterium diphtheriae***, is most prevalent in fall and winter.

- The **incubation** period is 2-7 days, possibly longer, and transmission is through direct contact with nasal, eye, and oral secretions.
- The **symptoms** are slight fever, nasal discharge, sore throat, feeling unwell, poor appetite, and swelling of the airway.
- If the disease is severe, death can result. The patient requires isolation, bed rest, fluids, antibiotics, medication for fever, and an antitoxin. The patient may also require oxygen therapy and tracheostomy if the airway is obstructed.

TETANUS

Tetanus, caused by **Clostridium tetani**, occurs all over the world. The spores formed by the bacillus are present in soil, dust, and the GI tracts of animals and humans.

- The **incubation** period is 3-21 days.
- **Symptoms** start with headache, irritability, jaw muscle spasms, and inability to open the mouth. This is followed by severe back muscle spasms, seizures, incontinence, and fever.
- **Treatment** requires human tetanus immune globulin, penicillin G, Valium, and placement on a ventilator. The environment should be kept quiet because the spasms are initiated by stimuli.

FUNGAL INFECTIONS

CRYPTOCOCCOSIS

Cryptococcosis is an infection resulting from inhaling the **fungus** *Cryptococcus neoformans,* which is found worldwide in soil (can be associated with bird droppings), or *Cryptococcus gattii,* which is associated with certain trees in the Northwest.

- Cryptococcosis is most often due to *C. neoformans*. It is often found among those with compromised immune systems and is an **AIDS-defining opportunistic infection**.
- Healthy patients may be asymptomatic and the only finding may be pulmonary lesions on CXR that resolve spontaneously. The fungus can disseminate and cause meningitis, encephalitis, cutaneous lesions, and affect long bones and other tissues. **Symptoms** are based on the area of involvement. Patients may experience cough, pleuritic chest pain, weight loss, and fever if there is pulmonary involvement; headache, double vision, light sensitivity, N/V, and confusion if CNS involvement; cutaneous lesions (papules, pustules, nodules, ulcers) if the skin is involved.
- **Diagnosis** includes microscopic analysis, culture (gold standard), or an antigen test (highly sensitive; good for detecting early infection) for *Cryptococcus* using CSF, tissue, sputum, blood, or urine. Check CSF by India ink (limited sensitivity) or culture so meningitis can be ruled out. Confirm that no mass lesion is present by CT or MRI before LP is performed.
- Mild cases may only require monitoring to ensure that the infection does not spread. In more advanced cases, the infection is treated with different antifungal medications (e.g., fluconazole for pulmonary infections, amphotericin B ± flucytosine for meningitis). The patient should also be monitored for CNS infection and medication side effects. AIDS patients may need lifelong antifungals.
- **Complications** include cryptococcal meningitis, neural deficits, optic nerve damage, and hydrocephalus.

HISTOPLASMOSIS

Histoplasmosis is an infection caused by inhalation of **spores** from the fungus *Histoplasma capsulatum* that is found in soil and is associated with bird and bat droppings (e.g., chicken coops, caves).

- Healthy patients are usually asymptomatic and those with symptoms are typically immunocompromised or those who've had a heavy exposure to spores. The primary **pulmonary infection** occurs 3-17 days after exposure and can present with flu-like symptoms. It is typically self-limited but may become chronic. Histoplasmosis can also spread through the **blood** and can cause progressive disseminated disease in the immunocompromised (high mortality rate); this is an **AIDS-defining illness**.
- **Diagnose** through antigen tests (urine, serum), histopathology, or cultures; order a CXR. Mild and even moderate acute pulmonary histoplasmosis may resolve on its own.
- If needed, **treat** mild to moderate infections with itraconazole and severe illness with amphotericin B.

PNEUMOCYSTIS

Pneumocystis jiroveci is a **fungus** (previously known as *Pneumocystis* carinii) that causes **pneumonia** (PJP, previously PCP) in the immunocompromised. Most people have been exposed to this by the age of 3 or 4.

- **Symptoms** of PJP include a dry nonproductive cough, fever, dyspnea, and weight loss.
- CXR may show diffuse bilateral infiltrates or it may be normal; and pulse oximetry may be low, especially on exertion. **Diagnosis** is confirmed with sputum histopathology using sputum induction or bronchoalveolar lavage.
- **Treat** immediately with TMP-SMX (trimethoprim/sulfamethoxazole) for 21 days if HIV + and for 14 days in other cases. Steroids may be added for HIV patients with severe PJP. HIV/AIDS patients with CD4 counts <200/µL should receive PJP prophylaxis with TMP-SMX. Dapsone and pentamidine are alternatives.
- **Complications** include ARDS and death.

CANDIDAL INFECTIONS

Candida is a type of yeast that may cause a variety of infections:

- **Oral thrush** is commonly seen in diabetic patients and those who are immunosuppressed (HIV or underlying neoplasm). Patients often complain of burning on the tongue or in the mouth, associated with "curd-like" white patches that can be scraped away leaving reddish tissue underneath. Diagnosis is with KOH prep. Treatment is with oral or topical antifungals, including nystatin (swish and swallow or troches).
- **Candida esophagitis** also occurs in the immunosuppressed population, and patients may complain of dysphasia, odynophagia, and chest pain. This is diagnosed on EGD and may be treated with oral or IV antifungals (ketoconazole).
- **Candidal intertrigo**, or diaper rash, presents with beefy-red lesions at skin fold areas as well as satellite lesions. Treatment is with topical antifungals.
- **Candidemia** is diagnosed with fungal blood cultures and may lead to osteomyelitis, endocarditis, and other complications. Treatment is with IV antifungals.

RINGWORM

Ringworm is caused by an infection from the ***Tinea* fungus**, which produces patches on the skin that have normal centers, giving the appearance of a ring.

- The fungus can cause hair loss and patches of scaly skin that may develop blisters that ooze or crust.
- It is **transmitted** by touching the affected skin or through objects that have touched the affected skin.
- Ringworm may be **diagnosed** by viewing the skin section under a Wood's lamp. Skin cultures may also be taken for examination to identify the fungus. A potassium hydroxide (KOH) exam involves scraping the affected skin and placing the skin sample in KOH to test for the presence of the fungus.

VECTOR-BORNE AND PARASITIC INFECTIONS

MALARIA

Malaria is a **blood-borne disease** caused by a **parasite** from the genus *Plasmodium and* found in tropical areas. There are 4 known to cause disease in humans (*P. malariae, P. vivax, P. ovale,* and *P. falciparum*). These protozoa are transmitted by the **female *Anopheles* mosquito**. They travel to the **liver** where they multiply, are released, and then infect the RBCs, where they continue to multiply. Incubation time can be as little as 9 days or as much as multiple years depending on the species of the infecting parasite.

- **Signs and symptoms** include headache, high fever with shaking chills and sweating (rigors; occurs when merozoites, an immature form of the parasite, are released from RBCs), jaundice, anemia, and hepatosplenomegaly. Take a thorough history including recent travel.

- **Diagnose** with 3 thin and thick blood smears (gold standard) stained with Giemsa (preferred) and obtained 12-24 hours apart. Labs typically show elevated LDH, thrombocytopenia, and atypical lymphocytes. Rapid antigen tests are also available as well as PCR.
- **Treat** with chloroquine. If travelling, chemoprophylaxis depends on the area of travel due to species and resistance patterns, and may include chloroquine, primaquine, mefloquine, Malarone, or doxycycline. Report infections to your local or state health department.
- **Complications** include severe anemia and hemolysis, organ failure (liver, spleen, kidneys), cerebral malaria, ARDS, and death.

LYME DISEASE

Lyme disease occurs from a bite from a **deer tick** (blacklegged tick) infected with the **spirochete bacterium** *Borrelia burgdorferi*. It is the most common tick-borne disease in the U.S. and is more prevalent in heavily wooded areas. Adult ticks are more active during colder times whereas the nymphs (<2 mm in size) are more active in the warm, spring or summer months. Once the tick bites, it stays attached; however, it takes about 36-48 hours for nymphs and about 48-72 hours for adult ticks before the spirochete is transmitted to the person. **Incubation** period is 3-30 days. There are 3 stages to this disease: early localized, early disseminated, and chronic disseminated.

- At **Stage 1**, 75% have the characteristic expanding red rash (erythema migrans; can be large, ~30cm) which can progress to have central clearing (bull's eye), headache, fever, chills, myalgias, and fatigue.
- **Stage 2** occurs weeks to months after initial infection and involves systemic symptoms (flu-like), neck stiffness, headaches, migrating pain in muscles and joints, rashes, paresthesias, Bell's palsy, confusion, fatigue, myocarditis, and heart palpitations.
- **Stage 3** occurs months to years after initial infection and involves neurologic (e.g., encephalitis) and rheumatologic issues, especially arthritis of large joints (e.g., knee).

DIAGNOSIS AND TREATMENT OF LYME DISEASE

Diagnose Lyme disease using 2-tiered testing: antibodies (IgM, IgG), then Western blot. Antibiotic treatment for localized Lyme disease involves 2-3 weeks of doxycycline, amoxicillin, or cefuroxime axetil is started immediately after diagnosis. IV antibiotics may be needed for severe disease (e.g., IV ceftriaxone). Prevention is key by wearing clothes covering the skin, using tick repellents, showering soon after being outdoors in tick-prone areas, and thoroughly checking for ticks (especially in hard to see areas by using a mirror). The Lyme vaccine is no longer available and previous vaccine recipients are still at risk of contracting the disease as protection decreases over time. Complications are prevalent with untreated Lyme disease and include chronic arthritis, fatigue, chronic musculoskeletal issues, acrodermatitis chronica atrophicans, and memory and concentration issues. Report cases to the local health dept.

ROCKY MOUNTAIN SPOTTED FEVER

Rocky Mountain spotted fever is a tick-borne illness caused by **Rickettsia rickettsii**. It tends to occur in spring and summer throughout the United States.

- **Incubation** period is about one week.
- **Symptoms** include headache, fever, nausea, vomiting, loss of appetite, muscle pain, and rash on the ankles and wrists.
- **Treatment** requires an antibiotic, usually Vibramycin.

ZIKA VIRUS IN PREGNANT WOMEN

Zika virus is a **flavivirus** that is transmitted by the *Aedes* mosquito and through sexual contact. This virus can be passed on to an unborn baby causing severe congenital defects while causing mild or no disease in the mother. It is advised that all pregnant women avoid traveling to areas with the Zika virus (e.g., Central and South America, Mexico, Caribbean, Africa).

- **Incubation** period is 3-14 days and symptoms may last 4-7 days. The virus has been found to remain longer in semen than in other body fluids.
- If **symptoms** are present, they may include fever, headache, myalgias, arthralgias, a maculopapular rash, and conjunctivitis. Congenital defects include severe microcephaly, severe brain abnormalities, macular scarring, hearing loss, motor disabilities (e.g., hypertonia), and contractures. Women should be screened for Zika exposure at each prenatal visit.
- **Diagnostic** testing is recommended for all asymptomatic pregnant women who have continued exposure to Zika and for all symptomatic pregnant women who have possibly been exposed to the Zika virus. Testing includes RNA NAT testing on serum and urine, and serum IgM Zika antibody testing. Prenatal ultrasound helps determine if the effects of Zika are present. Report cases to the state health department; and the CDC can be consulted.
- There is **no treatment** or cure for the Zika virus.

HELMINTH INFESTATIONS

Helminth infestations (worms) include **roundworms** [nematodes: *Ascaris*, hookworms (cause anemia), **filariae** (cause elephantiasis)] and **flatworms** [tapeworms (cause weight loss); **flukes** (intestinal or liver)]. **Pinworms** are a type of roundworm that cause enterobiasis and is the most common helminth infestation. Pinworms are more prevalent in warmer areas of the country and infestations occur more frequently in children. The worms lay eggs within the digestive tract and then travel to the anal area where they are usually found. Pinworms are highly contagious. As a patient itches the anal area where the eggs are located, the eggs cling to the fingers and can easily be transmitted to other people either directly or through food or surfaces. The eggs can survive for 2-3 weeks on inanimate objects.

- Patients may be asymptomatic or have intense anal itching that is usually worse at night and can cause insomnia. Abdominal pain, nausea, and vomiting can also occur.
- **Diagnose** with the "tape test" which involves pressing cellophane tape over the perianal area to pick up eggs or worms and examine under the microscope. Most other helminth infestations can be diagnosed with a stool sample for ova and parasites; filariasis requires a blood smear or antigen test.
- Anthelmintic medications are given in a single dose and repeated in 2 weeks to kill the pinworms and their larvae (mebendazole, albendazole, or pyrantel pamoate). The entire family and close contacts should be treated simultaneously since pinworms are so contagious.

GIARDIA LAMBLIA

Giardia lamblia is a **protozoan** that infects water supplies and spreads to children through the fecal-oral route. It is the most common cause of non-bacterial diarrhea in the United States, causing about 20,000 cases of infection each year in all ages.

- Children often become infected after swallowing recreational waters (pools, lakes) while swimming or putting contaminated items into the mouth. *Giardia* live and multiply within the small intestine where cysts develop.
- **Symptoms** occur 7-14 days after ingestion of 1 or more cysts and include diarrhea with greasy floating stools (rarely bloody), stomach cramps, nausea, and flatulence, lasting 2-6 weeks. A chronic infection may develop that can last for months or years.
- **Treatment** includes Furazolidone 5-8 mg/kg/day in 4 doses for 7-10 days or Metronidazole 40 mg/kg/day in 3 doses for 7-10 days. Chronic infections are often very resistant to treatment.

TOXOPLASMOSIS

Toxoplasmosis is an infection caused by the **parasite *Toxoplasma gondii***, which is commonly found in soil. It is widespread and transmitted through cat feces; however, it also may be contracted by eating undercooked meat (especially pork, lamb, or venison) or poorly washed vegetables. Toxoplasmosis can cause serious disease and can affect various organs; and immunocompromised and pregnant women and their unborn babies are especially likely to have side effects of the disease (the "T" in congenital TORCH infections).

- Healthy patients are usually asymptomatic; however, once infected the parasite can remain latent until the patient becomes immunocompromised and the parasite is reactivated causing **symptoms**. The disease can cause a flu-like illness with fever, myalgias, and lymphadenopathy. More serious effects include retinochoroiditis, brain lesions, and encephalitis. Congenital toxoplasmosis may cause retinochoroiditis, microcephaly, hydrocephalus, intellectual disability, and possibly miscarriage or stillbirth.
- **Diagnose** with serology for *Toxoplasma* antibodies IgM and IgG. Also, PCR may be used to test amniotic fluid, CSF, or tissue.
- **Treat** with pyrimethamine (preferred) plus folinic acid or sulfadiazine plus folinic acid. Pregnant women should avoid high-risk practices like changing the cat litter and should avoid sand boxes.

Pharmacologic Pain Management

WHO PAIN LADDER

The WHO pain ladder was developed as an algorithm for treating pain through medications with progressively increasing potency. The approach can be used effectively with both adult and pediatric patients. Beginning with the least potent medication option, each step adds a stronger analgesic until optimum pain relief is reached.

The **WHO pain ladder** has three steps.

- **Step 1**: The patient is given a non-opioid medication which may be used alone or in conjunction with other adjuvant therapies.
- **Step 2**: If the patient reports no change in the pain level, mild- to moderate-level pain-relieving opioids are introduced along with adjuvants if they have not been previously introduced.
- **Step 3**: Uncontrolled pain is then treated with opioids for moderate to severe pain. Adjuvants may also be continued.

SCHEDULING OF PAIN MEDICATIONS

For mild to moderate pain, patients may take **acetaminophen** alternating with an **NSAID** such as ibuprofen on a regularly scheduled basis or as needed (PRN) at the onset of pain or when pain is anticipated (such as before a dressing change). However, for severe chronic pain, long-acting **opioid pain medications**, such as time-released MS Contin, Duragesic, and OxyContin, should be given regularly around the clock, because these medications help not only control but also prevent pain. The patient should not skip a dose when free of pain, because this makes control more difficult when the pain recurs. In addition to **time-scheduled medications**, the patient may need **short-acting supplementary medications**, such as Percocet, to take on a PRN basis. When taking short-acting medications, the patient should take the medication at the onset of pain, before anticipated pain, or at the onset of increased pain, rather than waiting until the pain is severe, because the goal should always be to keep the pain under control.

ACETAMINOPHEN

Acetaminophen remains one of the safest analgesics for **long-term use**. It can be used to treat mild pain or as an adjuvant with other analgesics for more severe pain. Nonspecific musculoskeletal pain and osteoarthritis are particularly responsive to acetaminophen therapy. Acetaminophen also has a limited **anti-inflammatory nature**.

Acetaminophen should, however, be used cautiously in persons with altered liver or kidney function, as well as those with a history of significant alcohol use, regardless of liver function compromise. It should be dosed separately from any opioid analgesic, which should be given separately as well. This allows for individual titration of each drug to assess the individual needs and side effects separately.

NSAIDs

NSAIDs act by inhibiting the cyclooxygenase (COX) enzyme, which controls prostaglandin formation. COX-1 affects platelet clumping, gastric blood flow, and mucosal integrity. COX-2 affects pain, inflammation, and fever. COX-1 and 2 inhibitors include aspirin and ibuprofen. Ibuprofen has a lower occurrence of side effects, such as gastric bleeding, than aspirin does. A COX-2 inhibitor, such as Celebrex, must be used with caution due to increased cardiovascular risks when used for over 18 months. NSAIDs are useful for both arthritis and bone cancer pain and work well with opioids for relief of postoperative and other severe pain. NSAIDs may increase the effects of antiseizure drugs and warfarin. Smaller doses are needed if kidney function is impaired.

LOCAL ANESTHETIC PAIN RELIEF

Local anesthetics block neural conduction of pain through the application of the anesthetic directly to the nerve endings in the area of pain. It can be injected prior to minor surgery or suturing. It can be injected intercostally for thoracic or high abdominal surgeries. The addition of a vasoconstrictor prolongs effectiveness of the anesthetic. A cream containing local anesthetics (EMLA) can be rubbed on the skin to decrease pain from IV starts or lumbar punctures. It should be applied 60-90 minutes prior to the procedure. A lidocaine 5% patch is approved to relieve pain from postherpetic neuralgia. The patient applies up to 3 patches for 12 hours at a time. Local anesthetics can be applied via the use of an epidural catheter to provide pain control for surgery, childbirth, or postoperative pain control. Opioids can be infused along with the anesthetic agent. Patients using an epidural catheter for postoperative pain tend to ambulate sooner, suffer fewer complications as a result, and go home more quickly.

OPIOIDS

GUIDELINES FOR OPIOID USE

Opioid analgesic therapy is a widely used method of chronic pain control. By adhering to clinical guidelines, pain control can be safely optimized. **Intramuscular administration** should be used as a last resort except in the presence of a "pain emergency" when no other treatment is readily available. Such cases are rare since subcutaneous delivery is almost always an alternative. Noninvasive routes such as **transdermal** and **transmucosal**, which bypass the enteral route, are optimal for continuous pain control and are often effective in eliminating breakthrough pain as well. Changing from one opioid to another, or altering the delivery method, may become necessary under the assumption that incomplete cross-tolerance among opioids occurs. Changing analgesics or method of delivery may result in a decreased drug requirement. When altering opioid delivery regimens, use **morphine equivalents** as the common factor for all dose conversions. This method will help reduce medication errors. Side effects such as sedation, constipation, nausea, and myoclonus should be anticipated in every care plan, and require both prevention and treatment methods.

SIDE EFFECTS OF OPIOID ANALGESICS

Examples of **opioid analgesics** are numerous and include morphine, hydromorphone, oxymorphone, methadone, meperidine, fentanyl, sufentanil, alfentanil, levorphanol, codeine, oxycodone, hydrocodone, propoxyphene, pentazocine, nalbuphine, and buprenorphine. Opioid analgesics have multiple effects on most of the organ systems of the body. Central nervous system (CNS) effects include respiratory depression, analgesia, euphoria, sedation, miosis, cough suppression, truncal rigidity, nausea, and vomiting. Cardiovascular effects are usually slight and include bradycardia, hypotension, reduced blood volume, and increased cerebral blood flow. Gastrointestinal effects can include constipation, decreased gastric motility, and decreased hydrochloric acid. Genitourinary effects are urinary retention and decreased renal function. Other effects are sweating, flushing, and histamine release with itching.

OPIOID USE DURING LAST FEW HOURS OF LIFE

Assessment of pain continues in the **last hours of life**, and medication is adjusted according to assessment. Pain does not necessarily increase as death approaches. It can be assumed that if pain was present prior to loss of consciousness it will continue in the patient's unconscious state. It should be assessed for and treated accordingly. Research has confirmed that administering opioids at the end of life does not hasten nor prolong the dying process. The patient's **prior medication regimen** should be continued. However, adjustments may be made in consideration of reduced renal or hepatic clearance. The **route of administration** should also be assessed for appropriateness and adjusted as needed (e.g., loss of consciousness, inability to swallow).

ORAL TRANSMUCOSAL FENTANYL CITRATE

Oral transmucosal fentanyl citrate consists of **fentanyl** on an oral applicator. The patient applies the dosage (starting at 200 mcg) to the **buccal mucosa** between the cheek and gum for rapid absorption and subsequent pain relief. This makes transmucosal fentanyl particularly useful for managing **breakthrough pain**. Pain relief generally begins within 5 minutes, but the patient should be instructed to wait 15 minutes after the previous dose has been completed before taking another dose. Swallowing even part of the dose rather than having it completely absorbed through the oral mucosa can affect the timing of pain relief onset. **Peak effect** occurs in 20 40 minutes with the total pain relief duration lasting 2-3 hours. Side effects can include somnolence, nausea, and dizziness. Consuming drinks such as coffee, tea, and juices that alter the oral secretion pH can also alter the absorption rate of transmucosal fentanyl.

METHADONE

Methadone is useful for treating **severe or chronic pain** and may be particularly helpful in the presence of **neuropathic pain**. It has a long-acting pain relief factor for a lower cost than many comparable medications. However, the exact dosing ratios with morphine remain unclear within the available research. Metabolism of methadone can also be swayed (either increased or decreased) by many other medications normally taken by patients with chronic conditions. Methadone can also be used to treat opioid addiction. US law for the prescription of methadone for addiction in detoxification or maintenance programs requires a special license and patient enrollment. The words "for pain" need to be clearly stated in the prescription. Methadone can cause drowsiness, weakness, headache, nausea, vomiting, constipation, sweating, and flushing, as well as sedation, decreased respirations, or an irregular heart rate.

OXYCODONE

Oxycodone, a synthetic formulation, is a long-acting opioid for **moderate to severe pain relief**. Side effects are similar to those of morphine. It has a similar pain relief ratio, with the possibility of less nausea and vomiting. Because if its **extended-release nature**, the medication cannot be cut or crushed for administration. Oxycodone does not carry any greater addiction risk than other types of opioids; however, public sensationalism related to this formulation may create hesitation for use among patients. Pharmacies may also limit the amount of this medication they will make available to an individual. Oxycodone should be used cautiously in patients with a history of hypothyroidism, Addison's disease, urethral stricture, prostatic hypertrophy, or lung or liver disease.

HYDROMORPHONE

Hydromorphone is available as tablets, liquid, suppository, and parenteral formulations. It offers the advantage of being synthetic, allowing for its use in the presence of a true **morphine allergy**. It is also helpful when significant side effects have occurred in the past or pain has been inadequately controlled with other medications. It may also be useful for controlling cough. However, neurotoxicity may occur, particularly myoclonus, hyperalgesia, and seizures. It should also be used cautiously in the presence of kidney, liver, heart, and thyroid disease, seizure disorders, respiratory disease, prostatic hypertrophy, or urinary problems. Common *side effects* include dizziness, lightheadedness, drowsiness, upset stomach if taken without food, vomiting, and constipation.

TITRATION OF MORPHINE FOR PAIN CONTROL

Morphine titration protocols vary according to the type of morphine used, the severity of pain, and the patient's tolerance:

Type	Peak	Duration (hours)
Short-acting	60 minutes	4-5
Long-acting	3-4 hours	8-24
IM	30-60 minutes	4-5
SQ	50-90 minutes	4-5
IV	20 minutes	4-5
Rectal	20-60 minutes	3-7

For example, **optimal dosage** is usually calculated by starting with short-acting oral morphine at 30 mg every 3-4 hours with doses increased by 25-50% for moderate pain or 50-100% for severe pain each time until the patient has at least 50% reduction in pain on a scale of 1-10 or a behavior scale. The dose may need to be reduced if excessive sedation occurs. Once the patient's pain is controlled on short-acting morphine and 24-hour dosage needs are calculated, the patient could be switched to extended-release. **Breakthrough pain** is usually treated with dosages that are 10% of the 24-hour dose. Dosages may be repeated or increased if there is inadequate relief of pain at the peak time. Increasing the dose prior to peak time will result in increased drowsiness.

MORPHINE USE FOR CHRONIC CANCER PAIN

One advantage of morphine for chronic cancer pain is that it has no **ceiling dose**. As tolerance to the medication increases or the disease progresses in severity, the dose can be gradually increased to an infinite level. It is also available in many different forms for administration, including intravenous, intramuscular, immediate release, sustained release, long-acting, liquid oral preparations, and suppositories. Morphine is often used as the **equivalency standard** for other opioid analgesics. Common *side effects* of morphine include sedation, respiratory depression, itching, nausea, chronic spasms or twitching of muscle groups, and constipation. Constipation is experienced by all patients receiving opioids. This inevitability should be planned for and treated aggressively. Hallucinations are common when morphine is initiated. After the first few days, most patients will overcome the respiratory depression, nausea, itching, and extreme sedation as tolerance for the medication is developed.

DOSAGES FOR MORPHINE, CODEINE, HYDROMORPHONE, AND LEVORPHANOL

The dosages for both the enteral and parenteral routes of morphine, codeine, hydromorphone, and levorphanol are as follows:

- **Morphine**: Enteral dosage is 30 mg (available as continuous and sustained-release formulations to last 12-24 hours); parenteral dosage is 10 mg.
- **Codeine**: Enteral dosage is 200 mg (not generally recommended); parenteral dosage is 130 mg.
- **Hydromorphone**: Enteral dosage is 7.5 mg (available as a continuous-release formula lasting 24 hours); parenteral dosage is 1.5 mg.
- **Levorphanol**: In acute pain episodes, enteral dosage is 4 mg; parenteral dosage is 2 mg. For chronic pain, dosage is equivalent for both enteral and parenteral at 1 mg. Levorphanol has a long half-life, increasing the chances of dosage accumulation over time.

Adhering to the statement "If the gut works, use it," as much as 90 percent of all patients will at least start out able to use oral medications instead of other routes.

CALCULATION FOR CONVERTING MEDICATION REGIMEN BETWEEN TWO OPIOIDS

Calculate the current 24-hour drug dose, or the total amount given in a 24-hour period. Multiply the current 24-hour dose times the ratio of the 24-hour equivalent dose for the new drug over the 24-hour equivalent of the old drug. This calculation provides the **equivalent 24-hour dose** for the new drug. Divide the new dose amount by the number of doses to be provided during the day. This amount equals the new **target dosage**.

$$\text{current 24 hr dose} \times \frac{\text{new drug 24 hr equiv dose}}{\text{current drug 24 hr equiv dose}} = \text{new 24 hr dose}$$

$$\frac{\text{new 24 hr dose}}{\text{doses per day}} = \text{new target dosage}$$

KETAMINE

Ketamine is a dissociative anesthetic that can provide pain relief as an alternate or complement to an opioid. The dissociative quality is an effective way to help the patient separate from the sensation of pain. Ketamine treatment begins with an initial bolus of 0.1 mg/kg IV. If there is no improvement, a second bolus with double the dosage is provided in 5 minutes. This can be repeated as needed. Boluses should be followed by a decrease in the patient's current opioid dose by 50% and an infusion of ketamine. **Infusion dosing** for ketamine is 0.015 mg/kg/min, or about 1 mg/min for a 70 kg person. If IV access cannot be attained, subcutaneous infusion is a possibility with dosing of 0.3-0.5 mg/kg. Consider concurrent treatment with a **benzodiazepine** to prevent hallucinations or frightful dreams and observe for increased secretions, as these are all possible side effects of ketamine. The secretions may be treated with glycopyrrolate, scopolamine, or atropine as needed.

TREATING BREAKTHROUGH PAIN

The three basic types of breakthrough pain, and their treatment measures are as follows:

- **Incident pain**: Pain that can be specifically tied to an activity or event, such as a dressing change or physical therapy. These events can be anticipated and treated with a rapid-onset, short-acting analgesic just prior to the painful event.
- **Spontaneous pain**: This type of pain is unpredictable and cannot be pinpointed to a relationship with any certain time or event. There is no way to anticipate spontaneous pain. In the presence of neuropathic pain, adjuvant therapy may be useful. Otherwise, a rapid-onset, short-acting analgesic is used.
- **End-of-dose failure**: Pain that specifically occurs at the end of a routine analgesic dosing cycle when medication blood levels begin to taper off. Careful evaluation of end-of-dose failure can help prevent it sooner. It may indicate an increased dose tolerance and the need for medication dose alterations.

TREATING NEUROPATHIC PAIN

Treatment options for neuropathic pain are often different from the methods used to treat other types of pain. The three drug classes most commonly used and proven effective for treating neuropathic pain are **anticonvulsants**, **anesthetics**, and **antidepressants**. Some are given on an as-needed basis, but most require consistent dosing with **24-hour symptom control**. Examples of the most common medications include amitriptyline, nortriptyline, duloxetine, gabapentin, topical lidocaine, opioids, and pregabalin. Medication choice is dependent on factors such as the type and progression of the disorder and the associated physical and emotional problems, such as nerve injury, muscle weakness or spasms, anxiety, depression, or sleep disturbances.

TREATING BONE PAIN

Treatment options for bone pain may depend on the causative agent related to the pain, such as the primary cancer site, severely weakened bones, or fractures. **Systemic treatment choices** include chemotherapy, radiation, and hormone therapy. **Hormone therapy** is used in the presence of estrogen and androgen receptors within the cancer cells. **Bisphosphonates**, such as ibandronate, zoledronate, and alendronate, may help strengthen the bones, slow damage, and prevent fractures; they can also help reduce pain. However, side effects can include fatigue, fever, nausea, vomiting, and anemia. **Surgery** may also be considered to remove cancerous cells or reinforce weakened areas of bone. **Opioids** and **NSAIDs/COX-2 inhibitors** are most often used for pain relief and need to be provided on a consistent basis.

Morphine combined with ibuprofen provides the benefit of a centrally acting opioid with a peripherally acting NSAID. Ibuprofen also acts as an effective adjuvant analgesic agent to enhance the relief provided by the opioid without increasing opioid side effects.

MEASURES TAKEN DURING PAIN CRISIS

During a pain crisis, assess for a change in the mechanism or location of the pain and attempt to differentiate between **terminal anxiety** or agitation and the **physical causes** of pain. Begin with a rapid increase in **opioid treatment**. If the pain is unresponsive to opioid titration, switching to **benzodiazepines**, such as diazepam and lorazepam, may produce a more effective response. If terminal symptoms remain unresponsive, assess for **drug absorption**. While invasive routes of medication delivery are generally avoided unless necessary, the only guaranteed route of drug delivery is the IV route. If there is any question about absorption, it is appropriate to establish parenteral access. IM delivery should be considered as a last resort. When all accessible resources have been exhausted, seek a pain management consultation as quickly as possible. Alternative methods of terminal pain control include radiotherapy, anesthetic, or neuroablative procedures.

Concerns Surrounding Use of Pain Medications with End-of-Life Patients

Common concerns surrounding the use of pain medications with end-of-life patients include:

- **Adequacy**: Patients are often concerned that medication may not be adequate to control pain and that chronic or breakthrough pain will occur. Patients may be concerned that if they take adequate pain medication, it will be less effective later when pain may be worse.
- **Sedation/addiction**: Some patients and family members are concerned about the risks of addiction, and others may be concerned about the effects of the medication on the patient's cognition, as some patients may become confused, disoriented, or sedated, depending on the medication or dosage.
- **Adverse effects**: Nausea and vomiting may be almost as debilitating to a patient as the pain it is intended to alleviate. Constipation, a common adverse effect, may be very uncomfortable for a patient. Some medications may result in itching and others may cause myoclonus, both of which are uncomfortable for the patient.

Prescribing Controlled Substances to Patients with Advanced Illness and Addiction Challenges

In the presence of **addiction challenges**, it becomes important to choose a **long-acting opioid** that can facilitate around-the-clock dosing and minimize the need for short-term medications used for breakthrough doses. **Short-term medication** use should be very limited or eliminated entirely if possible. Whenever possible, **nondrug adjuvants** such as relaxation techniques, distraction, biofeedback, TNS, and therapeutic communication should be used in place of short-term medications. When short-term medication therapy is needed, a **nonopioid** is best. Limit the amount of medication available to the patient at any given time and monitor for compliance with pill counts and urine toxicology screens as necessary. In some instances, a referral to an addictions specialist is recommended.

Tolerance and Pseudotolerance

Tolerance is the adaptation of the body to continued exposure to a drug or chemical. The effects of the drug at the same level of exposure are minimized over time. Additional dosing is required to maintain the same outcomes.

Pseudotolerance is the misguided perception of the health care provider that a patient's need for increasing doses of a drug is due to the development of tolerance, when the reality is that disease progression or other factors are responsible for the increase in dosing needs.

Addiction and Pseudoaddiction

Addiction is a primary and constant neurobiologic disease with genetic, psychosocial, and environmental factors that create an obsessive and irrational need or preoccupation with a substance. Addictive behaviors include unrestricted, continued cravings, as well as compulsive and persistent use of a drug despite harmful experiences and side effects.

Pseudoaddiction is an assumption that the patient is addicted to a substance when in actuality the patient is not experiencing relief from the medication. It is prolonged, unrelieved pain that may be the result of undertreatment. This situation may lead the patient to become more aggressive in seeking medicated relief, thus resulting in the inappropriate "drug seeker" label.

Physical Dependence

Physical dependence occurs when the body adapts to a drug, requiring increasing dosages over time to gain the same effect, and withdrawal of that drug then will result in an **abstinence syndrome** (withdrawal). Physical dependence can be described as a form of **addiction**. While physical dependence was commonly thought of as being related to narcotic drugs (such as morphine, methadone, fentanyl), many different types of drugs may cause some degree of physical dependence. For example, abruptly stopping a beta-blocker may result in cardiac arrhythmias or cardiac arrest. Abruptly stopping SSRIs may result in severe depression and anxiety. Thus, when considering stopping a patient's drugs near the end of life, physical dependence must be considered as many drugs should be **tapered** to avoid withdrawal effects. Drugs that affect the **central nervous system**, such as ethanol, barbiturates, and benzodiazepines, pose considerable risk of dependence and may result in severe withdrawal symptoms.

Geriatric Pathophysiology

GERIATRIC SYNDROMES

Geriatric syndromes represent a category of illnesses that is comprised of the most common non-disease conditions that are seen amongst the geriatric community. It is the responsibility of the nurse to be competent in these critical areas:

- **Falls**: As individuals age, their senses dull, leaving them vulnerable to falls due to a combination of sensory decline and chronic disease. Patients and caregivers should be provided with recommendations for fall prevention, and health care providers should create safe inpatient environments with proper fall prevention protocols.
- **Frailty**: A syndrome characterized by decreased stamina, strength, weight, and speed. This combination of issues results from the natural decline of aging and presents specific risks (falls, confusion, and depression) that must be assessed amongst the geriatric population.
- **Incontinence**: Urinary incontinence is an especially common ailment amongst the elderly population due to neurological conditions, physical limitations, and cognitive decline. This particular ailment is not only physically limiting and introduces risks for skin breakdown and infection, but it is socially limiting and can lead to psychological issues as well.
- **Delirium**: Confusion is the most common manifestation of any physical ailment amongst the elderly, along with the prevalence of dementia amongst the elderly. Delirium should never be cast aside in an elderly individual. Though common, it may be an indication of other more serious issues.
- **Functional Decline**: Functional decline is the diminished ability of an individual to carry out the activities of daily living to sustain independence and perform self-care. With this, comes the consideration for additional support, be it live-in care, nursing homes, or assisted living communities.

ADDITIONAL HEALTH ISSUES FOR THE ELDERLY

The following are additional health issues for the elderly:

- **Antibodies and Immunity**: An elderly patient can react to an infection with antibodies that have been created by the body before, but if the infection is new, it is more difficult for the body to respond appropriately. Cells in the immune system cannot proliferate as easily in an older patient as in a younger one. The number of T-cells is stable, but they do not work as well and can have less cytotoxicity. Additionally, there is not as much thymus-gained immunity because the thymus gland is smaller. This also means it is harder for an older patient to make antibodies.
- **Allergies**: Identify the type of allergic response the patient has and to what allergens, especially when getting the patient history. Determine if the response is actually an allergy to a medication or an adverse effect of it.
- **Driving**: An elderly patient senses change with age. A decreased ability to hear does not mean a patient cannot drive, but sight is very important, including binocular sight, ability to see color, and ability to see in the dark.
- **REM**: Rapid eye movement starts approximately 120 minutes after going to sleep, and happens again in 3–4 evenly spread out increments that last 10–15 minutes. It is linked to skeletal muscle atonia, rapid eye movements, and dreaming. REM sleep occurs less frequently as one gets older. With aging, the patient is more likely to wake up, which affects their sleep quality.

URINARY INCONTINENCE

Urinary incontinence (UI) is the involuntary loss of urine. Incidence increases with age and is more common in women. There are several **types of urinary incontinence**:

- **Transient**: Adverse medication reaction, urinary tract infection, severe constipation, immobility, mental disorders.
- **Urge or Reflex**: Detrusor muscle spasms cause an urgent desire to urinate because of neurological impairment in Parkinson's, stroke, Alzheimer's, and sitting. Can be triggered by drinking, or hearing or seeing running water.
- **Stress (SUI)**: Increased intra-abdominal pressure from sneezing, coughing, laughing, pregnancy, childbirth damage to the detrusor muscle and pelvic floor fascia, and menopausal hormone changes. Twice as common in women as men.
- **Enuresis**: Bedwetting while asleep.

Decreased bladder strength, diminished ability to concentrate urine, and decreased urethral closing pressure following menopause are common causes of incontinence in the elderly. Incontinence is also influenced by depression, less mobility, decreased vision, and less awareness of feeling a full bladder. Voiding routines are helpful in managing incontinence among the elderly. The typical voiding routine for a fully-grown adult patient is as follows: The initial urge to go to the bathroom happens at the point of the bladder having 200-300 mL in it. Grown patients generally void 4-6 times daily, and most will not need to go during the night except when there is a condition that makes it so or if the patient is using diuretic medication. The sensation of the bladder beginning to fill up begins at 90-150 mL, and the need to go starts at 200-300 mL. Usually, an hour or two will elapse between the first feeling of needing to go and the bladder being at full capacity. Full, easy capacity is around 300-600 mL. There should not be any leaking if going to the bathroom has to be postponed.

AGE-RELATED CHANGES IN RESPIRATORY SYSTEM

As a patient ages, the respiratory system changes in the following ways:

- **Rib cage becomes more rigid**. There will be more width measured across the anteroposterior chest. When a patient gets old, the number of alveoli decreases. They get inflexible and can no longer draw back. This means that the patient cannot breathe out as well, leading to more residual volume. There is less basilar inflation and the patient cannot get foreign bodies out as well. This condition also happens to someone who has kyphosis.
- **Decreased ability for the chest wall to work** so that it is harder to take a deep inhalation.
- **Trachea and bronchi increase in measurement** so that there is more unused area and lessened air volume that gets to the alveoli. Small airway shutting means there is less vital capacity and more residual volume.
- **Lung parenchyma is not as elastic** so that the alveoli do not function as effectively.
- **Breaths are not as deep and coughs are not as forceful** because the muscles are not as strong.

CHRONIC DIARRHEA

Chronic diarrhea is more than three bowel movements per day, with watery stools lasting more than two weeks. It is more common and potentially more serious for the elderly population. The most common cause is infectious, but **chronic diarrhea** in the elderly population can also be caused by inflammatory bowel disease, diverticulitis, colon cancer, medication side effects, and irritable bowel syndrome. Take a careful history, including a list of travel destinations. Look for these signs and **symptoms of dehydration** in the physical exam:

- Flushed, dry skin
- Dark, scanty urine
- Fast pulse and respiration
- Fever

- Vomiting or nausea
- Head rushes
- Thirst
- Dry mouth
- Anorexia
- Chills
- Tingling
- Cramps
- Exhaustion
- Confusion
- Seizures
- Unconsciousness

Send stools to the lab for culture, ova and parasites, occult blood, fecal leukocytes, and *C. difficile* toxin, especially if the patient was recently hospitalized. Collect blood for a CBC and electrolytes. Order an abdominal x-ray, and follow up with a barium enema or colonoscopy, if indicated. Treat the underlying cause. Significantly dehydrated patients require hospital admission for IV therapy.

FRACTURES

Fractures are a common cause of disability in the elderly population. The elderly population is at higher risk for sustaining **fractures** due to decreased bone mass and strength, and increased risk for falls due to poor vision and balance. The most common locations for fractures in the elderly are the distal radius, proximal humerus, proximal femur and tibia, vertebrae, hip, and pubic ramus. Most fractures are the result of minor trauma. Fractures are slightly more common in women. Make the diagnosis based on the history, physical exam, and x-ray results. Immobilize the fracture above and below the break. Administer analgesics. Refer the patient to a physiotherapist, an orthopedic surgeon, and a PSW. The goal of treatment is as rapid a return to normal activity as is possible. The elderly population is more vulnerable to complications, such as permanent functional impairment, bedsores, and pulmonary embolism. The aide, nurse, or caregiver must turn the patient every two hours to minimize complications.

AGE-RELATED CATARACTS

The lens is the clear part of the eye behind the pupil that focuses light on the retina. **Cataracts** are categorized by gradual clouding or opacification of the lens. One or both eyes can be affected, and cataracts can be congenital. Incidence increases with age and affects 70% of people over the age of 75. Risk factors include trauma, radiation, diabetes, family history, smoking, alcoholism, sun exposure, steroid use, and previous eye surgery. Signs and symptoms for cataracts include gradual lens clouding; blurry vision; decreased night vision; brown tint or color fading; halo or glare around lights; diplopia (double vision); trouble distinguishing blue and purple. An ophthalmologist makes the diagnosis by slit lamp exam and retinal exam. Cataracts are followed until they cause significant visual loss and then are treated by surgical removal of the clouded lens and replacement with a permanent intraocular or removable external lens.

HEARING LOSS

Approximately 25% of adults over the age of 65 have varying degrees of hearing loss. Risk factors for hearing loss include:

- A positive family history
- Chronic exposure to loud noises, especially if hearing protection was not worn
- Use of ototoxic drugs, like Gentamicin, NSAIDs, loop diuretics, or cancer chemotherapy

Hearing loss can be either peripheral or central. **Peripheral hearing loss** results when the ear canal is obstructed by impacted wax, a foreign object, or damage to the middle or inner ear. **Central hearing loss** is the result of damage to the portions of the brain that are needed for hearing: Vestibulocochlear nerve, brain stem, contralateral inferior colliculus, superior olivary nucleus, inferior colliculi, ipsilateral medial geniculate nucleus of the thalamus, and primary auditory cortex below the superior temporal gyrus in the temporal lobe.

MUSCLE WASTING OR ATROPHY

Sarcopenia describes the process of progressive muscle wasting that is seen in the elderly population. Muscle protein production decreases with age, resulting in a loss of muscle mass, and eventually a loss of physical functional ability. Decreased activity and a lack of exercise contribute to the process of muscle wasting. As sarcopenia progresses, it leads to decreased mobility and puts patients at higher risk for developing other health problems. The process of muscle wasting can be slowed, halted, or reversed with treatment. The most effective treatment is exercise, specifically resistance training. Adequate nutrition, including sufficient amounts of Vitamin B_{12}, protein, and calcium is an important part of the treatment regimen. Use of growth hormone, estrogen or testosterone is controversial. Sarcopenia differs from **cachexia**, which is wasting from a chronic disease, most often cancer.

SINUSITIS

Elderly individuals are at higher risk for the development of **sinusitis**. Causes include the drying out of the nasal passages, weakened nasal cartilage leading to obstruction, and a weakened immune system. The elderly population is also at increased risk for more severe infections and complications. Sinusitis can be acute or chronic. It is considered acute if symptoms have been present for less than four weeks. Patients usually present with fever, cough, facial pain, headache, mouth breathing, and nasal discharge. The diagnosis is generally made clinically; however, occasionally a CT scan and nasal swab for culture and sensitivity can be helpful. Treatment includes antibiotics and decongestants. Chronic sinusitis requires a referral to an ENT specialist (otorhinolaryngologist).

HYPOGONADISM

Male **hypogonadism** means that the testes do not produce sufficient quantities of testosterone. The patient will be impotent, infertile, and have little or no sex drive. Male hypogonadism can be present at birth from Klinefelter or Kallmann syndromes, and may present also with a micropenis and/or undescended testicles. Hypogonadism can occur later in life from pituitary or testicular tumors, especially if the man must be castrated (orchiectomy) to slow advancing prostate cancer. Hypogonadism results from aging in 30% of men over the age of 50 as **andropause**. Patients present with beard and body hair loss, decreased muscle mass, osteoporosis, gynecomastia (female pattern breast growth), and complain of erectile dysfunction (ED), emotional lability, fatigue, inability to concentrate, and decreased libido. Patients may also have hot flashes. The diagnosis is made based on the clinical picture and the serum testosterone level. Treatment is testosterone replacement therapy, but it can cause polycythemia. A good serum testosterone target level for seniors is 250-1,000 ng/dL.

MENOPAUSE

Menopause is cessation of menstrual cycles and childbearing. It is diagnosed after a woman has no periods for 12 *consecutive* months. Perimenopausal women skip periods for months but are not infertile. Menopause is usually a natural process of normal ageing. However, many women experience instant menopause through complete hysterectomy (TAHBSO), cancer chemotherapy, radiation exposure, early ovarian failure, or another pathological condition. The average age of menopause is 51; normal age range is 45-55. Late menopause is 60 and is a risk for uterine cancer. Symptoms of impending menopause include irregular periods, hot flashes, emotional lability, and difficulty sleeping because of night sweats. Diagnosis is made clinically, and confirmed with blood tests for LH, FSH, estrogen, and thyroid panel. The onset of menopause produces an elevated follicle-stimulating hormone level and a decreased estradiol level. Treatment is combined estrogen and progesterone replacement therapy, antidepressants, gabapentin, and clonidine. Do not use estrogen alone if the woman still has her uterus, because it predisposes her to cancer.

COMMON COMORBIDITIES SEEN AMONGST THE ELDERLY POPULATION

Geriatric comorbidities are combinations of chronic or acute illnesses that significantly increase the mortality rate amongst this population and are also associated with faster rates of disability exacerbation and functional decline. Understanding these comorbidities not only help the nurse manage these specific comorbidities, but also aid in the guidance of health promotion and disease prevention efforts to decrease the rates of comorbidity amongst their elderly patients. A 2010 study clustered comorbidities most commonly found in the elderly population into 3 groups (Ross, 2010). The three most common comorbidity patterns amongst the geriatric population include:

- **Cardiovascular/metabolic disorders**: Heart disease, MI, coronary artery disease and congestive heart failure often coincide with metabolic issues such as hypertension, diabetes, obesity, and gout.
- **Anxiety/depression/somatoform disorders and pain**: Pain (systemic, localized, or joint related) often coincide with psychological conditions such as anxiety, depression, and cognitive decline. Gastrointestinal issues also seem to coincide with these psychological conditions.
- **Neuropsychiatric disorders**: Psychiatric conditions such as Parkinson's and dementia, are often tied to neurological issues such as incontinence, vascular issues, and/or nerve pain.

COMMON PSYCHOLOGICAL RESPONSES TO CHRONIC ILLNESS

Chronic illness not only effects the physical health of individuals, but often has many **psychological manifestations** as well. This psychological stress is tied to the most basic needs that are engrained in individuals as children, and therefore can cause the regression of the patient to adapt more childlike responses to chronic illness over time. Often these psychological responses to chronic illnesses are based on general concepts of fear, self-esteem, and loss of control.

- **Fear**: Chronic illness, when debilitating with possibly severe consequences, forces patients to face common fears of death, loss, and pain. Remaining in a constant state of fear (stress) can lead to depression, anxiety, and anger.
- **Self-esteem**: While in the early stages of chronic illness many patients find strength and determination to conquer the disease. But, after time, the inability to do so wears on the individual's sense of strength and capability. With a loss of self-esteem, can come feelings of despair and hopelessness, which often result in an increasing rate of decline. Patients with strong support systems and positive outlooks often fare better with chronic disease.
- **Loss of control**: When chronic disease dictates an individual's life and abilities, the patient loses a sense of control over their own life. Losing one's independence can be extremely difficult mentally and emotionally, especially when the patient was previously active and healthy. By providing the patient with treatment options and educating the patient on self-care the nurse can attempt to return some elements of control to the patient, which can motivate them to own their fight against disease and find a new normal in their life that is manageable and fulfilling.

Geriatric Pharmacology

MEDICATION CONSIDERATIONS FOR ELDERLY PATIENTS

An elderly patient has an increased chance of adverse effects from medications. Approximately 1/3 of hospitalizations that are related to side effects of drugs and 1/2 of drug-associated fatalities happen in patients that are at least 60 years of age. In the United States, expenses for prescriptions for elderly patients make up 30% of every prescription filled and 40–50% of non-prescription drugs. Elderly patients spend more than $3 billion annually on these medications. Most elderly individuals have at least one ongoing health condition, including arthritis, high blood pressure, heart problems, diabetes, or other conditions, often requiring more than one drug for treatment. There are more adverse drug reactions (ADR) amongst elderly patients, 10% of whom require hospitalization for treatment for the side effects. Frequently seen adverse reactions include edema, queasiness, vomiting, anorexia, vertigo, loose stools, infrequent and difficult stools, bewilderment, and urinary retention. Be careful not to misidentify these as another condition or symptom of aging.

PHARMACOKINETICS OF OLDER ADULTS

Pharmacokinetics involves four steps: Absorption, distribution, metabolism, and elimination. All of these steps are affected by the age of the patient as the organs involved degenerate from wear and tear:

1. **Absorption** of most drugs occurs in the small intestine. Drug absorption in older adults may be delayed or decreased due to decreased blood flow to the small intestine. This could change the blood levels of drugs achieved in the geriatric patient.
2. **Distribution** of the drug is altered due to a change in body composition. Elderly patients have decreased total body water and lean muscle mass. This relative increase in total body fat may increase the duration of action of lipid-soluble drugs.
3. Most drugs are **metabolized** by either the liver or the kidneys. Decreased function of these organs leads to delayed metabolism and elimination of certain medications.
4. **Renal function** and **elimination effectiveness** diminish with age, often decreasing the kidney's ability to remove toxins and medications from the body. For this reason, drugs may remain in the body longer, therefore requiring smaller doses among the elderly.

BEERS CRITERIA

The Beers Criteria, also called the Beers List, identifies inappropriate medication use among older adults. The list is used to determine which medications are beneficial compared to those that impose risks for older adults. Because older adults are at risk of polypharmacy and inappropriate medication use, the Beers Criteria helps healthcare providers identify which medications are truly necessary and are in the patient's best interests to use. All medications that the patient takes are identified, and indications are given as to whether the medications should be avoided among those older than age 65. The recommendations are then rated for strength, and the quality of the research supporting the recommendations is identified.

DIFFICULTIES THE ELDERLY POPULATION MAY ENCOUNTER WITH MEDICATION USE

Common difficulties with medication use amongst the elderly include:

- Overuse of prescription medications
- Medication adherence and compliance issues (e.g., providing incorrect or incomplete past medical history to the professional, or using medicine that is out of date, changing dose without practitioner's orders to do so)
- Misunderstanding of how the medicine is supposed to be used due to problems with comprehension, hearing, or proper education style
- Not remembering the reason, amount, or how often the drug should be used (may result in repeating the medicine when it has already been taken)
- Difficulty affording the medication
- Vision issues resulting in misreading the label and taking the wrong dosage

- Problems getting the bottle open, dealing with small pills, cutting pills in half, and using inhalers
- More than one medical worker or more than one pharmacy can lead to inadvertent redundancy of the same medication, as can using the generic and brand name of the same thing at the same time

COMMON ADVERSE OUTCOMES OF FREQUENTLY USED PRESCRIPTION MEDICATIONS

Certain physical and psychological states may be an adverse outcome resulting from a prescribed medication:

- **Bewilderment:** Digoxin, cimetidine, dopamine agent, antihistamine, hypnotic, sedative, anticholinergic, anticonvulsant
- Anorexia: Digoxin
- **Low energy or weakness:** Diuretic, antidepressant, antihypertensive
- Absentmindedness: Barbiturate
- Difficult bowel movements: Anticholinergic
- **Loose stool:** Oral antacid
- **GI upset:** Iron, NSAID, salicylate, corticosteroid, estrogen, alcohol
- Ringing in the ears (tinnitus): Analgesic
- **Urinary retention:** Anticholinergic, alpha-agonist
- **Orthostatic low blood pressure:** Antihypertensive, sedative, diuretic, antidepressant
- **Depression:** Benzodiazepine
- **Vertigo:** Sedative, antihypertensive, anticonvulsant, diuretic

ADVERSE OUTCOMES OF HISTAMINE BLOCKERS, IBUPROFEN, AND BETA-BLOCKERS

Histamine blockers in the elderly can cause paradoxical central nervous system provocation that has an outcome of ataxia in this population. Antihistamines may cause problems with vision and walking, leading to falls, which may cause unforeseen hospital visits or require a nursing home. Antihistamines can also interfere with the effectiveness of other medications or enhance other medications' negative side effects.

Some elderly patients are already dealing with decreased renal functioning. **Ibuprofen** has the ability to worsen these issues leading to nephrosis, cirrhosis, and congestive heart failure.

If the patient is older, a **beta-blocker** is not a good option for treating hypertension due to their decreased beta-adrenergic receptor sensitivity for the elderly patient. Elderly patients need smaller amounts of calcium entry antagonists, ACE inhibitors, or diuretics. Too high a dose (in the elderly) will cause moodiness, impotence, weariness, and lessened ability to think clearly. Elderly patients are particularly prone to congestive heart failure and peripheral vascular insufficiency due to beta-adrenergic toxins.

POLYPHARMACY

Polypharmacy is a term used to describe inappropriate use of multiple medications at one time. It occurs when medications are taken that are not indicated, medications that have adverse interactions with one another are taken together, and patients take contraindicated medications. Polypharmacy is a common problem in the geriatric population. Most office visits result in new prescriptions being written and patients may accumulate many different medications in their home. Polypharmacy greatly increases the patient's risk of having an adverse drug reaction.

To manage polypharmacy and prevent complications, obtain a detailed drug history at each visit. This should include nonprescription medications and herbal remedies. Educating patients about the problem of polypharmacy is very important. This can occur in the clinician's office or with a community education program. Assist elderly patients with medication identification, recommending pill boxes to help the patient divide medications and minimize risks for medication misuse.

MASTER Rules for Rational Drug Therapy

Although drugs are often very useful and effective in treating illnesses, there is a point when it becomes dangerous to the patient. Drug resistance, drug interactions, and drug intolerances are all common problems, especially among elderly patients, because an iatrogenic illness can develop. For these reasons, it is important to limit drugs to only those that are absolutely necessary. To help the practitioner decide whether a drug should be used or not, they must remember the **MASTER rules**.

- **M** is for **minimizing** the number of drugs a patient is taking.
- **A** is for considering **alternate** treatments that may be as or more effective than using a drug.
- **S** is for **start** low and increase slowly. Only give the patient the minimum amount, and be careful when increasing doses.
- **T** is for **titration** of drugs; tailor the amount given over time to the individual patient.
- **E** is for **education** of the patient about the drugs he or she is taking.
- **R** is for **regular** reviewing of drugs and doses.

Psychosocial Pathophysiology

DEVELOPMENTAL DELAYS AND INTELLECTUAL DISABILITY

Developmental delays occur when a patient does not progress mentally at the same rate as the general population. Intellectual disability is a condition in which individuals may have difficulty adapting to changing environments, need guidance in decision-making, and have self-care or communication deficits. Behaviors range from shy and passive to hyperactive and aggressive. Intellectual disability may be inherited (Tay-Sachs), toxin-related (maternal alcohol consumption), perinatal (hypoxia), environmental (lack of stimulation/neglect), or acquired (encephalitis, brain injury). **Diagnosis** involves performance results from standardized tests with behavior analysis. Intellectual disability classifications are based on IQ:

- **55-69 (mild, 85% of cases):** Educable to about 6th grade level. May not be diagnosed until adolescence. Usually able to learn skills and be self-supporting but may need assistance and supervision.
- **40-54 (moderate, 10% of cases):** Trainable and may be able to work and live in sheltered environments or with supervision.
- **25-39 (severe, 3-4% of cases):** Language usually delayed and can learn only basic academic skills and perform simple tasks.
- **≤25 (profound, 1-2% of cases):** Usually associated with neurological disorder with sensorimotor dysfunction. Require constant care and supervision.

Nursing considerations: Always treat patients according to their developmental level, not their physical age. This is especially important when considering education and consent. People with developmental delays are at increased risk for injury and abuse.

PERSONALITY DISORDER

A personality disorder is a fixed and enduring set pattern or traits of behavior that **deviate from expected behaviors within a culture**. These disorders inhibit the individual's ability to have meaningful interpersonal relationships, to be fulfilled, or to enjoy life. Onset usually occurs during adolescence or early adulthood. A personality disorder is an attitude directed toward the whole world including one's own self. This attitude is expressed through thoughts, feelings, and behaviors. Many times, the behaviors will become less extreme as the person gets older.

DSM CLASSIFICATION GROUPINGS

The DSM-5 lists 10 personality disorders grouped into three clusters: A, B, and C.

- **Cluster A** includes disorders that are characterized by odd or eccentric behaviors and a tendency for social awkwardness and withdrawal.
- **Cluster B** includes disorders that are characterized by erratic, highly emotional, dramatic, or impulsive behaviors.
- **Cluster C** includes disorders that are characterized predominantly by fearful or anxious symptoms.

SPECIFIC DIAGNOSES INCLUDED IN CLUSTER A FOR PERSONALITY DISORDERS

Cluster A: The classification of Cluster A for personality disorders includes the diagnoses of paranoid, schizoid, and schizotypal personality disorders.

- The **paranoid** individual is very distrustful and suspicious of others. They believe that other people are up to no good, are keeping secrets, and may intend to harm them. There is usually no basis or evidence to support this belief.

- The **schizoid** individual exhibits a consistent social detachment. Many of their behaviors indicate a restricted emotional response and can include appearing cold and indifferent, having no desire for close personal relationships, having no desire for intimacy, choosing solidarity over socializing, and usually having no close friends or relatives.
- Like the schizoid individual, the **schizotypal** individual tends to lack intimate relationships, but this is due to social ineptitude and fear rather than a lack of interest in relationship. They also experience cognitive and perceptual distortions, seeing or hearing things that are not there, and hold odd or superstitious beliefs.

Specific Diagnoses Included in Cluster B for Personality Disorders

Cluster B: The classification of Cluster B for personality disorders includes the diagnoses of antisocial, borderline, histrionic, and narcissistic personality disorders.

- The **antisocial** individual exhibits a blatant disregard for other people. They frequently lie, manipulate, exploit, and commit illegal acts.
- The **borderline** individual has a markedly unstable self-image. They are very impulsive, self-destructive, have unstable and intense interpersonal relationships, mood instability, inappropriate and intense anger, and may have recurrent suicidal or self-mutilating behaviors.
- The **histrionic** individual is extremely emotional and desires to be the center of attention. They often perform attention-seeking behaviors and have frequent, intense, and short-lived relationships.
- The **narcissistic** individual has a great sense of self-importance and is often arrogant. They lack empathy for others and can be exploitative and manipulative, and they tend to react violently if they perceive disrespect or opposition.

Specific Diagnoses Included in Cluster C for Personality Disorders

Cluster C: The classification of Cluster C for personality disorders includes the diagnoses of avoidant, dependent, and obsessive-compulsive personality disorders.

- The **avoidant** individual is socially inhibited and consequently avoids interaction with others. They are very sensitive to criticism or rejection and often have feelings of inadequacy.
- The **dependent** individual has very low self-esteem and will be submissive and dependent in behaviors and relationships, making them susceptible to being taken advantage of. If they lose their primary supportive relationship, they will quickly seek to establish another one.
- The **obsessive-compulsive** individual will have an extreme preoccupation with minute details, and will possess an inflexible perfectionism and desire for control. They also exhibit cold, unfeeling, and superior attitudes towards others.

Bipolar Disorder

Bipolar disorder causes severe mood swings between hyperactive states and depression, accompanied by impaired judgment because of distorted thoughts. The hypomanic stage may allow for creativity and good functioning in some people, but it can develop into more severe mania, which may be associated with psychosis and hallucinations with rapid speech and bizarre behavior, and then into periods of profound depression. While most cases are diagnosed in late adolescence, there is increasing evidence that some children present with symptoms earlier; especially at risk are children with a bipolar parent. Bipolar disorder is associated with high rates of suicide, so early diagnosis and treatment is critical.

Symptoms may be relatively mild or involve severe rapid cycling between mania and depression.

Treatment includes both medications (usually given continually) to prevent cycling and control depression and psychosocial therapy, such as cognitive therapy, to help control disordered thought patterns and behavior. Psychiatric referral should be made.

OBSESSIVE-COMPULSIVE DISORDER

Anxiety disorders also include the diagnosis of obsessive-compulsive disorder (OCD). OCD involves either **obsessions** or **compulsions** that are persistent impulses or thoughts that are uncontrollable by the person. These thoughts lead to an **abnormally elevated anxiety response**. Some examples of obsessions can include fear of dirt, germs, robbery, contracting a medical disease, unintentional discarding of important information, having images of a sexual nature, or things not being symmetrical or completed. Compulsions are when the individual is driven to perform certain repetitive behaviors in ritualistic order with the outcome being resolution of the anxiety caused by the obsession.

Some examples of **compulsive repetitive behaviors** can include hand washing, checking locks, counting objects found routinely within their normal day, hoarding, ordering or arranging items, or saying words silently.

COMORBIDITIES

When an individual has two or more disorders occurring at the same time, these disorders are considered to share **comorbidity**. Obsessive-compulsive disorder (OCD) is often found sharing comorbidity with other psychological disorders. Many times, individuals with OCD also have Tourette's syndrome, depression, panic attacks, mood disorders, social and specific phobias, eating disorders, or personality disorders. It has been found that Tourette's syndrome and OCD actually cause similar brain dysfunctions. Depression is commonly seen in patient's suffering from OCD due to the isolating effects it can have upon their lifestyle. It is also common for these individuals to have substance abuse problems due to trying to self-medicate to solve their struggles with OCD.

DEPRESSION

Depression is a mood disorder characterized by profound feelings of sadness and withdrawal. It may be acute (such as after a death) or chronic with recurring episodes over a lifetime. The cause appears to be a combination of genetic, biological, and environmental factors. A major depressive episode is a depressed mood, profound and constant sense of hopelessness and despair, or loss of interest in all or almost all activities for a period of at least two weeks. Some drugs may precipitate depression: diuretics, Parkinson's drugs, estrogen, corticosteroids, cimetidine, hydralazine, propranolol, digitalis, and indomethacin. Depression is associated with neurotransmitter dysregulation, especially serotonin and norepinephrine. Major depression can be mild, moderate, or severe.

Symptoms include changes in mood, sadness, loss of interest in usual activities, increased fatigue, changes in appetite and fluctuations in weight, anxiety, and sleep disturbance.

Treatment includes tricyclic antidepressants (TCAS) and SSRIs, but SSRIs have fewer side effects and are less likely to cause death with an overdose. Counseling, undergoing cognitive behavioral therapy, treating underlying cause, and instituting an exercise program may help reduce depression.

ANXIETY AND DEPRESSION DUE TO INTENSIVE CARE STAYS

Anxiety and depression affect over half of patients who are treated in intensive care not only during the stay but also after discharge, especially if care is long-term or if their needs for moderate or high care continue. Additionally, studies have shown that those who suffer depression during and after ICU stays have increased risk of mortality over the next two years. Patients with anxiety may appear restless (thrashing about the bed), have difficulty concentrating, exhibit tachycardia and tachypnea, experience insomnia and feelings of dread, and complain of various ailments, such as stomach ache and headache. Symptoms of depression may overlap (and patients may have both anxiety and depression) and may also include fatigue, insomnia, withdrawal, appetite change, irritability, pessimistic outlooks, feelings of worthlessness, sadness, and suicidal ideation. Brief screening tools for anxiety and depression should be used with all ICU patients and interventions per psychological referral made as needed.

ANXIETY DISORDERS

Anxiety is a human emotion and experience that everyone has at some point during their life. Feelings of uncertainty, helplessness, isolation, alienation, and insecurity can all be experienced during an **anxiety response**. Many times, anxiety occurs without a specific known object or source. It can occur because of the unknown. Anxiety occurs throughout the life cycle, and therefore anxiety disorders can affect people of all ages. Populations that are most commonly affected include women, smokers, people under the age of 45, individuals that are separated or divorced, victims of abuse, and people in the lower socioeconomic groups. An individual can have one single anxiety disorder, experience more than one anxiety disorder, or have other mental health disorders all occurring at the same time.

GENERALIZED ANXIETY DISORDER

Generalized anxiety disorder can be very insidious and occurs when an individual consistently experiences **excessive anxiety and worry**. This anxiety and worry will be present almost every day and lasts for a period of at least six months. The worry and anxiety will be uncontrollable, intrusive, and not related to any medical disease process. It will pertain to real-life events, situations, or circumstances and may occur along with mild depression symptoms. The individual will also experience three or more of the following symptoms: fatigue, inability to concentrate, irritability, insomnia, restlessness, loosing thought processes or going blank, and muscle tension. The continued anxiety and worry will eventually affect daily functioning and cause social and occupational disturbances.

COMORBIDITIES

Individuals with generalized anxiety disorder (GAD) will often have **other mental health disorders**. When a person has more than one psychological disorder occurring at the same time, these disorders are considered to be **comorbid**. Most patients suffering from GAD will have at least one more psychiatric diagnosis. The most common comorbid disorders can include major depressive disorder, social or specific phobias, panic disorder, and dysthymic disorder. It is also common for these individuals to have substance abuse problems, and they may look to alcohol or barbiturates to help control their symptoms of anxiety.

LEVELS OF ANXIETY

There are four main levels of anxiety that were named by Peplau. They are as follows:

1. **Mild anxiety** is associated with normal tensions of everyday life. It can increase awareness and motivate learning and creativity.
2. **Moderate anxiety** occurs when the individual narrows their field of perception and focuses on the immediate problem. This level decreases the perceptual field; however, the person can tend to other tasks if directed.
3. **Severe anxiety** leads to a markedly reduced field of perception and the person focuses only on the details of the problem. All energy is directed at relieving the anxiety and the person can only perform other tasks under significant persuasion.
4. **Panic** is the most extreme level of anxiety and associated with feelings of dread and terror. The individual is unable to perform any other tasks no matter how strongly they are persuaded to do so. This level can be life-threatening with complete disorganization of thought occurring.

PHYSICAL SYMPTOMS

Anxiety produces a very physical response and effects the largest body systems, such as cardiovascular, respiratory, GI, neuromuscular, urinary tract, and skin. Symptoms vary and can increase upon a continuum depending upon the level of anxiety the person is experiencing.

- **Cardiovascular symptoms** can include palpitation, tachycardia, hypertension, feeling faint or actually fainting, hypotension, or bradycardia.
- **Respiratory symptoms** can include tachypnea, shortness of breath, chest pressure, shallow respirations, or choking sensation.
- **GI symptoms** can include revulsion toward food, nausea, diarrhea, and abdominal pain or discomfort.

Even though anxiety occurs psychologically, it can produce extreme **physical responses** from the neuromuscular system, urinary tract, and skin. These symptoms can range from mild to severe depending upon the degree of anxiety the person is experiencing.

- **Neuromuscular symptoms** can include hyperreflexia, being easily startled, eyelid twitching, inability to sleep, shaking, fidgeting, pacing, wobbly legs, or clumsy movements.
- **Urinary tract symptoms** can include increased frequency and sensation of need to urinate.
- **Skin symptoms** can include flushed face, sweaty palms, itching, sensations of being hot and/or cold, pale facial coloring, or diaphoresis.

BEHAVIORAL AND AFFECTIVE RESPONSES

Behavioral and affective symptoms along with a multitude of physical symptoms are observable in anxious patients. The effects of these responses can affect the person experiencing the anxiety along with their relationships with others.

- Some **behavioral responses** can include restlessness and physical tension, hypervigilance, rapid speech, social or relationship withdrawal, decreased coordination, avoidance, or flight.
- **Affective responses** are the patient's emotional reactions and can be described subjectively by the individual. Patients may describe symptoms such as edginess, impatience, tension, nervousness, fear, frustration, jitteriness, or helplessness.

COGNITIVE RESPONSES

Anxiety not only produces physical and emotional symptoms, but it can also greatly affect the individual's intellectual abilities. **Cognitive responses** to anxiety occur in three main categories. These include sensory-perceptual, thought difficulties, and conceptualization. Responses that affect the patient's **sensory-perceptual fields** can include feeling that their mind is unclear or clouded, seeing objects indistinctly, perceiving a surreal environment, increased self-consciousness, or hypervigilance. **Thinking difficulties** can include the inability to remember important information, confusion, inability to focus thoughts or attention, easily distracted, blocking thoughts, difficulty with reasoning, tunnel vision, or loss of objectivity. **Conceptual difficulties** can include the fear of loss of control, inability to cope, potential physical injury, developing a mental disorder, or receiving a negative evaluation. The patient may have cognitive distortion, protruding scary visual images, or uncontrollable repetition of fearful thoughts.

PANIC ATTACKS

Panic attacks are short episodes (peaking in 5-10 minutes) of intense anxiety that can result in a wide variety of **symptoms** that include:

- Dyspnea
- Palpitations
- Hyperventilation
- Nausea and vomiting

- Intense fear or anxiety
- Pain and pressure in the chest
- Dizziness and fainting
- Tremors

Panic attacks may be associated with agoraphobia, depression, or intimate partner violence and abuse (IPVA), so a careful history is important. Typically, patients believe they are dying or having a heart attack and require reassurance and treatment, such as diazepam or lorazepam, in the ED for the acute episode. In severe cases, ASA may be given and EKG done to rule out cardiac abnormalities. Patients should be referred for psychiatric evaluation for ongoing medications such as SSRIs (sertraline, paroxetine, fluoxetine) to prevent recurrence. Panic attacks become chronic panic disorders if they are recurrent, with each attack each followed by at least a month of fear of another attack.

PTSD

Patients that experience a traumatic event may re-experience the trauma through distressing thoughts and recollections of the event. In addition, psychological effects of the trauma may include difficulty sleeping, emotional lability and problems with memory and concentration. Patients may also wish to avoid places or activities that remind them of their trauma. These are all characteristics of **post-traumatic stress disorder (PTSD)** and may cause patients extreme distress and significantly impact their quality of life.

Signs and symptoms: Nightmares, flashbacks, insomnia, symptoms of hyperarousal including irritability and anxiety, avoidance, and negative thoughts and feelings about oneself and others.

Diagnosis: PTSD is diagnosed through psychological assessment and criteria defined in the Diagnostic and Statistical Manual of Mental Disorders, Fifth Edition (DSM-5).

Treatment: Pharmacologic therapy may be utilized to help control the symptoms of PTSD. Non-pharmacologic therapy options include group and individual/family therapy, cognitive behavioral therapy, and anxiety management/relaxation techniques. Hypnosis may also be utilized.

STRESS
RELATIONSHIP BETWEEN STRESS AND DISEASE

Stress causes a number of physical and psychological changes within the body:

- Cortisol levels increase
- Digestion is hindered and the colon stimulated
- Heart rate increases
- Perspiration increases
- Anxiety and depression occur and can result in insomnia, anorexia or weight gain, and suicide
- Immune response decreases, making the person more vulnerable to infections
- Autoimmune reaction may increase, leading to autoimmune diseases

The body's **compensatory mechanisms** try to restore homeostasis. When these mechanisms are overwhelmed, pathophysiological injury to the cells of the body result. When this injury begins to interfere with the function of the organs or systems in the body, symptoms of dysfunction will occur. If the conditions are not corrected, the body changes the structure or function of the affected organs or systems.

ADAPTATION OF CELLS TO STRESS

The most common stressors to cells include the lack of oxygen, presence of toxins or chemicals, and infection. **Cells react to stress** by making the following changes:

- **Hypertrophy**: Cells swell, leading to an overall increase in the size of the affected organ.
- **Atrophy**: Cells shrivel and the overall organ size decreases in size.
- **Hyperplasia**: The cells divide and overgrowth and thickening of the tissue results.
- **Dysplasia**: The cells are changed in appearance as a result of irritation over an extended period of time, sometimes leading to malignancy.
- **Metaplasia**: Cells change type as a result of stress.

If the stress that caused the cells to change continues, the cells become injured and die. When enough cells die, organ and systemic failure occur.

PSYCHOLOGICAL RESPONSE TO STRESS

When stress is encountered, a person **responds** according to the threat perceived to compensate. The threat is evaluated as to the amount of harm or loss that has occurred or is possible. If the stress is benign (such as with marriage), then a challenge is present that demands change. Once the threat or challenge is defined, the person can gather information, resources, and support to make the changes needed to resolve the stress to the greatest degree possible. Immediate psychological response to stress may include shock, anger, fear, or excitement. Over time, people may develop chronic anxiety, depression, flashbacks, thought disturbances, and sleep disturbances. Changes may occur in emotions and thinking, in behavior, or in the person's environment. People may be more able to adapt to stress if they have many varied experiences, a good self-esteem, and a support network to help as needed. A healthy lifestyle and philosophical beliefs, including religion, may give a person more reserve to cope with stress.

IMPACT OF DIFFERENT KINDS OF STRESS

Everyone encounters **stress** in life and it **impacts** each person differently. There are the small daily "hassles," major traumatic events, and the periodic stressful events of marriage, birth, divorce, and death. Compounded stress experienced on a daily basis can impact health status over time. Stressors that occur suddenly are the hardest to overcome and result in the greatest tension. The length of time that a stressor is present affects the impact with long-term, relentless stress, such as that generated by poverty or disability, resulting in disease more often. If there is **ineffective coping**, a person will suffer greater changes resulting in even more stress. The nurse can help patients to recognize those things that induce stress in their lives, find ways to reduce stress when possible, and teach effective coping skills and problem-management.

VIOLENCE AND AGGRESSION

Violence and aggression are sometimes seen in critical care settings. The nurse must be aware of signs of impending violence or aggression in order to intervene and prevent injury to self or staff.

- **Violence** is a physical act perpetrated against an inanimate object, animal, or other person with the intent to cause harm. Violence often results from anger, frustration, or fear. It often occurs because the perpetrator believes that he is threatened in some way. Violence may occur suddenly without warning or following an escalating pattern of aggressive behavior.
- **Aggression** is the communication of a threat or intended act of violence that often occurs before the act of violence is carried out. This communication can occur verbally or nonverbally. Gestures, shouting, increasing volume of speech, invasion of personal space, and prolonged eye contact are all examples of aggression. The nurse should promptly recognize all forms of aggression and redirect or remove the patient from the situation to avoid an act of violence.

MANAGEMENT OF PATIENTS WITH VIOLENT BEHAVIOR

Patients may exhibit **violent behavior** for a number of reasons, including metabolic disorders (hypoglycemia), neurological disorders (brain tumor), psychiatric disorders (schizophrenia), or substance abuse (drugs and alcohol). Patients who make threats or have a history of violent behavior should be approached with caution.

Diagnosis includes history, physical exam, CBC and chemistry panel, toxicology screening, ECG, and, in some cases, CT scans or lumbar punctures. Violent behavior tends to escalate from anxiety to defensiveness to aggression, so identifying these signs and providing support through information, setting limits, using restraints, and seclusion can avoid injuries. Handcuffs should not be removed in the ED, and patients who are so violent they must be restrained should not be allowed to leave the ED against medical advice.

Pharmacologic treatment includes:

- **Antipsychotic drugs**: Haloperidol 5 mg IM (1-2 mg for elderly patients)
- **Benzodiazepines**: Lorazepam 2-4 mg IM/IV (often in conjunction with antipsychotic drugs)
- **Hypnotics**: Droperidol 2.5 mg IM/IV

HOMICIDAL IDEATION

Homicidal ideation, the intention to kill another person, can occur for a variety of reasons:

- **Sociopathy/psychopathy**: These patients usually appear quite normal and may even seem charming, but they can be very dangerous because they lack empathy for others. Some are involved in gangs in which violent behavior is expected and valued.
- **Psychosis**: Uncontrolled schizophrenia and paranoia may result in a patient behaving in a homicidal manner. In some cases, these changes may be brought about by pathology, such as TBI or brain tumor.
- **Medications**: Medications such as antidepressants, SSRIs, and antipsychotics as well as interferon have been associated with homicidal ideation in some patients. Patients on multiple medications may experience an involuntary intoxication that results in rage reactions and sometimes even the death of others.

Indications of homicidal ideation may include verbal threats, use of weapons, and violent behavior. Patients who express homicidal ideation or have attempted homicide require immediate psychiatric referral and may require restraint. The nurse should conduct a complete review of medications and notify security personnel if the patient poses a danger.

PSYCHOSIS

Psychosis is a severe reaction to stressors (psychological, physical) that results in alterations in affect and impaired psychomotor and behavioral functions, including the onset of hallucinations and/or delusions. Psychosis is not a diagnosis but is a symptom that may be caused by a mental disorder (such as schizophrenia or bipolar disease) or a physical disorder (such as a brain tumor or Alzheimer's disease). Psychosis may also be induced by some prescription drugs (muscle relaxants, antihistamines, anticonvulsants, corticosteroids, antiparkinson drugs), illicit drugs (cocaine, PCP, amphetamines, cannabis, LSD), and alcohol. Treatment depends on identifying the underlying cause of the psychosis and initiating treatment. For example, if caused by schizophrenia, then antipsychotic drugs and hospitalization in a mental health facility may be indicated. In most cases of drug-induced psychosis, stopping the drug alleviates the symptoms although some may benefit from the addition of a benzodiazepine or antipsychotic drug until symptoms subside.

SUICIDAL IDEATION

Patients may attempt suicide for many reasons, including severe depression, social isolation, situational crisis, bereavement, or psychotic disorder.

Suicidal indications are as follows:

- Depression or dysphoria
- Hostility to others
- Problems with peer relationships, and lack of close friends
- Post-crisis stress (divorce, death in family, graduation, college)
- Withdrawn personality; quiet or lonely appearance or behavior
- Change in behavior (dropping grades, unkempt appearance, change in sleeping patterns)
- A sudden increase in positive mood may indicate patient has a plan
- Co-morbid psychiatric problems (bipolar, schizophrenia)
- Substance abuse

The following are indicators of **high risk for repeated suicide attempt**:

- Violent suicide attempt (knives, gunshots)
- Suicide attempt with low chance of rescue
- Ongoing psychosis or disordered thinking
- Ongoing severe depression and feeling of helplessness
- History of previous suicide attempts
- Lack of social support system

Nursing considerations: Take all suicidal ideations seriously; do not minimize them. Suicidal patients should be watched continuously, given plastic utensils, break-away wall rails/shower heads, no cords/sharp instruments.

SUBSTANCE ABUSE

Substance abuse is the abuse of drugs, medicines, or alcohol that causes mental and physical problems for the abuser and family. Abusers use substances out of boredom, to hide negative self-esteem, to dampen emotional pain, and to cope with daily stress. As the abuse continues, abusers become unable to take care of daily needs and duties. They lack effective coping mechanisms and the ability to make healthy choices. They can't identify and prioritize stress or choose positive behavior to resolve the stress in a healthy way. Some family members may act as codependents because of their desire to feel needed by the abuser, to control the person, and to stay with him or her. The nurse can help the family to confront an individual with their concerns about the person and their proposals for treatment. Family members can enforce consequences if treatment is not sought. Family members may also need counseling to learn new behaviors to stop enabling the abuser to continue substance abuse.

PATHOPHYSIOLOGY OF ADDICTION

Genetic, social, and personality factors may all play a role in the development of **addictive tendencies**. However, the main factor of the development of substance addiction is the pharmacological activation of the **reward system** located in the central nervous system (CNS). This reward systems pathway involves **dopaminergic neurons**. Dopamine is found in the CNS and is one of many neurotransmitters that play a role in an individual's mood. The mesolimbic pathway seems to play a primary role in the reward and motivational process involved with addiction. This pathway begins in the ventral tegmental area of the brain (VTA) and then moves forward into the nucleus accumbens located in the middle forebrain bundle (MFB). Some drugs enhance mesolimbic dopamine activity, therefore producing very potent effects on mood and behavior.

INDICATORS OF SUBSTANCE ABUSE

Many people with substance abuse (alcohol or drugs) are reluctant to disclose this information, but there are a number of **indicators** that are suggestive of substance abuse:

Physical signs include:

- Burns on fingers or lips
- Pupils abnormally dilated or constricted, eyes watery
- Slurring of speech, slow speech
- Lack of coordination, instability of gait, tremors
- Sniffing repeatedly, nasal irritation, persistent cough
- Weight loss
- Dysrhythmias
- Pallor, puffiness of face
- Needle tracks on arms or legs
- Odor of alcohol/marijuana on clothing or breath

Behavioral signs include:

- Labile emotions, including mood swings, agitation, and anger
- Inappropriate, impulsive, or risky behavior
- Lying
- Missing appointments
- Difficulty concentrating, short term memory loss, blackouts
- Insomnia or excessive sleeping; disoriented, confused
- Lack of personal hygiene

ALCOHOL WITHDRAWAL

Chronic abuse of ethanol (alcoholism) can lead to physical dependency. Sudden cessation of drinking, which often happens in the inpatient setting, is associated with **alcohol withdrawal syndrome.** It may be precipitated by trauma or infection and has a high mortality rate, 5-15% with treatment and 35% without treatment.

Signs/Symptoms: Anxiety, tachycardia, headache, diaphoresis, progressing to severe agitation, hallucinations, auditory/tactile disturbances, and psychotic behavior (delirium tremens).

Diagnosis: Physical assessment, blood alcohol levels (on admission).

Treatment includes:

- Medication: IV benzodiazepines to manage symptoms; electrolyte and nutritional replacement, especially magnesium and thiamine.
- Use the CIWA scale to measure symptoms of withdrawal; treat as indicated.
- Provide an environment with minimal sensory stimulus (lower lights, close blinds) & implement fall and seizure precautions.
- Prevention: Screen all patients for alcohol/substance abuse, using CAGE or other assessment tool. Remember to express support and comfort to patient; wait until withdrawal symptoms are subsiding to educate about alcohol use and moderation.

Psychosocial Interventions

BEHAVIOR MODIFICATION

Behavior modification is a type of systematic therapy that works toward the goal of replacing **maladaptive behaviors** with **positive behaviors**. This type of therapy can be utilized with individuals, groups, or entire communities. The hope of this approach is to get rid of the unwanted behaviors by utilizing positive reinforcement directed toward the desired behaviors. After experiencing **positive reinforcement**, the participant will want to repeat the good behaviors to gain the reward. These new behaviors will then become habits over time and will replace the old behaviors. This type of therapy can be very effective with eating disorders, smoking cessation, or addictions.

COGNITIVE-BEHAVIORAL THERAPY

Cognitive-Behavioral Therapy (CBT) focuses on the impact that thoughts have on behavior and feelings, encouraging the individual to use the power of rational thought to alter perceptions. CBT centers on the concept of unlearning previous behaviors and learning new ones, questioning behaviors, and doing homework. This approach to counseling is usually short-term, about 12-20 sessions. The first sessions obtain a history, middle sessions focus on the problems, and the last sessions review and reinforce newly learned habits and thought patterns. Individuals are assigned homework during the sessions to practice new ways of thinking and to develop new coping strategies. The therapist helps the individual identify goals and then find ways to achieve those goals. CBT acknowledges that all problems cannot be resolved, but one can deal differently with problems. The therapist asks questions to determine the individual's areas of concern and encourages the individual to question his or her own motivations and needs. CBT is goal-centered, so each counseling session is structured toward a particular goal, such as coping techniques.

AARON BECK'S COGNITIVE THERAPY

Aaron Beck discovered that during psychotherapy patients often had a second set of thoughts while undergoing free association. Beck called these **automatic thoughts**, which were labeled and interpreted, according to a personal set of rules. Beck called dysfunctional automatic thoughts **cognitive disorders**. Beck identified a triad of negative thoughts regarding the self, environment, and world. The key concepts in **Aaron Beck's cognitive therapy** include the following:

- **Therapist/patient relationship**: Therapy is a collaborative partnership. The goal of therapy is determined together. The therapist encourages the patient to disagree when appropriate.
- **Process of therapy**: The therapist explains the following: one's perception of reality is not reality. The interpretation of sensory input depends on cognitive processes. The patient is taught to recognize maladaptive ideation, identifying the following: observable behavior, underlying motivation, his or her thoughts and beliefs. The patient practices distancing the maladaptive thoughts, explores his or her conclusions, and tests them against reality.
- **Conclusions**: The patient makes the rules less extreme and absolute, drops false rules, and substitutes adaptive rules.

RECOVERY MODEL

The Recovery Model approach to mental health shifts control of treatment options to the patient rather than the physician deciding the plan of care. This has been effective in those patients who have the capacity to make decisions to allow them to be more independent and take a more active role in the decision-making regarding their treatment plan. The goal of this model is to allow the patient to be more **autonomous** so that they may achieve the ultimate goals of gaining employment, finding housing, and living independently. The more independent the patient can become, the more they progress to making independent decisions about the treatment of their mental health issues. This model is not appropriate for those patients who are so incapacitated by their illness that they do not understand they are ill. The amount of independence and decision-making that is turned over to the patient should increase as they become more stable.

ACCEPTANCE COMMITMENT THERAPY

Acceptance commitment therapy (ACT) approaches behavioral change from a different perspective than conventional CBT. Patients are encouraged to examine their thought processes (**cognitive defusion**) when undergoing episodes of anxiety or depression. They identify a thought, such as, "People think I am ugly," and then analyze whether or not this is true, listing evidence, and then evaluating whether or not the anxiety is decreased after this evaluation process. Eventually, this process becomes automatic, eliminating the need to write everything down. Mindfulness is a basic concept of ACT, and patients are encouraged to examine their values and control those things that are under their control, such as their facial expression or actions. ACT represents (A) **accepting** reactions, (C) **choosing** a direction, and (T) **taking** action to effect change.

SINGLE-SESSION THERAPY

Single-session therapy is the **most frequent form of counseling** because individuals often attend only one session for various reasons even if more are advised. Individuals may not have insurance or believe that one session is sufficient. Sessions typically last 1 hour. The goal is to identify a problem and reach a solution in one session. The therapist serves as a facilitator to motivate the individual to view the problem as part of a pattern that can be changed and to identify a solution. The therapist may use a wide range of techniques that culminates in a **plan for the individual** (e.g., homework exercises) so the individual can begin to make changes.

SOLUTION-FOCUSED THERAPY

Solution-focused therapy aims to **differentiate methods** that are effective from those that are not, and to identify areas of strengths so they can be used in problem solving. The premise of solution-focused therapy is that change is possible but that the individual must identify problems and deal with them in the real world. This therapy is based on questioning to help the individual establish goals and find solutions to problems:

- **Pre-session**: The patient is asked about any differences he or she noted after making the appointment and coming to the first session.
- **Miracle**: The patient is asked if any miracles occurred or if any problems were solved, including what, if anything, was different and how this difference affected relationships.
- **Exception**: The patient is asked if any small changes were noted and if there were any problems that no longer seemed problematic and how that manifested.
- **Scaling**: The patient is asked to evaluate the problem on a 1–10 scale and then to determine how to increase the rating.
- **Coping**: The patient is asked about how he or she is managing.

NONVIOLENT CRISIS INTERVENTION AND DE-ESCALATION TECHNIQUES

Nonviolent crisis intervention and de-escalation techniques begin with self-awareness because the normal response to aggression is a stress response (freezing, fight/flight, fear). The nurse must control these responses in order to deal with the situation. The nurse should recognize signs of impending conflict (clenched fists, and sudden change in tone of voice or body stance, and change in eye contact). Steps include:

- Maintain social distance (≥12 feet) if possible and stay at the same level as the person (sitting or standing).
- Speak in a quiet calm tone of voice, limiting eye contact and avoiding changes in voice tone, facial expression, and gestures (especially avoid pointing or waving a finger at the person).
- Ask the person's name (if necessary) and use the name when addressing the person.
- Validate the person by acknowledging their issue: "I can see that you are angry about the changes in your treatment."
- Show empathy without being judgmental: "I'm sorry you are upset."
- Ignore questions that are challenging and avoid arguing.

- Practice active listening by paraphrasing and clarifying.
- Assist the person to explore options and the results of those options: "What is it that you would like to do?"

PHYSICAL RESTRAINTS

Restraints are used to restrict movement and activity when other methods of controlling patient behavior have failed and there is a risk of harm to the patient or others. There are two primary types of **physical restraints**: violent (behavioral) and non-violent (clinical). Violent restraints are more commonly used in the psychiatric unit or when individuals exhibit aggressive behavior. More commonly, non-violent restraints are used to ensure that the individual does not interfere with safe care. Non-violent restraints are commonly used in the confused elderly or intubated patient to prevent pulling out lines/removing equipment. The federal government and the Joint Commission have issued strict **guidelines** for temporary restraints or those not part of standard care (such as post-surgical restraint):

- Each facility must have a written policy and restraints are only used when ordered by a physician (usually require written/signed order every 24hrs and within 4 hours of restraint initiation).
- An assessment must be completed frequently, including circulation, toileting, and nutritional needs (generally every 1-2 hours).
- All alternative methods should be tried before applying a restraint and the least restrictive effective restraint should be used.
- A nurse must remove the restraint, assess, and document findings at least every 2 hours, every hour for violent restraints.

Key: Least restrictive option for the least amount of time.

CHEMICAL RESTRAINTS

Chemical restraints involve the use of pharmacological sedatives to manage an individual's behavior problems. This type of restraint is indicated only when severe agitation/violence puts the patient at risk for injury to themselves or others. **Chemical restraints** inhibit the individuals' physical movements, making their behavior more manageable. It is important to realize that medication used on an ongoing basis as part of treatment is not legally considered a chemical restraint, even though the medications may be the same. There is little consensus about the use of chemical restraints, although benzodiazepines and antipsychotics are frequently used to control severe agitation (haloperidol, lorazepam, etc.). Oral medications should be tried first before injections, as oral medication is less coercive. It is important for the nurse to realize that chemical restraints are used as a last resort when other measures (such as de-escalation and environmental modification) have failed and there is an immediate risk of harm to the patient or others.

Psychosocial Pharmacology

ANTIPSYCHOTIC MEDICATIONS

FIRST-GENERATION

There are a variety of first-generation antipsychotics available, though their use is becoming less prominent now that atypical antipsychotic agents are available. Some **first-generation antipsychotics** include:

- Chlorpromazine (Thorazine)
- Thioridazine hydrochloride (Mellaril)
- Haloperidol (Haldol)
- Pimozide (Orap)
- Fluphenazine hydrochloride (Prolixin)
- Molindone hydrochloride (Moban)
- Trifluoperazine hydrochloride (Stelazine)

Possible side effects include photosensitivity, sexual dysfunction, dry mouth, dry eyes, nasal congestion, blurred vision, constipation, urinary retention, exacerbation of narrow-angle glaucoma, various cardiac effects, extrapyramidal effects, dyskinesia, sedation, cognitive dulling, amenorrhea, menstrual irregularities, hyperglycemia or hypoglycemia, increased appetite, and weight gain. The most common extrapyramidal symptom caused by antipsychotic agents is tardive dyskinesia, in which clients are unable to control their movements, such as tics, lip-smacking, and eye blinking. The extrapyramidal system is a group of neural connections outside of the medulla that control movement. **Extrapyramidal effects** are the result of drug influence on the extrapyramidal system and include:

- Akinesia (inability to start movement)
- Akathisia (inability to stop movement)
- Dystonia (extreme and uncontrolled muscle contraction, torticollis, flexing, and twisting)

SECOND-GENERATION

Second-generation antipsychotics (SGAs), also called atypical antipsychotics, are used for bipolar disorders, schizophrenia, and psychosis, and include aripiprazole (Abilify), clozapine (Clozaril), olanzapine (Zyprexa), quetiapine (Seroquel), risperidone (Risperdal), and ziprasidone (Geodon). Females report more side effects than males, but the recommended doses for males and females are identical. Women were underrepresented when SGAs were clinically tested, because researchers feared teratogenic effects on fetuses:

- Side effects include constipation, increased appetite, weight gain, urinary retention, various sexual side effects, increased prolactin, menstrual irregularities, increased risk of diabetes mellitus, decreased blood pressure, dizziness, agranulocytosis, and leucopenia.
- Atypical antipsychotics may interact with fluvoxamine, phenytoin, carbamazepine, barbiturates, nicotine, ketoconazole, phenytoin, rifampin, and glucocorticoids.
- The use of atypical antipsychotic agents correlates with significant weight gain. Overweight and obese clients are likely to develop insulin resistance and glucose intolerance, which may lead to diabetes mellitus. Data show clozapine and olanzapine as the greatest offenders. Ziprasidone seems to present the lowest risk.

> **Review Video: Anti-Psychotic Drugs: Clozapine, Haloperidol, Etc.**
> Visit mometrix.com/academy and enter code: 369601

ANTIDEPRESSANTS

INDICATIONS FOR TREATMENT WITH ANTIDEPRESSANT

The main **indicator** for use of an antidepressant is simply **depression**. This can be further expanded to include major depression, atypical depression, and anxiety disorders. Depression-type symptoms commonly include loss of interest in usual or pleasurable activities, decreased levels of energy, having a depressed mood, decreased ability to concentrate, loss of appetite, or suicidal thoughts. Antidepressants are also commonly used to treat **anxiety disorders** that include panic attacks, obsessive-compulsive disorder (OCD), social phobias, and post-traumatic stress disorder. They may also be beneficial in treating chronic pain syndromes, premenstrual syndrome, insomnia, attention deficit hyperactivity disorder, or bed-wetting.

SSRIS

Selective serotonin reuptake inhibitors (SSRIs) prevent the reuptake of serotonin at the presynaptic membrane. This increases the amount of serotonin in the synapse for neurotransmission. This class of antidepressants has been shown to reduce depression and anxiety symptoms. Common side effects are usually short in duration and include headache, GI upset, and sexual dysfunction. They do not cause significant anticholinergic, cardiovascular, or significant patient sedation side effects. Examples of SSRIs include citalopram (Celexa), escitalopram (Lexapro), fluoxetine (Prozac), Fluvoxamine (Luvox), paroxetine (Paxil), and sertraline (Zoloft). These drugs are not highly lethal in overdose.

MONITORING

SSRI monitoring includes the following:

- Monitor for increased depression and suicidal ideation, especially in adolescents.
- Inform patients of the following:
    - Smoking decreases effectiveness.
    - Fatal reactions may occur with monoamine oxidase inhibitors.
    - Taking SSRIs with benzodiazepines or alcohol has an additive effect.
    - Some drugs, such as citalopram, may increase the effects of β-blockers and warfarin.
- Avoid cimetidine, which is prescribed for ulcers and gastroesophageal reflux disease, and St. John's wort.
- Inform patients of possible decreased libido and sexual functioning.
- Monitor for insomnia and gastrointestinal upset.

TRICYCLIC ANTIDEPRESSANTS

Tricyclic antidepressants not only block the reuptake of serotonin and norepinephrine, they also act to block muscarinic cholinergic receptors, histamine H1 receptors, and alpha1 noradrenergic receptors. These receptors do not affect depression symptoms, but their blockade is implicated in some of the side effects associated with tricyclics. The blockade of the muscarinic receptors produces anticholinergic side effects such as dry mouth, blurred vision, constipation, urinary retention, and tachycardia. The blockade of the histamine receptors is associated with drowsiness, low blood pressure, and weight gain. The alpha1 noradrenergic receptor blocking action produces the side effects associated with orthostatic hypotension, vertigo, and some memory disturbances.

MECHANISM OF ACTION AND NECESSARY EVALUATIONS

Most of the tricyclic antidepressants have very similar mechanisms of action and side effects. Although their exact **mechanism of action** is unknown, they are believed to act to inhibit the reuptake of both serotonin and norepinephrine. These drugs have a high **first-pass rate of metabolism** and are excreted by the kidneys. A complete **physical and history** should be obtained before starting a patient on tricyclic drugs. Because this class of antidepressants can cause death with an overdose, an initial **suicide risk assessment** must be obtained, and continued assessments for this risk are necessary. This class of drug can cause a prolongation in the electrical conduction of the heart. Therefore, a **baseline ECG** should be performed in children, young teenagers, anyone with cardiac electrical conduction problems, and adults over age 40.

MONITORING

Tricyclics monitoring includes the following:

- Observe for toxicity.
- Inform patients not to take with monoamine oxidase inhibitors.
- Observe for decreased therapeutic response to hypertensives (e.g., clonidine, guanethidine).
- Monitor other medications; the patient should avoid other central nervous system depressants, including alcohol. Some medications potentiate the effects of tricyclics, including bupropion, cimetidine, haloperidol, selective serotonin reuptake inhibitors, and valproic acid.
- Inform the patient to avoid prolonged exposure to sunlight or sunlamps.
- Administer major dosage of the drug at bedtime if the patient experiences drowsiness.
- Monitor for sedation, cardiac arrhythmias, insomnia, gastrointestinal upset, and weight gain.

MAOIs

The **mechanism of action** for monoamine oxidase inhibitors (MAOIs) is exactly what their name indicates. These drugs act to inhibit the enzyme **monoamine oxidase (MAO)**. There are actually two of these enzymes, **MAO-A** and **MAO-B**, and this class of medication inhibits both. These enzymes act to metabolize serotonin and norepinephrine. By inhibiting the production of these enzymes, there are increased levels of **serotonin** and **norepinephrine** available for neurotransmission. Medications that selectively inhibit MAO-B have no antidepressant effects and can be used to treat disease processes such as Parkinson's.

SIDE EFFECTS

Side effects associated with the use of monoamine oxidase inhibitors (MAOIs) are similar to antipsychotic medications. They can include symptoms such as GI upset, vertigo, headaches, sleep disturbances, sexual dysfunction, dry mouth, visual disturbances, constipation, peripheral edema, urinary hesitancy, weakness, increased weight, or orthostatic hypotension. The elderly population is at greatest risk for problems with **orthostatic hypotension** and should have lying, sitting, and standing blood pressure checks to monitor for this side effect. Orthostatic hypotension can lead to injuries related to falls, such as fractures. The most dangerous side effect can be an extreme **elevation in blood pressure** or **hypertensive crisis**. Hypertension can develop due to the presence of increased levels of **tyramine**. These levels increase because **monoamine oxidase**, which normally metabolizes tyramine, is inhibited. Increased levels of tyramine produce a vasoconstrictive response by the body that leads to increased blood pressure. Symptoms associated with hypertensive crisis can include severe occipital headache, palpitations, chest pain, diaphoresis, nausea and vomiting, flushed face, or dilated pupils. Complications associated with hypertensive crisis include hemorrhagic stroke, severe headache, or death. It is vital that patients receive in-depth education about the symptoms of hypertension, the need for close monitoring of blood pressure, and methods for sustaining a low-tyramine diet.

DIET RESTRICTIONS

Monoamine oxidase inhibitors can lead to increased levels of **tyramine** in the nerve cell. These increased levels can lead to a dangerous and possibly fatal increase in **blood pressure**. Certain **foods that contain tyramine** should be avoided to help prevent hypertensive episodes. Foods high in tyramine include strong or aged cheeses, cured meats, smoked or processed meats, pickled or fermented foods, sauces, such as soy or teriyaki sauce, soybeans, snow peas or broad beans, dried or overripe fruits, meat tenderizers, products containing monosodium glutamate, yeast-extract spreads, alcoholic beverages, and improperly stored foods or spoiled foods.

ANTI-ANXIETY MEDICATIONS

BENZODIAZEPINES

Benzodiazepines are the most commonly prescribed medications for **anxiety**. Some of the more commonly prescribed include chlordiazepoxide, lorazepam, diazepam, flurazepam, and triazolam. Benzodiazepines act to enhance the neurotransmitter **GABA**. This neurotransmitter inhibits the firing rate of neurons and therefore leads to a decline in anxiety symptoms. Indications for their use can include anxiety, insomnia disorders, alcohol withdrawal, seizure control, skeletal muscle spasticity, or agitation. They can also be utilized to reduce the anxiety symptoms preoperatively or before any other type of medical procedure such as cardiac catheterization or colonoscopy. This class of drug is also the treatment of choice for alcohol withdrawal.

SIDE EFFECTS

There are several common side effects associated with the use of benzodiazepines. One of the most common is the effect of **drowsiness**. Patients should be advised to use caution when operating motor vehicles or machinery. Activity will help decrease this effect. Other side effects include feelings of detachment, irritability, emotional lability, GI upset, dependency, or development of tolerance. The elderly population is at high risk for the development of **dizziness** or **cognitive impairment**, which places them at high risk for falls with associated injuries. When discontinuing a benzodiazepine after long-term use, the drug should be weaned off to prevent withdrawal side effects.

TREATMENT OF INSOMNIA

Benzodiazepines are used to treat **insomnia** because of their **sedative-hypnotic effects**. There are three different types of insomnia, which include the inability to fall asleep, inability to stay asleep, or the combination of both. Many times, insomnia can be helped by a change in habits or talking about worries or stress the patient may be experiencing. When using a sedative-hypnotic to treat sleep disturbances, the medication should have rapid onset and allow the patient to wake up feeling refreshed instead of tired and groggy. When administered at bedtime, most benzodiazepines will produce a sleep-inducing effect and should be used on a short-term basis.

USE OF BUSPIRONE FOR TREATMENT OF ANXIETY

Due to the addictive potential of benzodiazepines, the use of **nonbenzodiazepines** to treat anxiety has increased. One of the most commonly used nonbenzodiazepine medications is the drug **buspirone**. This medication is highly effective in treating anxiety and its associated symptoms such as insomnia, poor concentration, tension, restlessness, irritability, and fatigue. Buspirone has no addiction potential, is not useful in alcohol withdrawal and seizures, and is not known to interact with other CNS depressants. Because it may take several weeks of continual use for the effects of this drug to be realized by the patient, it cannot be used on an as-needed basis. Buspirone does not increase depression symptoms and therefore is useful in treating anxiety associated with depression. Side effects associated with medication can include GI upset, dizziness, sleepiness, excitement, or headache.

Education Topics

BANDURA'S THEORY OF SOCIAL LEARNING

In the 1970s, Bandura proposed the theory of social learning, in which he posited that learning develops from observing, organizing, and rehearsing behavior that has been modeled. Bandura believed that people are more likely to adopt the behavior if they value the outcomes, if the outcomes have functional value, and if the person modeling the behavior is similar to the learner and is admired because of status. Behavior is the result of observation of behavioral, environmental, and cognitive interactions. There are **four conditions** required for modeling:

- **Attention**: The degree of attention paid to modeling can depend on many variables (physical, social, and environmental).
- **Retention**: People's ability to retain models depends on symbolic coding, creating mental images, organizing thoughts, and rehearsing (mentally or physically).
- **Reproduction**: The ability to reproduce a model depends on physical and mental capabilities.
- **Motivation**: Motivation may derive from past performances, rewards, or vicarious modeling.

TRANSTHEORETICAL MODEL OF CHANGE

The transtheoretical model of change puts forth concepts applicable to the process of educating patients and their family members. The **stages** of the transtheoretical model of change include the following:

1. The first stage is **precontemplation**. At this point, the patient is not aware of any need for a change in the health behavior.
2. In the next stage, **contemplation**, the patient begins to realize why the change may be necessary after recognizing that the health behavior in question is unhealthy and weighing the consequences of continuing this behavior.
3. During the stage of **preparation**, the patient imagines making the change at a future time and starts to formulate a plan to do so.
4. The **action** stage occurs when the patient makes specific modifications in health behavior and begins to note the resulting positive changes.
5. During the **maintenance** stage, the patient is able to implement the change over time by utilizing strategies to prevent a return to previously unhealthy behaviors.
6. **Termination** is the stage at which a patient has incorporated the changed behavior into daily functioning, and the patient will not resume the previous unhealthy behavior.

KURT LEWIN

FORCE FIELD ANALYSIS

Force field analysis was designed by Kurt Lewin, a social psychologist, to analyze both the driving forces and the restraining forces for change:

- **Driving forces** instigate and promote change, such as leaders, incentives, and competition.
- **Restraining forces** resist change, such as poor attitudes, hostility, inadequate equipment, or insufficient funds.

The educator can use this force field analysis diagram to discuss variables related to a proposed change in process:

- Write the proposed change in the center column.
- Brainstorm and list driving forces and opposed restraining forces. Score the forces. (When driving and restraining forces are in balance, this is a state of equilibrium or the status quo.)
- Discuss the value of the proposed change.
- Develop a plan to diminish or eliminate restraining forces.

Lewin's Model of Change Theory

Lewin's model of change theory may be used to help some patients make decisions for change. Patients can be educated about the need for change and can be assisted with making alterations in behavior or thoughts in order to better facilitate change; however, only the patient can truly implement the change permanently. Lewin's concept of change theory involves a three-part process:

- **Unfreezing** is the part of the model in which the patient becomes open to change, sees a need for it, and removes the boundaries inhibiting change.
- The patient then makes the **actual change** according to expected outcomes and goals.
- Finally, **refreezing** is the process of maintaining the change so that it becomes a habit, and one that the patient is likely to uphold for a long period of time.

Lewin's theory also involves either driving forces or restraining forces. Driving forces are those outside measures that support the change, while restraining forces inhibit success in implementing the change.

Principles of Adult Learning

Adults have a wealth of life and/or employment experiences. Their attitudes toward education may vary considerably. There are, however, some **principles of adult learning** and typical characteristics of adult learners that an instructor should consider when planning strategies for teaching parents, families, or staff.

- Practical and goal-oriented:
  - Provide overviews or summaries and examples.
  - Use collaborative discussions with problem-solving exercises.
  - Remain organized with the goal in mind.
- Self-directed:
  - Provide active involvement, asking for input.
  - Allow different options toward achieving the goal.
  - Give them responsibilities.
- Knowledgeable:
  - Show respect for their life experiences/education.
  - Validate their knowledge and ask for feedback.
  - Relate new material to information with which they are familiar.
- Relevancy-oriented:
  - Explain how information will be applied.
  - Clearly identify objectives.
- Motivated:
  - Provide certificates of professional advancement and/or continuing education credit for staff when possible.

> **Review Video: Adult Learning Processes and Theories**
> Visit mometrix.com/academy and enter code: 638453

Learning Styles

Not all people are aware of their preferred **learning style.** A range of teaching materials and methods that relate to all three major learning preferences (visual, auditory, and kinesthetic) and that are appropriate for different ages should be available. Part of assessment for teaching involves choosing the right approach based on observation and feedback. Often, presenting learners with different options gives a clue to their preferred learning style. Some people have a combined learning style.

Visual learners learn best by seeing and reading:

- Provide written directions or picture guides, or demonstrate procedures. Use charts and diagrams.
- Provide photos or videos.

Auditory learners learn best by listening and talking:

- Explain procedures while demonstrating and have the learner repeat.
- Plan extra time to discuss and answer questions.
- Provide audio recordings.

Kinesthetic learners learn best by handling, doing, and practicing:

- Provide hands-on experience throughout teaching.
- Encourage handling of supplies and equipment.
- Allow the learner to demonstrate.
- Minimize instructions and allow the person to explore equipment and procedures.

APPROACHES TO TEACHING

There are many approaches to teaching, and the educator must prepare, present, and coordinate a wide range of educational workshops, lectures, discussions, and one-on-one instructions on any chosen topic. All types of classes will be needed, depending upon the purpose and material:

- **Educational workshops** are usually conducted with small groups, allowing for maximal participation. They are especially good for demonstrations and practice sessions.
- **Lectures** are often used for more academic or detailed information that may include questions and answers but limits discussion. An effective lecture should include some audiovisual support.
- **Discussions** are best with small groups so that people can actively participate. This is a good method for problem solving.
- **One-on-one instruction** is especially helpful for targeted instruction in procedures for individuals.
- **Online learning modules** are good for independent learners.

Participants should be asked to evaluate the presentations in the forms of surveys or suggestions, but ultimately the program is evaluated in terms of patient outcomes.

READINESS TO LEARN

The patient/family's readiness to learn should be assessed because if they are not ready, instruction is of little value. Often, readiness is indicated when the patient/family asks questions or shows an interest in procedures. There are a number of factors related to readiness to learn:

- **Physical factors:** There are a number of physical factors that can affect ability. Manual dexterity may be required to complete a task, and this varies by age and condition. Hearing or vision deficits may impact a person's ability to learn. Complex tasks may be too difficult for some because of weakness or cognitive impairment, and modifications of the environment may be needed. Health status, age, and gender may all impact the ability to learn.
- **Experience:** People's experience with learning can vary widely and is affected by their ability to cope with changes, their personal goals, motivation to learn, and cultural background. People may have widely divergent ideas about what constitutes illness and/or treatment. Lack of English skills may make learning difficult and prevent people from asking questions.
- **Mental/emotional status:** The external support system and internal motivation may impact readiness. Anxiety, fear, or depression about one's condition can make learning very difficult because the patient/family cannot focus on learning, so the nurse must spend time to reassure the patient/family and wait until they are emotionally more receptive.

312

- **Knowledge/education:** The knowledge base of the patient/family, their cognitive ability, and their learning styles all affect their readiness to learn. The nurse should always begin by assessing what knowledge the patient/family already has about their disease, condition, or treatment and then build from that base. People with little medical experience may lack knowledge of basic medical terminology, interfering with their ability and readiness to learn.

BLOOM'S TAXONOMY

Bloom's taxonomy outlines behaviors that are necessary for learning and that can be applied to healthcare. The theory describes three types of learning.

Cognitive: Learning and gaining intellectual skills to master six categories of effective learning.

- Knowledge
- Comprehension
- Application
- Analysis
- Synthesis
- Evaluation

Affective: Recognizing 5 categories of feelings and values from simple to complex. This is slower to achieve than cognitive learning.

- **Receiving phenomena**: Accepting need to learn
- **Responding to phenomena**: Taking active part in care
- **Valuing**: Understanding the value of becoming independent in care
- **Organizing values**: Understanding how surgery/treatment has improved life
- **Internalizing values**: Accepting the condition as part of life, being consistent and self-reliant

Psychomotor: Mastering 7 categories of motor skills necessary for independence. This follows a progression from simple to complex.

- **Perception**: Uses sensory information to learn tasks
- **Set**: Shows willingness to perform tasks
- **Guided response**: Follows directions
- **Mechanism**: Does specific tasks
- **Complex overt response**: Displays competence in self-care
- **Adaptation**: Modifies procedures as needed
- **Origination**: Creatively deals with problems

TEACHING TECHNIQUES

There are many teaching techniques the nurse can utilize when educating patients. The nurse can demonstrate skills repeatedly when teaching and then allow the patient as much time as needed to practice the skill. The nurse should use equipment that will be available in the home and provide written instructions that can be referred to later if needed. Encouraging discussion of the information helps the patient understand and clarify. Discussion also allows the patient to vent emotions about the disease and the learning process, and to assimilate the information so that a change in behavior can result. Discussion provides feedback to the patient and encouragement to continue learning. Teaching groups of people may be appropriate when there are others who require the same information. The members can support each other with encouragement, empathy, and camaraderie, although some patients will not learn well in groups and will need individual teaching. Groups must be followed up with on an individual basis to give the chance to clarify information, to evaluate the level of learning and goal achievement, and to alter the learning plan as needed for each person.

INSTRUCTION GROUP SIZES

Both one-on-one instruction and group instruction have a place in patient/family education.

- **One-on-one instruction** is the most costly for an institution because it is time intensive. However, it allows the patient and family more interaction with the nurse instructor and allows them to have more control over the process by asking questions or having the instructor repeat explanations or demonstrations. One-on-one instruction is especially valuable when patients and families must learn particular skills, such as managing dialysis, or if confidentiality is important.
- **Group instruction** is the less costly because the needs of a number of people can be met at one time. Group presentations are more planned and usually scheduled for a particular time period (an hour, for example), so patients and families have less control. Questioning is usually more limited and may be done only at the end. Group instruction allows patients/families with similar health problems to interact. Group instruction is especially useful for general types of instruction, such as managing diet or other lifestyle issues.

RESOURCES TO USE WHEN TEACHING PATIENTS AND THEIR FAMILIES

Many hospitals that find the need to repeatedly teach the same information to patients and families prepare brochures or other written materials or teaching videos that are available for use. The nurse should review material first and make notes specific to the patient. The nurse should also watch the video with the patient and discuss it afterwards. Written materials can augment lecture and demonstrations and are useful for the patient to keep for later reference.

There are also commercial materials that can be used, provided by various drug or equipment companies. **Teaching resources** are available online from the National Institutes of Health and other reputable sources. The nurse can use these prepared materials whenever possible to save time for actual teaching but must remember to customize them to the patient. They help provide pictures, colors, and interesting features that keep the patient's interest in learning alive. There are also many books, groups, and websites that the patient should be made aware of for resources after discharge.

READABILITY

Studies have indicated that learning is more effective if oral presentations and/or demonstrations are supplemented with reading materials, such as handouts. **Readability** (the grade level of the material) is a concern because many patients and families may have limited English skills or low literacy, and it can be difficult for the nurse to assess people's reading level. The average American reads effectively at the 6th to 8th grade level (regardless of education achieved), but many health education materials have a much higher readability level. Additionally, research indicates that even people with much higher reading skills learn medical and health information most effectively when the material is presented at the 6th to 8th grade readability level. Therefore, patient education materials (and consent forms) should not be written at higher than 6th to 8th grade level. Readability index calculators are available on the internet to give an approximation of grade level and difficulty for those preparing materials without expertise in teaching reading.

VIDEOS

Videos are a useful adjunct to teaching as they reduce the time needed for one-on-one instruction (increasing cost-effectiveness). Passive presentation of **videos**, such as in the waiting area, has little value, but focused viewing in which the nurse discusses the purpose of the video presentation prior to viewing and then is available for discussion after viewing can be very effective. Patients and/or families are often nervous about learning patient care and are unsure of their abilities, so they may not focus completely when the nurse is presenting information. Allowing the patients/families to watch a video demonstration or explanation first and allowing them to stop or review the video presentation can help them to grasp the fundamentals before they have to apply them, relieving some of the anxiety they may be experiencing. Videos are much more effective than written materials for those with low literacy or poor English skills. The nurse should always be available to answer questions and discuss the material after the patients/families finish viewing.

LEARNING CONTRACT

In order to be compliant with a therapeutic regimen, the patient needs information about the disease, the purpose of medications and treatments, and side effects and complications to watch for. A written **learning contract** organizes this information into specific learning goals, demonstrates the importance of the information, and ensures that all pertinent information is taught. Others on the healthcare team can note patient progress and easily determine what to teach next. The patient has a written plan to follow as well.

The learning contract should take into consideration the patient's age, sex, cultural and religious values, and educational level achieved. One must consider the patient's financial status, socio-economic status, living situation, and support network. The complex nature of a therapeutic regimen combined with distracters such as side effects, pain, denial, and fear can weaken the patient's resolve to maintain compliance. One must evaluate the patient's attitudes towards healthcare, coping mechanisms, and motivation and provide reinforcement as needed.

EDUCATIONAL GOALS, OBJECTIVES, AND PLANS

Once a topic for performance improvement education has been chosen, then goals, measurable objectives with strategies, and lesson plans must be developed. A class should stay focused on one topic rather than trying to cover many. For example:

Goal: Increase compliance with hand hygiene standards in ICU.

Objectives:

- Develop series of posters and fliers by June 1.
- Observe 100% compliance with hand hygiene standards at 2 weeks, 1-month, and 2-month intervals after training is completed.

Strategies: Conduct 4 classes at different times over a one-week period, May 25-31.

- Place posters in all nursing units, staff rooms, and utility rooms by January 3.
- Develop slide show presentation for class and provide online access to the presentation for all staff by May 25.
- Utilize handwashing kits.

Lesson plans: Discussion period: Why do we need 100% compliance?

- Slide show: The case for hand hygiene
- Discussion: What did you learn?
- Demonstration and activities to show effectiveness
- Handwashing technique

LEARNER OUTCOMES

When the quality professional plans an educational offering, whether it be a class, an online module, a workshop, or educational materials, the professional should identify **learner outcomes,** which should be conveyed to the learners from the very beginning so that they are aware of the expectations. The subject matter of the educational material and the learner outcomes should be directly related. For example, if the quality professional is giving a class on decontamination of the environment, then a learner outcome might be: "Identify the difference between disinfectants and antiseptics." There may be one or multiple learner outcomes, but part of the assessment at the end of the learning experience should be to determine if, in fact, the learner outcomes have been achieved. A survey of whether or not the learners felt that they had achieved the learner outcomes can give valuable feedback and guidance to the quality professional.

IMPLEMENTATION AND EVALUATION OF TEACHING PLAN

Implementation and evaluation of the teaching plan includes:

- Follow teaching plan but be flexible and alter plan to suit the patient's learning needs.
- Work with a healthcare team to follow the teaching plan and ensure consistency in teaching methods as well as coordinate efforts and take responsibility for altering the plan and evaluating learning to meet goals.
- Monitor patient's motivational level, encourage with positive feedback as needed, and record patient responses to teaching and changes in behaviors as a result of all teaching sessions.
- Use tools, such as checklists, rating scales, observed behavior, written tests, and the nature of the questions from the patient when evaluating the effectiveness of the teaching plan in reaching the patient's goals for learning.
- Evaluate the plan after each session and at the end.

Communicate information taught and patient learning to any home health or community nurses involved. They can then continue the patient's teaching by evaluating behavior in the home and continuing to address learning needs as they arise.

EVALUATING EFFECTIVENESS OF EDUCATION

Education, like all interventions, must be evaluated for **effectiveness**. Two determinants of effectiveness include:

- **Behavior modification** involves thorough observation and measurement, identifying behavior that needs to be changed and then planning and instituting interventions to modify that behavior. The nurse can use a variety of techniques, including demonstrations of appropriate behavior, reinforcement, and monitoring until new behavior is adopted consistently. This is especially important when longstanding procedures and habits of behavior are changed.
- **Compliance rates** are often determined by observation, which should be done at intervals and on multiple occasions, but with patients, this may depend on self-reports. Outcomes is another measure of compliance; that is, if education is intended to improve patient health and reduce risk factors and that occurs, it is a good indication that there is compliance. Compliance rates are calculated by determining the number of events/procedures and degree of compliance.

TEACHING ELDERLY PATIENTS

The elderly patient's level of functioning must be assessed before teaching. Cognitive abilities and mental functioning may be affected by illness and aging:

- Short-term memory loss can affect the amount of material retained.
- Concentration may be decreased.
- Reaction time is delayed.
- Color discrimination, general vision, and hearing may be decreased.

The nurse should **pace** the teaching accordingly and **tailor** materials for any deficits. Family should be present for teaching if possible, to help the patient to remember key points after discharge. Large print on non-glare paper that is easy to read should be used. The nurse should use color-coding cues only if colors are easily perceived. The learning environment must be quiet and comfortable with no distractions or interruptions.

- Repeat information numerous times and allow the patient as much practice time as needed.
- Use audio-visual aids to reinforce information given verbally.
- Face the patient when speaking and encourage him/her to use hearing devices if used.
- Make sure the lighting in the room is adequate.

TEACHING PATIENTS WITH LEARNING DISABILITIES

Determine the type of learning disability in order to design teaching:

- When a patient has a **visual problem**, the nurse should use **verbal teaching**, repeated several times as needed and record the session for the patient to hear later if possible or use prepared audiotapes or CDs containing the information. The patient should verbalize learning to show attainment of the learning goal.
- When **auditory perception** is a problem, learning materials should be **visual** with as few words as possible. Demonstration, role-playing, and practicing the procedure will be useful to the patient. Printed materials should employ pictures, and computer use can be useful.
- If the patient has an **expressive problem**, he/she needs time to process the input and to ask questions. **Hand gestures, demonstrations, and the senses** should be utilized for teaching when appropriate.

A developmental disability will require information presented in a format that is appropriate for the person's developmental level. The nurse should keep explanations simple, and use gestures, demonstrations, activities, and repetition to teach.

TEACHING TO DISABLED PATIENTS AND FAMILIES

The teaching of disabled patients and their families begins with an assessment of the family's willingness and preparation for the heavy duty of care that will be required. The nurse must teach information about diseases or disabilities as well as medications, procedures, diet, and physical therapies. The patients must be taught to perform ADLs as well as possible and caregivers taught how to assist when needed:

- Give patients enough information to understand and manage the disabilities and to empower them with a sense of control and coping.
- Don't overwhelm them with information.
- Plan the teaching to provide information according to learning readiness and priorities but be flexible and change the plan if needed.
- Utilize checklists of skills to help keep track of all that has been learned.
- Give praise, continued feedback, support, and empathy with every teaching session.
- Provide resources that patients and family can use after discharge and refer to home health for continuing support and teaching.

IMPORTANCE OF PATIENT'S CULTURE IN DESIGN OF TEACHING PLAN

The nurse must always assess the individual's cultural beliefs and values and not assume that they are the same as the culture on a whole. These beliefs determine what information the patient feels that they can pursue. Teaching that conflicts with these beliefs will be rejected. The patient's perception of health and the healthcare system must be determined because a lack of confidence in the teacher can impair motivation to learn. The nurse must **assess the patient's beliefs** about the following to develop a personalized teaching plan:

- Body image, self-esteem
- Abilities and level of knowledge
- Principles of living
- Diet, activity, health practices
- Involvement of family and support persons
- Physical and mental health and disease
- Causes of disease
- Aging

- Gender issues
- Spirituality, customs, rituals, religious precepts

Patient Safety Measures

JOINT COMMISSION'S PATIENT SAFETY GOALS

The Joint Commission has a set of **goals that impact patient safety** for each type of healthcare facility. Within the hospital environment, there are several goals that pertain:

- Each facility must have a way to identify patients that will avoid errors of identification.
- Caregivers are to give careful, accurate communications about patients and their care so that mistakes are not made.
- A system to avoid medication errors must be in place.
- Medications must be reconciled when the patient moves from place to place within the hospital or is discharged to other caregivers.
- The risk of infection must be decreased so that patients are at less risk for hospital-related infections.
- The facility must have a fall prevention program and evaluate its effectiveness.

All patients and family must be encouraged to be active in their own care to help to avoid errors. They must also know how to make sure their concerns for safety of care are heard and acted upon.

ASPECTS OF PATIENT SAFETY IN THE HOSPITAL

Deliberate decisions by the health care providers/facility can help create an environment conducive for patient safety. Some of those aspects include:

- **Educating the patient on signaling staff**: The patient must be educated about the use of the call light, and the call light placed within easy reach. If the patient is unable to use the call light, then an alternative means of calling for help, such as a handheld bell, should be available. If the patient is unable to manage any type of signaling system, then the nurse should check on the patient at least every hour.
- **Protecting from falls and electrical hazards**: All clutter should be removed from floors and cords secured away from walkways. All electrical appliances should be checked to ensure they are working properly and have no frayed cords. Patients should be provided assistive devices, such as walkers, if necessary, to improve stability.
- **Making appropriate room assignments**: Patients with the greatest need for supervision should be placed closest to the nursing desk and within the line of sight whenever possible. In environments such as critical care, each nurse should be able to visualize their patient assignment from their nursing station.

MEDICATION ERRORS

There are about 7,000 deaths yearly in the United States attributed to **medication errors.** Studies indicate that there are errors in 1 in 5 doses of medication given to patients in hospitals. Patient safety must be ensured with proper handling and administering of medications:

- **Avoid error-prone abbreviations or symbols**. The Joint Commission has established a list of abbreviations to avoid, but mistakes are frequent with other abbreviations as well. In many cases, abbreviations and symbols should be avoided altogether or restricted to a limited approved list.
- **Prevent errors due to illegible handwriting or unclear verbal orders**. Handwritten orders should be block printed to reduce chance of error; verbal orders should be repeated back to the physician.
- **Institute barcoding and scanners** that allow the patient's wristband and medications to be scanned for verification.
- **Provide lists of similarly-named medications** to educate staff.
- Establish an **institutional policy** for the administration of medications that includes protocols for verification of drug, dosage, and patient, as well as educating the patient about the medications.

ASSESSING PATIENTS FOR ALLERGIES

When assessing patients for **allergies** it's important to determine the type of symptoms they have, when the initial reaction occurred, and what type of treatment they have used in the past to manage this complication (including antihistamines). Allergies of particular interest include:

- **Food**: Ask patients about any specific foods that cause an adverse reaction as some foods may have cross-reactivity to latex (such as kiwi, papaya, avocado, and bananas), so patients may be at risk of developing latex allergy and should avoid contact with latex. Some medications may contain substances derived from food, such as eggs, fish, gelatin, lactose, and soy.
- **Latex**: Sensitivity to latex can result in mild reactions, such as itching and rash, to severe anaphylactic reactions, and is common among those with repeated contact with healthcare environments, such as those with spina bifida or multiple surgeries, so it should be suspected with these clients. While non-latex options are more readily available in most hospitals (non-latex gloves and Foley catheters, for instance), latex continues to be used in hospital materials, therefore this allergy must be assessed immediately upon arrival so that appropriate materials can be substituted if necessary.
- **Environmental**: The most common environmental allergies include pollens, dust mites, animals, cigarette smoke, cockroaches, and mold/mildew, so the nurse should be sure to ask about these as well as any other environmental allergies. Some patients are sensitive to strong colognes and perfumes, so the use of these is often regulated by hospital dress codes on units with immunocompromised patients.

NON-PHARMACOLOGIC PRESCRIPTION PRECAUTIONS

Some non-pharmacologic prescriptions may contribute to accident or injury, including the following:

- **Oxygen supplies**: Oxygen may be administered at the wrong level of liters (too much or too little), and the oxygen supply may be inadvertently obstructed or disconnected. Oxygen concentrators may not have backup batteries and may fail to function if electricity goes off. If people smoke around oxygen, this increases the risk of fires. Nasal cannulas and face masks that delivery oxygen, when used over prolonged periods of time, can cause pressure injuries, therefore appropriate assessment and skin care is also necessary.
- **Assistive devices**: If equipment, such as canes and walkers, are improperly fitted, they may increase risk of falls.
- **Dialysis equipment**: Contamination of equipment is always a concern and can result in peritonitis (peritoneal dialysis) and sepsis (hemodialysis). If the lines become separated, the client may exsanguinate.
- **Hot/cold compresses**: If cold compresses are placed directly on the skin, they may damage the tissue, especially if left in place for too long. Hot compresses may cause burns if temperature is too high and may damage wounds if placed directly over them.

SEIZURE PRECAUTIONS

Seizure disorders are broadly categorized as partial seizures (which begin locally) or generalized seizures (which are bilateral and symmetrical and may be convulsive or non-convulsive):

- **Partial seizures** include *simple partial* (with motor, sensory, and/or autonomic symptoms but without impaired consciousness), *complex partial* (with cognitive, affective, psychosensory, and/or psychomotor symptoms, as well as impaired consciousness), or *partial secondarily generalized*.
- **Generalized seizures** include seizures that are bilateral and symmetric without local onset and may be convulsive or non-convulsive. These seizures include *tonic-clonic, tonic, clonic, absence* (petit mal), *atonic*, and *myoclonic seizures*, as well as *unclassified seizures*.

Seizure precautions are a standard set of safety protocol that ensure patient safety in those patients with a high risk or history of seizures. Generally, these precautions include padding the siderails, keeping the bed at the lowest position, and maintaining suctioning at the bedside Precautions also include ensuring privacy and providing supportive care in the event of a seizure, such as easing the patient to the floor and providing padding to protect the head. Side rails should be raised and pillow removed if the patient is in bed. The patient should be placed on one side with the head flexed so the tongue does not block the airway. The patient should *not* be restrained or a padded tongue-blade inserted between the teeth.

PATIENT DEFICITS THAT IMPEDE CLIENT SAFETY

Certain patient deficits can inherently impede client safety, including the following:

- **Visual impairment**: Patients are at risk of trips, slips, falls, burn injuries, poisoning (mistaken containers, ingredients), and medication errors because of taking the wrong medication or wrong dosage.
- **Hearing impairment**: Patients are at increased risk of falls and may not hear danger signals, such as fire alarms, smoke detectors, police/fire sirens, and tornado warning sirens, and may, therefore, not be aware that they are in danger. Most smoke detectors emit a high-frequency alarm that cannot always be detected by those with high-frequency hearing loss.
- **Sensory/Perceptual impairment**: Patients (such as those with stroke or brain injury) may exhibit a wide variety of impairments so safety concerns may vary. For example, those with one-sided neglect may have injuries to the neglected side, such as from running into doors or other things. Those with face blindness may easily get lost if away from familiar places or people.

R.A.C.E. ACRONYM FOR FIRE SAFETY

RACE is an acronym used for fire safety on the hospital unit:

- **R**escue: Remove all patients from area of danger
- **A**ctivate alarm: Pull fire alarm/call 9-1-1
- **C**onfine the fire: Close doors to unit/place
- **E**vacuate/Extinguish (NFPA/OSHA fire safety): Use **PASS** for fire extinguisher
  - **P**ull
  - **A**im at the base of the flames
  - **S**queeze the trigger
  - **S**weep: Use a sweeping motion across the flames

ERGONOMICS

Ergonomics is the study of preventing workplace injury and stress. In nursing, it refers to the way in which a nurse can prevent injury to self and others due to the stressors and strains required in the nursing field. Some important **ergonomic principles** include:

- **Body Mechanics:** The body should be kept in proper alignment during tasks, with a wide base of support and center of gravity low. Use larger muscles (buttocks, thighs, shoulders) for activities rather than smaller when possible. Avoid twisting or jerking movements. Maintain 90° angle in elbows and knees when sitting, elbows at the side, with back straight and looking straight ahead.
- **Lifting:** Use appropriate transfer devices; use as many people as necessary. Manual lifting should be avoided. Bend at the knees, tighten core, and keep weights close to the body – *never* bend or twist when lifting.
- **Repetition**: Avoid repetitive movements/stressors and use proper safety equipment when needed (earplugs for loud noises, etc.).

NOSOCOMIAL INFECTIONS

Nosocomial infections are those that are healthcare-associated or hospital-acquired. The following is a list of common nosocomial infections.

- *Enterococci* infections include urinary infections, bacteremia, endocarditis as well as infections in wounds and the abdominal and pelvic areas.
- *Enterobacteriaceae* cause about half of the urinary tract infections and a quarter of the postoperative infections.
- *Escherichia coli* primarily causes urinary tract infections (especially related to catheters), diarrhea, and neonatal meningitis but it can also lead to pneumonia, and bacteremia (usually secondary to urinary infection).
- Group B β-hemolytic *Streptococci* (GBS) has increasingly been a cause of infections in neonatal units, causing pneumonia, meningitis, and sepsis. GBS infections may occur as wound infections after Cesarean sections, especially in those immunocompromised.
- *Staphylococcus aureus* is a major cause of nosocomial post-operative infections, both localized and systemic, and from indwelling tubes and devices.
- Methicillin-resistant *Staphylococcus aureus (MRSA)* is a common cause of surgical infections.
- *Clostridium difficile* causes more nosocomial diarrhea cases than any other microorganism.
- *Candida*, a yeast fungal pathogen, can overgrow and lead to mucocutaneous or cutaneous lesions and sepsis.
- *Aspergillus* spp., filamentous fungi, produce spores that become airborne and can invade the respiratory tract, causing pneumonia.

CATHETER-RELATED INFECTIONS

Intravenous catheter-related infections are a significant cause of morbidity and mortality in the hospital setting. Usually, these infections are due to *Staphylococcus aureus*, *enterococcus*, or fungal infection such as *Candida*. These infections are important because they may progress and eventually lead to bacteremia, infective endocarditis, septic pulmonary emboli, septic shock, osteomyelitis, or superficial thrombophlebitis. Therefore, vigilance should be maintained to prevent these infections. The patient may exhibit fevers, chills, and discomfort around the catheter site. The site itself may show purulence or erythema. The subclavian vein is the preferred intravenous site and the femoral is the least-preferred site due to high infection rates. Infections are diagnosed with blood cultures and catheter tip cultures. Initial treatment includes removal of the catheter and antibiotic treatment. Antibiotics should be empiric at first, then directed toward culture results. Treatment duration should be 2 weeks at first, but 4-6 weeks if there is a complicated infection.

INFECTION CONTROL MEASURES

Standard infection control measures are designed to prevent transmission of microbial substances between patients and/or medical providers. These measures are indicated for everyone and include frequent handwashing, gloves whenever bodily fluids are involved, and face shields and gowns when splashes are anticipated. For more advanced control with tuberculosis, SARS, vesicular rash disorders (such as VZV), and most recently COVID-19, **airborne precautions** should be instituted to prevent the spread of tiny droplets that can remain suspended in the air for days and travel throughout a hospital environment. Therefore, negative pressure rooms are essential, and providers and patients should wear high-efficiency N95 masks and be fitted in advance. For disorders such as influenza or other infections spread by droplets (spread by cough or sneeze) basic surgical masks should be worn (**droplet precautions**). For **contact precautions** in the setting of fecally-transmitted infection or vesicular rash diseases, gowns/gloves should be used and contact limited. White coats are not a substitute for proper gowning. In the case of a *Clostridium difficile* infection, contact precautions should be used in addition to washing hands with soap and water (rather than alcohol-based hand sanitizer) after patient contact.

INFECTION CONTROL PLAN

The purpose of an infection control/surveillance plan should be clearly outlined and may be multifaceted, including the following elements:

- **Decreasing rates of infection**: The primary purpose of a surveillance plan is to identify a means to decrease nosocomial infections, including a notification system and laboratory surveillance.
- **Evaluating infection control measures**: Surveillance can evaluate effectiveness of infection control measures. (Surgical checklists, handwashing, housekeeping, ventilation).
- **Establishing endemic threshold rates**: Establishing threshold rates can help to enact control measures to reduce rates.
- **Identifying outbreaks**: About 5-10% of infections occur in outbreaks, and comparing data with established endemic threshold rates can help to identify these outbreaks if analysis is done in a regular and timely manner.
- **Achieving staff compliance**: Objective evidence may convince staff to cooperate with infection control measures.
- **Meeting accreditation standards**: Some accreditation agencies require reports of infection rates.
- **Providing defense for malpractice suits**: Providing evidence that a facility is proactive in combating infections can decrease liability.
- **Comparing infection rates with other facilities**: Comparing data helps focus attention and resources.

PROTOCOL FOR NEEDLESTICK INJURY AND POSTEXPOSURE PROPHYLAXIS

If the healthcare provider experiences a **needlestick injury**, the individual's initial response should be to irrigate the wound with soap and water. As soon as possible, the incident must be reported to a supervisor and steps taken according to established protocol. This may include testing and/or prophylaxis, depending on the patient's health history. In some cases, the patient may also be tested for communicable diseases, such as HIV, in order to determine the risk to the healthcare provider. PEP (post-exposure prophylaxis) is available for exposure to HIV (human immunodeficiency virus) and hepatitis B virus (hepatis B immune globulin). However, no PEP is available for HCV (hepatitis C virus) although the CDC does provide a plan for management. PEP should be initiated within 72 hours of exposure. All testing and treatments associated with the needlestick injury must be provided free of cost at a hospital or medical facility.

Non-Pharmacologic Treatments

COMPLEMENTARY THERAPY

Complementary therapies are often used, either alone or in conjunction with conventional medical treatment. These methods should be included if this is what the patient/family chooses, empowering the family to take control of their plan of care. Complementary therapies vary widely and most can easily be incorporated. The **National Center for Complementary and Alternative Medicine** recognizes the following:

- **Whole medical systems**: Chinese medicine (acupressure, acupuncture), naturopathic and homeopathic medicines, and Ayurveda
- **Mind-body medicine**: Prayer, artistic creation, music and dance therapy, biofeedback, focused relaxation, and visualization
- **Biological medicine**: Aromatherapy, herbs, plants, trees, vitamins and minerals, and dietary supplements
- **Manipulation**: Massage and spinal manipulation
- **Energy medicines**: Magnets, electric current, pulsed fields, Reiki, qi gong, and laying-on of the hands

PRECAUTIONS

The use of alternative and complementary therapies should be thoroughly discussed by patients and their physician. Patients should be encouraged to use therapies that are shown to have a beneficial, complementary effect on conventional medical treatment. These therapies include the use of massage, superficial stimulation, relaxation, distraction, hypnosis, and guided imagery.

- Encourage patients to practice the techniques until they are proficient in their use to give them a chance to prove their value.
- Teach the patient how the therapies work to encourage the patient to believe in them to contribute to the placebo effect.
- Caution the patient against abandoning current medical treatment.
- Inform the patient of the high cost of alternate therapies that can divert needed funds and result in little or no benefit.
- Provide the patient with resources in the form of books, pamphlets, and informative websites that prove the results of scientific research so that they can evaluate alternative therapies for themselves.

WHOLE MEDICAL SYSTEMS

Whole medical systems are different philosophies and methods of explaining and treating health and illness. Some systems include:

- **Homeopathic medicine**: This European system uses small amounts of diluted herbs and supplements to help the body to recover from disease by stimulating an immune response.
- **Naturopathic medicine**: This is a European system that uses various natural means (herbs, massage, acupuncture) to support the natural healing forces of the body.
- **Chinese medicine**: Centers on restoring the proper flow of life forces within the body to cure disease by using herbs, acupressure and acupuncture, and meditation.
- **Ayurveda**: This is an Indian system that tries to bring the spirit into harmony with the mind and body to treat disease via yoga, herbs, and massage.

ESSENTIAL OILS AND CUPPING

Essential oils (concentrated oils from plants) are either inhaled (aromatherapy) or diluted and applied to the skin. Essential oils are believed to reduce stress, aid sleep, improve dermatitis, and aid digestion. Commonly used essential oils include eucalyptus, lavender, lemon, peppermint, rosemary, rose, and tea tree. Oils may cause skin irritation when applied to the skin.

Cupping is an ancient practice still used in Southeast Asia and the Middle East to reduce pain, promote healing, and improve circulation. With dry cupping, cups are heated by placing something flammable (such as paper or herbs) inside the cup and setting it on fire to heat the cup, which is then immediately placed on the back along the meridians (generally on both sides of the spine) to form a vacuum that draws blood to the skin and causes circular bruises believed to heal that part of the body. Wet cupping includes leaving the heated cup in place for three minutes, removing it, making small cuts in the skin, and then applying suction cups again to withdraw blood. Cupping should be avoided in children under 4 and limited to short periods in older children.

ACUPUNCTURE

Alternative systems of medical practice include acupuncture, homeopathy, and naturopathy. **Acupuncture**, an ancient Oriental practice, uses stainless steel or copper needles inserted into superficial skin layers at points where energy or life force called *qi* is believed to occur. The needles are supposed to restore balance and the flow of *qi*. The NIH has recognized the effectiveness of acupuncture for certain side effects of other cancer treatments, such as nausea, vomiting, and pain. However, there is no documented scientific evidence to support the principles expounded. Acupuncturists are certified through either formal coursework or apprenticeships, and there is also board certification in this area for physicians. The needles used are classified as class II, which means they have manufacturing and labeling requirements.

HERBAL REMEDIES AND REGULATIONS

In the United States, most **herbal preparations** are classified as dietary supplements. That means that they are not subject to the same rigorous manufacturing, safety, efficacy, and control practices as pharmaceutical drugs. Herbal supplements are only governed by the Dietary Supplement and Health Education Act (DSHEA). As long as no specific disease treatment or curative claims are made, the supplement can be marketed without limitation and safety concerns must be pursued by the FDA after the fact. Nevertheless, some herbal remedies have been undergoing clinical trials in the U.S. to substantiate their health-enhancing or traditional/historical or international use claims. However, the focal point of these studies is still only on the effectiveness of the specific supplement. In Europe, there has been some movement toward greater regulation and licensing of herbal products, but not to the extent of formal drug regulations.

TOXICITIES ASSOCIATED WITH HERBAL REMEDIES

Use of herbal preparations has been associated with a variety of **toxicities**, primarily in categories such as cardiovascular problems, hypersensitivity reactions, disorientation, gastrointestinal problems, and liver malfunction. Because quality control measures are relatively lax for these remedies, contamination from infectious agents and toxic metals can potentially cause other side effects. Many of these herbal medicines **interact with conventional drugs**, thus altering their pharmacodynamics. For example, St. John's wort, which is primarily used for depressive disorders or as a sedative, interacts with a wide range of traditional pharmacologic agents and suppresses their levels in the bloodstream. Kava kava, made from dried roots of a type of pepper bush, is used as a sedative, but it also has been associated with hepatic failure and via interactions with several other drugs can actually induce a comatose state. Ginseng is an Asian remedy touted for its curative properties in a number of diseases. However, it can react with steroidal drugs and induce shaking and manic episodes. These are just a few examples of potential dangers.

NON-PHARMACEUTICAL PAIN RELIEF

Non-pharmaceutical methods to relieve pain that can be used exclusively or combined with medications include massage, heat, cold, electrical stimulation, distraction, relaxation, imagery, visualization, and music. Other **alternatives or adjuncts to pain medication** include hypnosis, magnets, acupuncture, acupressure, and therapeutic touch. Herbs, aromatherapy, reflexology, homeopathic medicine, and prayer may also be accepted by the patient. Any method that the patient feels may help that isn't harmful should be used to help get relief.

MIND-BODY MEDICINE FOR PAIN AND DISEASE

Mind-body medicine (prayer, artistic creation, music and dance, biofeedback, relaxation, and visualization) can help distract people from pain or other symptoms if they are able to concentrate on the method. This can result in the transfer of less painful stimuli to the brain by stimulating the **descending control system**. These methods work if the patient can use them to create alternate sensations in the brain, but will not work if the patient is unable to concentrate due to intense pain.

Relaxation that occurs as a result of using these methods helps to reduce muscular tension that can make pain worse and reduces fatigue caused by chronic pain. Relaxation has been proven to be the most helpful after surgery. Postoperative patients report a greater feeling of control over their pain and tend to request fewer opioids to control pain. Biofeedback can help patients to recognize the feelings of both tension and relaxation and provide a way to indicate their success in managing muscle tension.

USE OF VISUALIZATION

There are a number of methods used for **visualization** to reduce anxiety and promote healing. Some include audiotapes with guided imagery, such as self-hypnosis tapes, but the patient can be taught basic **techniques** that include:

- Sit or lie comfortably in a **quiet place** away from distractions.
- Concentrate on **breathing** while taking long slow breaths.
- **Close the eyes** to shut out distractions and create an image in the mind of the place or situation desired.
- Concentrate on that **image**, engaging as many senses as possible and imaging details.
- If the mind wanders, breathe deeply and **bring consciousness back** to the image or concentrate on breathing for a few moments and then return to the imagery.
- End with positive imagery.

Sometimes, patients are resistive at first or have a hard time maintaining focus, so **guiding** them through visualization for the first few times can be helpful.

STIMULATION OF THE SKIN TO REDUCE PAIN

Skin, muscles, fascia, tendons, and the cornea contain **nociceptors** that are nerve endings that respond to painful stimuli. Massage, transcutaneous electrical nerve stimulation (TENS), heat and cold provide stimulation to other nerves that transfer only sensation, not pain. These signals block some of the transfer of the nociceptor impulses:

- **Massage** not only sends alternate sensation to the brain, but also results in relaxation that decreases the muscular tension that contributes to pain.
- **TENS** works well on incisional and neuromuscular pain by providing a gentle electrical stimulation that overrides the painful impulses from the area and may stimulate endorphins.
- **Heat therapy** increases blood flow and oxygen to promote healing and stimulates neural receptors, decreasing pain. Heat also helps loosen tense muscles that may be contributing to pain.
- **Cold therapy** decreases circulation and reduces production of chemicals related to inflammation, thereby reducing pain.

TEMPERATURE-CONTROLLED THERAPIES

METHODS OF HEATING AND COOLING

There are a number of different ways to **heat** (thermotherapy) or **cool** (cryotherapy) for **healing**:

- **Conduction**: Conveyance of heat, cold, or electricity through direct contact with the skin, such as with hot baths, ice packs, and electrical stimulation.
- **Convection**: Indirect transmission of heat in a liquid or gas by circulation of heated particles, such as with whirlpools and paraffin soaks.
- **Conversion**: Heating that results from converting a form of energy into heat, such as with diathermy and ultrasound.
- **Evaporation**: Cooling caused by liquids that evaporate into gases on the skin with a resultant cooling effect, such as with perspiration or vapo-coolant sprays.
- **Radiation**: Heating that results from transfer of heat through light waves or rays, such as with infrared or ultraviolet light.

SUPERFICIAL HEAT

Superficial heat with externally applied heat sources penetrates only the superficial layers of the skin (1-2 cm after about 30 minutes), but it is believed to relax deeper muscles by reflex, decrease pain, and increase metabolisms (2-3 times for every 10 °C increase in skin temperature). Therapeutic temperature range is 40-45 °C. **Superficial heat modalities** include:

- **Moist heat packs** placed on the skin and secured by several layers of towels to provide insulation, applied for 15-30 minutes.
- **Paraffin baths** (52-54 °C) with the hand, foot, or elbow dipped 7 times, cooling between dippings, and then wrapping with plastic and towels for 20 minutes.
- **Fluidotherapy** uses hot-air warmed (38.8-47.8 °C) cellulose particles into which a hand or foot is submerged for 20-30 minutes.

Passive and active range of motion exercises are done after superficial heat treatment. Contraindications include cardiac disease, peripheral vascular disease, malignant tumor, bleeding, and acute inflammation.

Deep heat differs from superficial heat in that the heat is generated internally using ultrasound, short wave, and microwave diathermy rather than applied to the surface of the skin. Deep heating has penetrance to 3-5 cm.

SHORTWAVE DIATHERMY

Shortwave diathermy uses radio waves (27.12 megahertz) to **increase the temperature in subcutaneous tissue** and is used along with passive and active range of motion exercises to **improve range** in painful conditions such as inflammation of the muscles, tendons, and bursae. The radio waves (eddy currents) are transmitted through a capacitor or inductor in a continuous or pulse waveform. Temperatures increase about 15 °C in fatty tissue and 4-6 °C in muscular tissue. Shortwave diathermy should not be used over any organs containing fluid, including the eyes, heart, head, or over pacemakers as the diathermy may disrupt the settings. Because this treatment may increase cardiac demand, it should be avoided in those with preexisting cardiac conditions and should not be used over malignancies. Additionally, it is contraindicated in areas of inflammation because heating the tissue increases inflammation. It cannot be used over prostheses as the metal may heat and damage tissue. Shortwave diathermy should avoid the epiphyses in children, as it may stimulate abnormal growth.

MICROWAVE DIATHERMY

Microwave diathermy is used similarly to shortwave diathermy but has a lower rate of heat increase and penetrance so it is used for muscles and joints near the surface rather than deep muscles, such as the hip. Heat is created by **electromagnetic radiation** (9.15-14.50 MHz) and raises temperature in fatty tissues by about

10-12 °C and in muscular tissue by 3-4 °C. **Treatment** is usually given for 15-30 minutes per session and is followed by range of motion exercises (passive and active) to increase flexibility. Contraindications are similar to those of shortwave diathermy in that this treatment should not be used where increase in temperature may be detrimental, such as over organs containing fluid, areas of inflammation, and epiphyses of children. Additionally, it should not be used over prostheses or pacemakers and should be avoided in those with cardiac disease.

CRYOTHERAPY

Cryotherapy uses therapeutic cold treatment to cool the surface of the skin and underlying subcutaneous tissues in order to decrease blood flow, pain, and metabolism. Initially response to cold therapy causes **vasoconstriction** to occur within the first 15 minutes but if the tissues are cooled to -10 °C, then the body responds with **vasodilation**. Cryotherapy affects sensory response so the person will at first feel cold, which progresses to burning, aching, and finally to numbness and tingling. Treatment is usually given for 15-30 minutes. **Treatment modalities** include:

- **Ice packs** such as refrigerated gel packs (-5 °C) or plastic bags filled with water and ice chips are applied directly to the skin for 10-15 minutes for superficial cooling and 15-20 minutes for greater penetrance.
- A **towel dipped in ice and water slurry** is wrapped around limb to provide cold therapy, but this is best used only for emergency situations when ice packs are unavailable, as the towel must be changed frequently as the skin warms the towel rapidly.
- **Ice massage** is applied directly to the affected area for 5-10 minutes, usually rubbing the ice in circular motions on the skin surface. An ice massager is easily made by filled a paper cup with water and freezing it with a tongue depressor or Popsicle stick (to use as a handle) inserted into the center as the water starts to freeze. Then, the paper can be torn away from the bottom and sides when the ice is solid. Ice massage is often followed by friction massage.
- **Ice baths** (13-18 °C) are used for limbs, such as the lower leg, foot, or hand. The body part is immersed for 20 minutes.

Cryotherapy is usually followed by **active and passive exercises**. Contraindications include impaired circulation or sensation, cardiac disease, Raynaud's disease, and nerve trauma.

WHIRLPOOL BATHS

Whirlpool baths are used to increase **circulation** and promote **healing**. They are tubs with a turbine that mixes air with water, which is pressurized and flows into the tub water to create turbulence. Tubs are usually large enough to accommodate the full body although smaller limb-sized whirlpool tubs are available. Water temperature is 95-104 °F (adjusted for the individual) and should be deep enough to completely submerge the affected part. The body part should be cleaned with soap and water before immersion or a shower taken. If the full body is treated, then the patient should wear a swimming suit. During the whirlpool treatment, the muscles relax from the heat and **range of motion exercises** can be done while in the water. Typically, treatments last about 20 minutes, but the patient should be monitored, especially for the first 5 minutes, as some people become lightheaded and can lose consciousness.

CONTRAST BATHS

Contrast baths (alternating hot and cold) are used in the sub-acute phase of healing (after edema begins to subside) for **strains and sprains**. It is believed that contrast baths increase the circulation and help to further decrease edema by a pumping action as the **vasoconstriction and vasodilation** alternate. Two containers are filled with water, one with hot and the other with cold. The hot water should be maintained at about 100-110 °F and the cold at 55-65 °F. The cycle begins and ends with immersion in cold water. Cold water immersions usually last about 1 minute and hot water immersions 4 minutes. Typically, the affected limb is immersed in the cold water for 1 minute, removed, and immediately immersed in hot water for 4 minutes. This cycle is repeated about 3-4 times.

THERAPEUTIC ULTRASOUND

Ultrasound treats soft-tissue injuries (such as myositis, bursitis, and tendinitis) with sound waves (frequency 0.8-3 MHz). Ultrasound utilizes a **piezoelectric crystal** that vibrates, producing sound waveforms, which are transmitted from the transducer through a gel substance into the tissue. The sound waves bounce off of the bone in an irregular pattern that causes an increase in temperature in the connective tissue, such as collagen fibers. Temperatures of the tissue may increase up to 43.5 °C, increasing metabolism in the area, neural conduction, as well as blood flow. Ultrasound is used to **decrease both contractures and scarring**. During treatment, the transducer passes in a circular motion about the skin surface, staying in contact with the gel medium. If a distal limb is submerged in water, the treatment is given with the head of the transducer 0.5-1.0 in from the skin surface. Treatment is followed by range of motion exercises, passive and active. Contraindications are similar to other heat-producing modalities and include peripheral vascular disease, but ultrasound may be used over metal prostheses.

TENS

Transcutaneous electrical nerve stimulation (TENS) uses electrical stimulation to stimulate **peripheral sensory nerve fibers** to reduce acute or recurrent pain. TENS machines may be 2-lead or 4-lead and have adjustments for both frequency (1-20 Hz) and pulse width (50-300 μs, 10-50 mA). Stimulation can be intermittent or continuous. TENS units are small and battery-powered with wires and adhesive electrodes attached so that they can be worn while the person goes about usual activities. The positioning of the electrodes and the settings depend upon the site and type of injury, following guidelines provided by the manufacturer. The TENS machine can be used for a number of hours, but if used for days at a time, it will be less effective. TENS treatment is contraindicated with demand pacemakers and should not be used on the head or neck or over irritated skin.

REHABILITATION

SAID PRINCIPLE OF REHABILITATION AND RECONDITIONING

The Specific Adaptation to Imposed Demands (SAID) principle suggests that when a person is injured or stressed, that person attempts to overcome the problem by **adapting** to the demands of the situation. This is based on **Wolff's law** (systems adapt to demands). For example, if one hand is not usable, the person adapts and uses the other hand. Unfortunately, this adaptation can lead to increasing disability, so when the SAID principle is applied to rehabilitation, it means that the person must do exercises that specifically aim to correct the problem. Thus, the functional needs of the person should always be considered when designing a specific exercise program for that individual (such as treadmill running for soccer players). The exercise activities should as closely mirror the functional activities as possible. For example, if the goal is increased strength rather than endurance, then the exercise program should rely more heavily on strengthening exercises.

MASSAGE FOR REHABILITATION AND RECONDITIONING

Massage therapy is commonly used in sports and may be employed before activities, at breaks during activities, and after the activity is completed. Many types of massage are used in sports, and some massage therapists specialize in sports massage, but all nurses who work with athletes of any age should know the basic techniques of **sports massage** as it is used to both treat and prevent injuries. Sports massage is based primarily on Swedish massage although the massage may be deeper and targeted toward a particular injury, and other types of massage may be incorporated into a sports massage program. Massage of an injured area is delayed for the first **48-72 hours** to prevent further injury to tissues. Different techniques include:

- **Compression**: Deep rhythmical compressions of the muscles are done to increase circulation and temperature and make muscles more pliable. It may be used prior to deeper massage techniques.
- **Effleurage**: This is usually the beginning massage and begins softly and increases in intensity with the hands gliding over the tissue, so it is done with some type of oil or emollient. Massage is done in rhythmical broad strokes with the palms of the hands. This massage helps to relax the athlete and identify areas of tightness or pain that may require additional attention.

- **Friction**: These are massages either in line with muscle fibers or across the muscle fibers to create stretching and to reduce adhesions and scarring during healing. The tissue is pressed firmly against the underlying tissue and then pressure moves the underlying tissue until resistance is felt. Friction massage may be done deeply, and this can be uncomfortable. Usually, the thumb or fingers are used for this type of massage.
- **Petrissage**: This is kneading massage and is usually used on large muscle areas, such as the calf or thigh. It increases circulation, so it is useful to relax and to improve circulation and drainage as well as to stretch muscles. The full hand is used for this massage with the heel and thumb stabilizing the tissue while the fingers squeeze the tissue.
- **Tapotement**: This type of massage uses quick rhythmic tapping, usually with the edge of the palm and little finger or the heel of the hand with the fingers elevated. It is done to increase circulation or relieve cramped muscles.
- **Vibration**: Vibratory massage is used for deep muscle relaxation and reduction of pain. Usually, the entire hand is placed against the skin, compressing the muscle and then vibrating the hand to cause movement.
- **Trigger point**: Pressure is applied with a finger or thumb to areas of point tenderness to reduce spasticity and pain.

PROGRESSION IN STRENGTHENING EXERCISES

Strengthening exercise progression includes the following exercises:

- **Isometric exercises** are done with the muscle and limb in static position with no movement of the joint or lengthening of the muscle. The muscle is contracted against resistance.
- **Isotonic exercises** include movement of the joint during exercise (such as running, weight lifting) and both shortening and lengthening of the muscles through eccentric or concentric contractions. Isotonic refers to tension, so the tension is constant during shortening and lengthening of the muscle.
- **Isokinetic exercises** utilize machines (such as stationary bicycles that can be set with various parameters) to control the rate and extent of contraction as well as the range of motion. Both speed and resistance can be set so the athlete is limited by the settings of the machine.
- **Plyometrics** is a particular type of exercise program that uses activities to allow a muscle to achieve maximal force as quickly as possible, and the sequence is a fast, eccentric movement (to stretch) followed quickly by a strong concentric movement (to contract).

Medication Interactions and Adverse Effects

DRUG CLASSIFICATION

The following are different ways to classify drugs:

- **Therapeutic classification**: The common uses for the drug will place it in a certain therapeutic classification.
- **Pharmacological classification**: The action of the drug determines which pharmacological category a drug will be in.

All drugs have a **chemical name** and a **generic name,** which is simpler. A company making the drug can give it a **trade or brand name**. The generic form of a drug is generally cheaper but may differ in efficacy from a brand name drug due to a difference in the amount of drug that is absorbed for use in the body. The Controlled Substances Act restricts usage of certain drugs and classifies them according to schedules that include:

- **Schedule I**: Ecstasy, LSD, marijuana, peyote, Quaalude, mescaline, psilocybin, heroin, and others
- **Schedule II**: Amphetamine, cocaine, codeine, fentanyl, Dilaudid, Demerol, Ritalin, morphine, opium, and others
- **Schedule III**: Anabolic steroids, barbiturates, codeine, Vicodin, and pentothal
- **Schedule IV**: Xanax, Librium, Klonopin, Tranxene, Redux, Darvocet, Valium, Ativan, Equagesic, Versed, phenobarbital, Restoril, Sonata, Ambien
- **Schedule V**: Lomotil and others

5 RIGHTS OF MEDICATION ADMINISTRATION

The 5 rights of medication administration are used to prevent/reduce medication errors in the hospital setting. Often these 5 rights are integrated into the scanning requirements of electronic documentation. The **5 rights of medication administration** must also be incorporated into the prescriber's order:

- **Right Patient**: Confirm the patient's identity using two identifiers, often being their full name and date of birth. Scanning will also confirm the patient's identity with their bar code and electronic health record.
- **Right Drug**: Check the name of the drug with the prescriber's order. By scanning the medication, the drug name will also be checked against the order.
- **Right Dose**: Check the dose of the drug with the prescriber's order. Some medications require a second nurse confirm any dosage calculations utilized before administration. Ensure the dosage is appropriate and contact the prescriber if there are any concerns.
- **Right route**: Routes include oral (PO), subcutaneous, intradermal, IV, or IM, amongst others. The route must also be confirmed with the prescriber's order.
- **Right time/frequency**: The drug may be administered as a one-time dose, PRN (as needed), or recurring administration (twice daily, every 8 hours, etc.).

CLINICAL SITUATIONS THAT HAVE IMPLICATIONS FOR MEDICATION ADMINISTRATION

It is quite important to recognize clinical situations involving patients that may have **implications for the administration of medications**. For example, many patients have co-morbid conditions that will impact decisions about their medication administration. A patient with non-insulin-dependent diabetes and coronary artery disease who is being treated for a hip fracture would require oral hypoglycemic medications, cardiovascular medications, pain medication, and anti-coagulants. Another example would be an insulin-dependent diabetic patient with concomitant hypertension and renal failure. This patient would require insulin, anti-hypertensive medications, and dosing adjustments of medications secondary to renal failure. The nurse who is responsible for the patient must ensure that the correct dosages of each prescribed medication are administered on time. Potential negative side effects and drug-drug interactions should be avoided, and the patient should be monitored for adverse reactions to newly prescribed drugs.

ROUTES OF DRUG ADMINISTRATION

The route of administration is the manner by which a drug is introduced into the body. The most **common routes of administration** are:

- Enteral (oral, rectal, or by feeding tube)
- Topical (on the skin, in the eyes or nose, vaginal, or inhaled)
- Parenteral (IV, subcutaneous, intramuscular, intracardiac, intraosseous, intradermal, intrathecal, intraperitoneal, transdermal, transmucosal, intravitreal, and epidural)

There are many variations on these three basic routes of administration. The FDA acknowledges 111 different routes of administration. When deciding on the route of administration, the doctor and pharmacist consider:

- How fast the patient requires the drug
- How effective it will be by a given route
- The likelihood of toxicity
- The discomfort it will cause
- How likely the patient is to comply with the route
- How likely the route is to play into the patient's addictive habits

INJECTIONS

The three most common types of injections and the preferred injection sites are as follows:

- **Subcutaneous Injection**: Deliver the drug under the skin with a ½ inch, 24- or 25-gauge needle held at a 45° angle to reach the fat. Choose the upper arm, abdomen, thigh, or lower back as the site. The maximum amount of subcutaneous medication is 0.5 ml. An example is insulin for a patient with diabetes.
- **Intramuscular Injection**: Deliver the drug into the muscle at a 90° angle to reach the deep tissue. Standard needle length is 1 to 1.5 inches depending on the weight of the individual. CDC guidelines recommend the use of a 22- to 25-gauge needle for adult intramuscular injections. Recommended sites for injection on the adult include deltoid (most recommended), vastus lateralis (thigh), ventrogluteal (hip), or dorsogluteal (buttocks). The maximum recommended amount of IM medication is 3 mL. An example is Vitamin B12 for a patient with pernicious anemia.
- **Intravenous Injection**: Deliver the drug into a vein of the arm, hand, leg, foot, scalp, or neck with an Angiocath, butterfly, or Insyte Autoguard needle. Use a size from 14 gauge to 26 gauge, depending on the fluid and the patient. The nurse sets the drip rate per minute by adjusting the clamp and monitoring the drip chamber. An example of a drug requiring intravenous injection is Zoledronate, which is given yearly to prevent bone fractures for individuals with osteoporosis.

> **Review Video: Calculating IV Drip Rates**
> Visit mometrix.com/academy and enter code: 396112

Two less frequently used forms of injection are: Intradermal (into the skin) for Mantoux TB test, and intraosseous access (IO) into the bone, which is used in emergency situations when other access sites are not available.

HERBAL-DRUG CONTRAINDICATIONS

Patients on certain medications should not take some herbals. Some **contraindications for common herbals** include:

- **Echinacea**: Anti-anxiety meds, antifungals, heart medications, HIV medications, anabolic steroids, methotrexate, NSAIDs
- **Gingko Biloba**: Anticoagulants, NSAIDs, aspirin, acetaminophen

- **Garlic**: Anticoagulants, oral hypoglycemics, NSAIDs
- **Licorice**: Diuretics, digoxin, antihypertensives
- **St. John's Wort**: Antidepressants, anticoagulants, Tamoxifen, oral contraceptives, HIV medications, anesthetics. Action is similar to MAO inhibitor
- **Valerian**: Sedatives, anti-seizure meds, anesthetics, alcohol, opioids
- **Feverfew**: Anticoagulants, migraine meds, NSAIDs
- **Ginger**: Anticoagulants, NSAIDs
- **Ginseng**: Anticoagulants, antihypertensives, NSAIDs, opioids. Do not take when pregnant or lactating
- **Goldenseal**: Antihypertensives, diabetic medications, meds for kidney diseases. Do not take when pregnant or lactating
- **Kava-kava**: Alcohol, anti-seizure meds, antidepressants, sedatives, anesthetics, antipsychotics, NSAIDS, opioids
- **Saw Palmetto**: Hormone therapy
- **Hawthorn**: Digoxin

Blood Drug Levels

Plasma drug levels are used for **therapeutic drug monitoring** because, although plasma is often not the site of action, plasma levels correlate well with therapeutic (effective) and toxic (dose-related adverse effects) responses to most drugs. The therapeutic range of a drug is that between the minimum effective concentration (level at which there is no therapeutic benefit) and the toxic concentration (level at which toxic effects occur). To achieve drug plateau (steady state), the drug half-life (time needed to decrease drug concentration by 50%) must be considered. Most drugs reach plateau with administration equal to four half-lives and completely eliminate a drug in 5 half-lives. Because drug levels fluctuate, peak (highest drug concentration) and trough (lowest drug concentration) levels may be monitored. Samples for trough levels are taken immediately prior to administration of another dose, while peak samples are taken at various times, depending on the average peak time of the specific drug, which may vary from 30 minutes to 2 hours or so after administration.

Side Effects of Medications

All drugs can have side effects, and some are toxic at certain levels or in combination with other drugs. Some side effects will be minor and may go away after a week or two. Others can be severe or life-threatening, such as anaphylaxis. Common side effects include nausea, vomiting, diarrhea, and rashes. Side effects may vary with individuals according to age, gender, and condition and may be related to non-compliance with treatment, incorrect dosage, polypharmacy, or drug interactions. Drug compendiums will list all possible side effects according to system or incidence. Pharmacologically similar medications usually have some common side effects among the drugs in that class. Nursing actions include:

- Always question the patient about allergies or previous drug reactions before administering medication.
- Educate the patient about possible side effects of all medications.
- Watch out for drug-drug and food-drug combinations that are dangerous.

Drug Interactions

Drug interactions occur when one drug interferes with the activity of another in either the pharmacodynamics or pharmacokinetics:

- With **pharmacodynamic interaction,** both drugs may interact at receptor sites causing a change that results in an adverse effect or that interferes with a positive effect.
- With **pharmacokinetic interaction**, the ability of the drug to be absorbed and cleared is altered, so there may be delayed effects, changes in effects, or toxicity. Interactions may include problems in a number of areas:

- o **Absorption** may be increased or (more commonly) decreased, usually related to the effects within the gastrointestinal system.
- o **Distribution** of drugs may be affected, often because of changes in protein binding.
- o **Metabolism** may be altered, often causing changes in drug concentration.
- o **Biotransformation** of the drug must take place, usually in the liver and gastrointestinal system, but drug interactions can impair this process.
- o **Clearance interactions** may interfere with the body's ability to eliminate a drug, usually resulting in increased concentration of the drug.

SPECIFIC INTERACTIONS

Some drugs will either increase or inhibit the actions of other drugs. They may interfere with receptor-site binding or the way in which the drug is metabolized or excreted. Certain drugs may cause drowsiness when taken together or with alcohol. Some foods will inhibit drug action, such as the inhibition of warfarin by vitamin-K-containing foods. Other foods may cause toxic levels of a drug to accumulate. Grapefruit juice, for example, is metabolized by the same enzyme that metabolizes about 50 drugs, including digoxin and statins, and this can prevent the liver from breaking down drugs and lead to severe reactions. The nurse should always obtain a complete medication list from the patient, including prescription and over-the-counter medications, herbals, vitamins, minerals, and dietary supplements that are taken regularly and occasionally. All medications taken should be checked for **potential interactions with drugs or foods**.

Health and Wellness Promotion

HEALTH PROMOTION

Nurses promote health when they assist individuals to change behavior in ways that help them to attain and maintain the highest level of wellbeing possible. Health promotion is a very popular way to control healthcare costs and reduce illness and early death. Health is increasingly the topic of newscasts and literature. The public is demanding more information pertinent to the maintenance of health and to the ways in which the average person can act independently to do so. Health promotion is centered on ideal personal habits, lifestyles, and environmental control that decrease the risk for disease. The US Public Health Service periodically identifies national health goals and most recently published a program called ***Healthy People 2030***, with measurable goals to increase the general quality and years of life for all and to increase the health status of all groups to an equal level of wellness. Health promotion programs in the community are now offered by workplaces, clinics, schools, and churches, not just by hospitals as in the past.

HEALTHY PEOPLE 2030

The 5 **main goals** of *Healthy People 2030* are

- Attaining healthy, thriving lives free of preventable disease, disability, injury, and premature death
- Eliminating health disparities, achieving health equality, and increasing health literacy
- Creating environments conducive to health-promotion
- Improving health in all life stages
- Collaborating with leadership and key stakeholders in policy design that improves the health and well-being of all

Healthy People 2030 has 62 topic areas with 355 total objectives divided across five sections:

- Health Conditions
- Health Behaviors
- Populations
- Settings and Systems
- Social Determinants of Health

MAIN COMPONENTS OF HEALTH PROMOTION

Health promotion efforts are concentrated in four areas:

- Individuals must be educated to realize that their **lifestyle and choices** have a large impact on their health. They must then be motivated to choose to modify their personal risk factors and take the responsibility to do so.
- The emphasis on **good nutrition** as the biggest factor that impacts health and the length of life must be brought into general awareness. This is occurring via the media through numerous books and articles educating people about the essential nutrients needed to maintain health.
- **Stress** is a constant in a production-driven society. Individuals must learn ways to manage and decrease stress to achieve and maintain health and to decrease the effects of stress upon chronic illness, risk of infections, and trauma.
- **Physical fitness** helps cardiovascular status, relieves stress, controls weight, delays aging, promotes strength and endurance, and improves appearance and performance. Individuals must have programs that increase activity gradually to prevent injury and are designed to meet individual needs.

HEALTH SELF-MANAGEMENT

Health self-management includes health maintenance, disease prevention, and health promotion. Health maintenance is defined as strategies that help maintain and/or improve health over time. Health maintenance is dependent on three factors, which include health perception, motivation for behavioral change, and compliance to set goals. Disease prevention is an effort to limit the development or progression of lifestyle-related illness. **Disease prevention** can be categorized into primary, secondary, and tertiary prevention.

- **Primary prevention** measures are employed prior to disease onset and are used in health populations.
- **Secondary prevention** measures are used to screen, detect, and treat disease in earlier stages to prevent further progression or development of other complications.
- **Tertiary prevention** measures are used to prevent the onset of other complications or comorbid conditions.

Health promotion strategies include risk reduction strategies applied to the general population.

INFLUENCES ON DECISION TO MODIFY BEHAVIOR TO ACHIEVE AND MAINTAIN HEALTH

Many factors have an influence on people's efforts to change behavior in a way that improves and maintains their health status. These factors include age, ethnicity, gender, lifestyle, level of education, self-esteem, motivation, and self-image. The patient's support network and the availability of health promotion programs and healthcare systems also have an influence on healthcare behaviors. Some people may be prevented from accessing health promotion programs because of lack of medical insurance. Financial status and employment are important as well. The presence of addictions and diseases, the length of illness, and the severity of disabilities are all factors to be considered. The value placed on health, the threat of potential losses, and the perceived benefits of behavior modification are important motivating factors.

STRATEGIES TO ENCOURAGE SMOKING CESSATION

The **health impact associated with smoking** varies among smokers and can be affected by the number of cigarettes used daily, exposure to smoking-associated stimuli, and educational level. The presence of stress and depression, psychosocial problems, lack of coping mechanisms, low income, and long-term habitual behavior are problematic for the quitter. Nurses can promote smoking cessation by taking every opportunity to bring up the subject, educating about the dangers of smoking and benefits of quitting, and providing **resources** to help patients quit. Strategies include:

- Educating about the personal effects of smoking upon that individual
- Encouraging patients to set a quit date
- Referring to programs and smoking cessation information
- Educating about the use of nicotine replacements including nicotine gum, lozenges, inhalers, transdermal patches, and nasal sprays
- Educating about the use of medications such as Zyban, Catapres, and Chantix
- Providing support via phone calls or office visits
- Discovering the reason for relapses
- Praising and rewarding any success in the quitting process

HEALTHY NUTRITION PRINCIPLES

Healthy nutrition principles include the following:

- Eating a range of different kinds of foods, and eating increased amounts fruits, vegetables, whole grains, poultry, and fish.
- Diets should consist of 55-60% **carbohydrates**, less than 30% **fat**, and the rest should be **protein** (0.8-1.0 g/kg).
- Restrict **saturated fat** to <10%. Restrict **cholesterol** to 300 mg/day.
- Utilize moderate amounts of sugar, salt, and sodium.
- Take a **multivitamin** including folic acid if the patient is female and able to have children. Get 200-800 IU/day of vitamin D in order to absorb calcium.

- **Calcium** intake should be: 1,300 mg/day for women age 13-18 or those who are pregnant/nursing; 1,000 mg/day for women age 19-50 years; 1,500 mg/day for age 51 years and older.
- Patients who are pregnant or having chemotherapy should not try to lose weight.
- **Weight loss** may improve diabetes, joint pain, inflammation, cardiovascular disease, hypothyroidism, or renal disease.

YOUNG ADULT HEALTH SCREENINGS

Health screening is encouraged for conditions that are very likely to occur and diseases that are likely to kill if they are not identified. The assessment should be trustworthy using proper techniques and proper follow-up.

Young adult (ages 20-39 years) screenings, according to the US Preventive Services Task Force (USPSTF), should include:

- A full head-to-toe physical (every 5-6 years)
- Blood pressure screening (every 3-5 years if range is within normal: <130/85 mmHg)
- Cholesterol screening (every 5 years; more frequently when total cholesterol is higher than 200 mg/dL)
- PPD test for tuberculosis when patient has had known contact with TB or is at increased risk (health care workers, prisoners, homeless, or immunocompromised)
- Dental check-up (annually)
- Thyroid palpation (every 3 years)
- Depression screening (at every visit)
- Men perform self-testicular exam every month
- Women conduct a self-breast exam every month; should receive a clinical breast exam every 3 years
- Pap smear and pelvic assessments every 3 years (or up to 5 years in conjunction with HPV testing)
- Screening for gonorrhea and chlamydia for all sexually active individuals
- Health education and promotion (every time patient is seen)
- Influenza vaccination (annually)
- Td immunization every 10 years

ADULT SCREENINGS

Adults (age 40 and older) screenings, according to the USPSTF, should maintain the same schedule as young adults (unless indicated below) in addition to the following:

- A full head-to-toe physical (annually)
- Blood pressure screening (annually)
- ECG (over 40, annually; only when there are cardiac risks)
- Clinical breast exam (annually in women over 40)
- Mammogram (biennially in women over 50)
- General colorectal cancer screening for risks (annually), and colorectal cancer screening via colonoscopy (every 10 years for those over 50 until age 75)
- Prostate-specific antigen screening (men over 50 with average risk, or younger if higher risk; upon the patient's informed request only)

DISEASE PREVENTION FOR THE ELDERLY

Although life spans are longer, **ongoing (chronic) diseases** are still the primary reason patients die. Elderly patients have more of an absolute chance of getting a disease, but they also react well to prevention. Keep good records of the elderly patient's history, including updating every year and following advice for patients over the age of 65 years. Evaluate nutrition, functional ability, alcoholic beverage intake (more than 2 alcoholic beverages a day constitutes abuse), smoking, illegal drugs, misuse of prescriptions, and exercise level.

- **Preventative measures** include a physical, screening assessments, and immunizations.
- Some **routine screenings** include: fasting glucose, papanicolaou smear, dipstick urinalysis, mammography, PPD, fecal occult blood/sigmoidoscopy, electrocardiogram, thyroid function, glaucoma and sight, hearing, and cholesterol.
- **Immunizations** include yearly flu shot, pneumococcal vaccine, and tetanus.

The following screens are controversial: depression for someone with no symptoms, dementia for someone with no symptoms, osteoporosis including bone densitometry for postmenopausal females (counsel females regarding hormone prophylaxis), colon and prostate cancer, and cholesterol for someone with no symptoms.

BENEFITS OF KNOWING EPIDEMIOLOGICAL PRACTICES

Epidemiology is important to nurses across all clinical settings, not just those in public health positions. Each and every nurse will treat a varied patient population during his or her career, and it is important for the nurse to create a plan of care that is tailored to the patient; the patient's age, race, career, and religion all represent different populations to which he or she belongs, and may affect clinical course, treatment, and outcome. Armed with **epidemiological knowledge** about his or her patients, the nurse can create a clinical decision-making framework, an effective care plan, and the means to share this information with his or her peers to aid in the care of other patients.

IMMUNIZATION VS. VACCINATION

Immunization refers to the body's buildup of defenses (antibodies) against specific diseases. It has an important role in preventing the spread of infection. Immunization prevents the individual from contracting a disease or lessens the severity of the disease, and can also prevent the complications (encephalitis, hearing loss, paralysis) associated with the infectious diseases. **Vaccination** is one method of creating immunity through the introduction of a small amount of the virus's or bacteria's antigen to the body, which then stimulates the body's creation of antibodies against that disease. Vaccination prevents the spread of infection to infants who are too young to have developed immunity and to those who are immunocompromised (cancer patients, transplantation recipients). Herd immunity results from a majority of the population being immune to a disease, therefore minimizing transmission. It is defined in terms of the percentage of the population that must be immunized in order to prevent outbreaks. This percentage may range from 80-85% for some disorders, but those that are highly contagious, such as measles, may require a herd immunity of 93-95%. Herd immunity can be obtained via widespread vaccination or widespread infection, though it is not recommended that individuals avoid immunization and rely on herd immunity for protection, as rates of immunization vary from one community to another.

TYPES OF VACCINES

There are a number of different types of vaccines:

- **Conjugated forms**: An organism is altered and then joined (conjugated) with another substance, such as a protein, to potentiate immune response (such as conjugated Hib).
- **Killed virus vaccines**: The virus has been killed but can still cause an immune response (such as inactivated poliovirus).
- **Live virus vaccines**: The virus is live but in a weakened (attenuated) form so that it doesn't cause the disease but confers immunity (such as measles vaccine).
- **Recombinant forms**: The organism is genetically altered and, for example, may use proteins rather than the whole cell to stimulate immunity (such as Hepatitis B and acellular pertussis vaccine).
- **Toxoid**: A toxin (antigen) that has been weakened by the use of heat or chemicals so it is too weak to cause disease but stimulates antibodies.

Some vaccines are given shortly after birth; others begin at 2 months, 12 months, or 2 years and some later in childhood.

DTaP AND Tdap VACCINES

Diphtheria and pertussis (whooping cough) are highly contagious bacterial diseases of the upper respiratory tract. Cases of diphtheria are now rare in the United States, although they still occur in some developing countries. There have, however, been recent outbreaks of pertussis in the United States. Tetanus is a bacterial infection contracted through cuts, wounds, and scratches. The **diphtheria, tetanus, and pertussis (DTaP) vaccine** is recommended for all children. DTaP is a newer and safer version of the older DTP vaccine, which is no longer used in the United States. **Tdap** is the DTaP booster shot meant to continue immunity to these diseases through adulthood, given every 10 years starting at age 11. DTaP requires 5 doses:

- 2 months
- 4 months
- 6 months
- 5-18 months
- 4-6 years (or at 11-12 years if booster missed between 4-6)

According to recent ACIP recommendations, DTap may now also be administered to children ages 7-9 as part of a catch-up series, but children will then require their routine Tdap dose at age 11-12. If DTap is administered to children ages 10-18 it can be counted as their adolescent Tdap booster. Adverse reactions can occur, but they are usually mild soreness, fever, and/or nausea. About 1 in 100 children will have high fever (>105 °F) and may develop seizures. Severe allergic responses can occur.

HPV VACCINE

Human papillomavirus (HPV) comprises >100 viruses. About 40 are sexually transmitted and invade mucosal tissue, causing genital warts, which are low risk for cancer, or changes in the mucosa, which can lead to cervical cancer. Most HPVs cause little or no symptoms, but they are very common, especially in those 15-25. Over 99% of cervical cancers are caused by HPV and 70% are related to HPVs 16 and 18. The HPV vaccine, Gardasil, protects against HPVs 6 and 11 (which cause genital warts), along with 16 and 18, which can cause cancer. Protection is only conveyed if the female has not yet been infected with these strains. The vaccine is currently recommended for females under 26 but studies have determined that those not adequately covered over the age of 26 and up to 45 can benefit. A series of 3 injections is required over a 6-month period:

- Initial dose 11-12 years (but may be given as young as 9 or ≥18)
- 2 months after first dose
- 6 months after first dose

PPV

Pneumococcal polysaccharide-23 vaccine (PPV) (Pneumovax and Pnu-Immune) is a vaccine that has been available since 1977 to protect against 23 types of pneumococcal bacteria. It is given to adults ≥65 and children ≥2 years in high-risk groups that include:

- Children with chronic heart, lung, sickle cell disease, diabetes, cirrhosis, alcoholism, and leaks of cerebrospinal fluid
- Children with lowered immunity from Hodgkin's disease, lymphoma, leukemia, kidney failure, multiple myeloma, nephrotic syndrome, HIV/AIDS, damaged or missing spleen, and organ transplant

Children ≤2 may not respond to this vaccine and should take PCV-7. Administration is as follows:

- One dose is usually all that is required although a second dose may be advised for children with some conditions, such as cancer or organ/bone marrow transplantations.
- If needed, a second dose is given 3 years after the first for children ≤10 and 5 years after the first for those ≥10.

INFANT IMMUNIZATION SCHEDULE SUMMARY

The recommended schedule for immunizations for the infant is summarized below:

- All newborns receive **ophthalmic drops or ointment**, to prevent blindness from possible gonorrhea infection, and an injection of vitamin K to prevent hemorrhagic disease.
- Before discharge, newborns are tested for **phenylketonuria** and **hypothyroidism**, and will possibly have their **hematocrit** and **hemoglobin** checked.
- **Hepatitis B vaccine** is given at birth, 1-2 months, and 6-18 months.
- **Diphtheria/tetanus/pertussis vaccine** is administered at 2 months, 4 months, 6 months, and 15-18 months.
- **Hib (Haemophilus influenza type b) vaccine** is given at 2 months, 4 months, and 12 months or later.
- **Poliovirus vaccine** is given at 2 months, 4 months, and 6-18 months.
- **MMR vaccine** is given at 12-18 months.
- **Varicella (chickenpox) vaccine** can be given at 12 months.

REQUIRED IMMUNIZATION HISTORY FOR CHILDREN UP TO 6 YEARS OF AGE

According to the Centers for Disease Control and Prevention, by 6 years of age, children in the United States should receive a three-part series of hepatitis B, three doses of rotavirus prevention; four injections protecting against diphtheria, tetanus, and pertussis; four doses of *Haemophilus influenzae* type b; four doses of pneumococcal vaccine; four doses of polio vaccine; two injections that protect against measles, mumps, and rubella; two varicella vaccinations; one hepatitis A vaccination; and a yearly influenza prevention injection.

VACCINATION OF CHILDREN WITH UNCERTAIN IMMUNIZATION HISTORIES

Children who have uncertain immunization histories may need vaccinations to meet guidelines. The number of vaccinations needed depends on the child's history. For children who are not up-to-date on immunizations, the necessary injections must be determined. These vaccinations can then be given on a schedule so that the child can catch up. For children with no immunization history or uncertain status, such as refugees or internationally adopted children, restarting the immunization series may be necessary to ensure adequate coverage with all vaccines, particularly measles, mumps, and rubella; varicella; hepatitis B; *Haemophilus influenzae* type b; and polio.

POSSIBLE SIDE EFFECTS

Immunization reactions can be minimized and the child made more comfortable by giving acetaminophen prior to the immunizations. Common reactions to immunizations include irritability, decrease in appetite, fever less than 102 °F, and swelling, redness and tenderness at injection site. These may last for the first 1-2 days and can be treated with acetaminophen every 4-6 hours for the first day. If more severe reactions occur, such as fever greater than 102 °F, severe prolonged irritability, or high-pitched crying, or the symptoms last more than 2 days, the parents should call the healthcare provider immediately.

IMPORTANT CONSIDERATIONS WHEN GIVING IMMUNIZATIONS

Every time a child comes into contact with the healthcare system, his **immunization status** should be assessed. Children are required, by all states, to be immunized before entering a licensed school or day care. Specific requirements will vary from state to state. Vaccines must be handled and stored according the manufacturers guidelines. Immunizations must be documented according to specific guidelines and parents must sign a consent form every time a vaccine is administered. Common illnesses such as colds, ear infections and diarrhea will not usually preclude giving vaccines. The MMR and varicella vaccines should not be given during pregnancy. There are two situations in which immunizations are contraindicated: a previous severe allergic reaction to a vaccine or one of its components and encephalopathy occurring within 7 days of giving a DTP or DTaP vaccine.

THE ANTI-VACCINATION MOVEMENT

While **opposition to vaccination** is not a new concept, it is a movement that has gained momentum with the power of information sharing via social media. Opposers to vaccination, often referred to as "Anti-Vaxxers," believe that vaccinations can cause complications such as autism and SIDS, especially when administered in infancy and early childhood, and believe that these risks far outweigh the benefits. There are also those who oppose such medical interventions due to religious beliefs.

While the therapeutic effects of vaccinations have been supported by evidence for both individuals and communities, it is important that healthcare professionals be equipped to respectfully inform and care for those that oppose vaccinations. Individuals should be educated regarding the evidence supporting vaccinations and the vaccinations required by law. The CDC offers a wealth of resources for healthcare workers and for individuals regarding vaccinations. The most notable resource is the CDC's Vaccine Information Statement, a living document that outlines the benefits and risks of vaccines, that healthcare workers can use to inform individuals and parents. If, despite efforts to educate, the individual or caregiver still refuses vaccination, there are ICD codes that providers are required to use to document this refusal (for example, ICD-10-CM: Z28.82: Immunization not carried out because of caregiver refusal). The healthcare worker must also document that preventive medical counseling was provided.

Professional Role

Therapeutic Communication

THERAPEUTIC COMMUNICATION
FACILITATING COMMUNICATION

Therapeutic communication begins with respect for the patient/family and the assumption that all communication, verbal and nonverbal, has meaning. Listening must be done empathetically. The following are some techniques that facilitate communication.

Introduction:

- Make a personal introduction and use the patient's name: "Mrs. Brown, I am Susan Williams, your nurse."

Encouragement:

- Use an open-ended opening statement: "Is there anything you'd like to discuss?"
- Acknowledge comments: "Yes," and "I understand."
- Allow silence and observe nonverbal behavior rather than trying to force conversation. Ask for clarification if statements are unclear.
- Reflect statements back (use sparingly): Patient: "I hate this hospital." Nurse: "You hate this hospital?"

Empathy:

- Make observations: "You are shaking," and "You seem worried."
- Recognize feelings:
  - o Patient: "I want to go home."
  - o Nurse: "It must be hard to be away from your home and family."
- Provide information as honestly and completely as possible about condition, treatment, and procedures and respond to the patient's questions and concerns.

Exploration:

- Verbally express implied messages:
  - o Patient: "This treatment is too much trouble."
  - o Nurse: "You think the treatment isn't helping you?"
- Explore a topic but allow the patient to terminate the discussion without further probing: "I'd like to hear how you feel about that."

Orientation:

- Indicate reality:
  - o Patient: "Someone is screaming."
  - o Nurse: "That sound was an ambulance siren."
- Comment on distortions without directly agreeing or disagreeing:
  - o Patient: "That nurse promised I didn't have to walk again."
  - o Nurse: "Really? That's surprising because the doctor ordered physical therapy twice a day."

342

Collaboration:

- Work together to achieve better results: "Maybe if we talk about this, we can figure out a way to make the treatment easier for you."

Validation:

- Seek validation: "Do you feel better now?" or "Did the medication help you breathe better?"

AVOIDING NON-THERAPEUTIC COMMUNICATION

While using therapeutic communication is important, it is equally important to avoid interjecting **non-therapeutic communication**, which can block effective communication. *Avoid the following:*

- Meaningless clichés: "Don't worry. Everything will be fine." "Isn't it a nice day?"
- Providing advice: "You should…" or "The best thing to do is…." It's better when patients ask for advice to provide facts and encourage the patient to reach a decision.
- Inappropriate approval that prevents the patient from expressing true feeling or concerns:
  - o Patient: "I shouldn't cry about this."
  - o Nurse: "That's right! You're an adult!"
- Asking for an explanation of behavior that is not directly related to patient care and requires analysis and explanation of feelings: "Why are you so upset?"
- Agreeing with rather than accepting and responding to patient's statements can make it difficult for the patient to change his or her statement or opinion later: "I agree with you," or "You are right."
- Making negative judgments: "You should stop arguing with the nurses."
- Devaluing the patient's feelings: "Everyone gets upset at times."
- Disagreeing directly: "That can't be true," or "I think you are wrong."
- Defending against criticism: "The doctor is not being rude; he's just very busy today."
- Changing the subject to avoid dealing with uncomfortable topics;
  - o Patient: "I'm never going to get well."
  - o Nurse: "Your family will be here in just a few minutes."
- Making inappropriate literal responses, even as a joke, especially if the patient is at all confused or having difficulty expressing ideas:
  - o Patient: "There are bugs crawling under my skin."
  - o Nurse: "I'll get some bug spray,"
- Challenging the patient to establish reality often just increases confusion and frustration:
  - o "If you were dying, you wouldn't be able to yell and kick!"

COMMUNICATING WITH PATIENTS WITH DISABILITIES

Guidelines for communicating with individuals with disabilities:

- Do not assume that the person with disabilities also has impaired cognition.
- Always treat the person with respect and dignity.
- Use first names with the patient if asked to do so, but start out formally as with any patient.
- Offer to shake hands even when a prosthesis is present.
- Be patient if communication is impaired.
- Offer assistance, but allow the patient to tell you what is helpful; otherwise don't assist.
- When a wheelchair is used, sit down so the patient does not have to strain their neck to speak with you.
- If providing directions, consider the obstacles that may be in the way and assist the person to find an appropriate way around them.

COMMUNICATION WITH PATIENTS WITH COGNITIVE DISABILITIES

The person with cognitive disabilities may be easily distracted, so verbal communication should be attempted in a quiet area:

- Address people with dignity and respect.
- Do not try to discuss abstract ideas but stick with concrete topics.
- Keep words and sentences very simple and try rephrasing when necessary. People may have difficulty in distinguishing your spoken words and deriving the meaning from them.
- Be very patient with people's attempts to speak to you since they may have difficulty in processing thoughts and changing them into spoken words.
- Use objects around you and gestures to illustrate your words since the patient may also use pointing and gesturing when unable to find the words to communicate with you. The person may prefer written communication, although some may be unable to read.
- Use touch to convey your regard during communication, as this is recognized by the patient as reassurance of your care and concern for them.
- Give a few instructions at a time as to not overwhelm them.

COMMUNICATING WITH DEAF OR HEARING-IMPAIRED PATIENTS

Communicating with a person with deafness or hearing impairment:

- Try to communicate in a quiet environment if possible.
- Wave or touch the person to let him or her know you are trying to communicate.
- Determine the method the person uses to communicate: sign language, lip reading, hearing devices, or writing.
- Fingerspell or use some signs if able to do so.
- Address the person directly when you speak even though the person may be looking at an interpreter or your lips.
- Look at the person as the interpreter tells you what was said.
- Speak slowly so the interpreter can keep up with you.
- If the person reads lips, face the person and speak clearly and normally, using normal volume.
- If writing a communication, do not speak while writing.
- Do not be afraid to check that the person understands you, and ask questions if you do not understand the person.

COMMUNICATION WITH PEOPLE WITH LOW VISION OR BLINDNESS

Communicating with a person with low vision or blindness:

- Greet the person with low vision or blindness, identifying yourself and others present.
- Always say goodbye when you are leaving.
- Alert the person to written communications, such as warning signs or printed notices.
- Face the person and touch briefly on the arm to let the person know you are speaking to him or her if you are in a group.
- Speak at normal loudness.
- Make any directions given specific in terms of the length of walk and obstacles, such as stairs.
- Use the position of hands on a clock face to give directions (potatoes at 3 o'clock) as well as using *right* or *left*.
- Mention sounds that the person may hear in transit or on arrival at a destination.
- Do not be afraid to use the word *see*, as the person will probably use it as well.

COMMUNICATING WITH A PATIENT ON A VENTILATOR

When a patient on a ventilator is conscious, he or she may still be able to communicate by blinking, nodding, shaking the head, or pointing to a picture or word board:

- If the person is able to write, try to reposition the IV line to leave the dominant hand free to communicate.
- Discuss the need for communication with the physician and ask if a valve or an electric larynx can be used to permit speech.
- Help the patient practice lip reading of single words.
- Remember the patient's glasses or hearing aids when attempting to communicate.
- Enlist the aid of a speech therapist if there is frustration on the part of the patient and family due to communication difficulty.

COMMUNICATING WITH PERSONS WITH SPEECH PROBLEMS DUE TO A STROKE

Methods to communicate with stroke patients with speech problems:

- **Dysarthria**: Patients have problems forming the words to speak them aloud. Give them time to communicate, offer them a picture board or other means of communicating, and give encouragement to family members who are frustrated with the difficulty of trying to communicate.
- **Expressive aphasia**: The patients' efforts at speech come out garbled when they try to say sentences, but single words may be clear. Encourage the patients to try to write and to practice the sounds of the alphabet. Resist the urge to finish sentences for the patients.
- **Receptive aphasia**: The patients have a problem comprehending the speech they hear. Communicate in simple terms and speak slowly. Test comprehension of the written word as an alternative method of communication.
- **Global aphasia**: The patient has both receptive and expressive aphasia. Use simple, clear, slow speech augmented by pictures and gestures.

COMMUNICATION PROBLEMS OF PATIENTS WITH PARKINSON'S DISEASE

Parkinson's disease causes problems with speaking in the majority (75-90%) of patients. The reason for this is not clear but may relate to increasing rigidity and changes in movement. Speech is often very low-pitched or hoarse, given in a monotone and with a soft voice. Speech production may decrease because of the effort required to speak. **Speech therapy** can develop exercises for the patient that can assist them in remembering to speak slowly and carefully, as patients are not always aware that their **communication** is impaired:

- Allow time for the patient to communicate, asking for repetition if you do not understand the message.
- Help family by teaching ways to facilitate communication with the patient and encouraging them to assist the patient to do the exercises provided by the therapist.
- If speech volume is very low, suggest amplification devices that can be obtained through speech therapy.

COMMUNICATION WITH PATIENTS WITH PSYCHIATRIC PROBLEMS

Persons with psychiatric disorders appreciate being addressed with respect, dignity, and honesty:

- Speak simply and clearly, repeating as necessary.
- Encourage patients to discuss their concerns regarding treatment and medications to improve compliance.
- Use good eye contact and be attentive to your body language messages.
- Be alert, but unless the person is known to be violent, try to relax and listen to them.
- Don't try to avoid words or phrases pertaining to psychiatric problems, but if you do say something inappropriate, apologize honestly to the patient.

- Offer patients outlets for their thoughts and feelings.
- Learn more about their disorder and ways to use therapeutic communication to help them with their problem, such as re-orienting them as needed.

CULTURAL COMPETENCE

Different cultures view health and illness from very different perspectives, and patients often come from a mix of many cultures, so the nurse must be not only accepting of cultural differences but must be sensitive and aware. There are a number of characteristics that are important for a nurse to have **cultural competence**:

- **Appreciating diversity**: This must be grounded in information about other cultures and understanding of their value systems.
- **Assessing own cultural perspectives**: Self-awareness is essential to understanding potential biases.
- **Understanding intercultural dynamics**: This must include understanding ways in which cultures cooperate, differ, communicate, and reach understanding.
- **Recognizing institutional culture**: Each institutional unit (hospital, clinic, office) has an inherent set of values that may be unwritten but is accepted by the staff.
- **Adapting patient service to diversity**: This is the culmination of cultural competence as it is the point of contact between cultures.

CULTURAL CHARACTERISTICS

HISPANIC PATIENTS

Many areas of the country have large populations of Hispanics and Hispanic Americans. As always, it's important to recognize that cultural generalizations don't always apply to individuals. Recent immigrants, especially, have cultural needs that the nurse must understand:

- Many Hispanics are Catholic and may like the nurse to make arrangements for a priest to visit.
- Large extended families may come to visit to support the patient and family, so patients should receive clear explanations about how many visitors are allowed, but some flexibility may be required.
- Language barriers may exist as some may have limited or no English skills, so translation services should be available around the clock.
- Hispanic culture encourages outward expressions of emotions, so family may react strongly to news about a patient's condition, and people who are ill may expect some degree of pampering, so extra attention to the patient/family members may alleviate some of their anxiety.

Caring for Hispanic and Hispanic American patients requires understanding of cultural differences:

- Some immigrant Hispanics have very little formal education, so medical information may seem very complex and confusing, and they may not understand the implications or need for follow-up care.
- Hispanic culture perceives time with more flexibility than American culture, so if parents need to be present at a particular time, the nurse should specify the exact time (1:30 PM) and explain the reason rather than saying something more vague, such as "after lunch."
- People may appear to be unassertive or unable to make decisions when they are simply showing respect to the nurse by being deferent.
- In traditional families, the males make decisions, so a woman waits for the father or other males in the family to make decisions about treatment or care.
- Families may choose to use folk medicines instead of Western medical care or may combine the two.
- Children and young women are often sheltered and are taught to be respectful to adults, so they may not express their needs openly.

MIDDLE EASTERN PATIENTS

There are considerable cultural differences among Middle Easterners, but religious beliefs about the segregation of males and females are common. It's important to remember that segregating the female is meant to protect her virtue. Female nurses have low status in many countries because they violate this segregation by touching male bodies, so parents may not trust or show respect for the nurse who is caring for their family member. Additionally, male patients may not want to be cared for by female nurses or doctors, and families may be very upset at a female being cared for by a male nurse or physician. When possible, these cultural traditions should be accommodated:

- In Middle Eastern countries, males make decisions, so issues for discussion or decision should be directed to males, such as the father or spouse, and males may be direct in stating what they want, sometimes appearing demanding.
- If a male nurse must care for a female patient, then the family should be advised that *personal care* (such as bathing) will be done by a female while the medical treatments will be done by the male nurse.

Caring for Middle Eastern patients requires understanding of cultural differences:

- Families may practice strict dietary restrictions, such as avoiding pork and requiring that animals be killed in a ritual manner, so vegetarian or kosher meals may be required.
- People may have language difficulties requiring a translator, and same-sex translators should be used if at all possible.
- Families may be accompanied by large extended families that want to be kept informed and whom patients consult before decisions are made.
- Most medical care is provided by female relatives, so educating the family about patient care should be directed at females (with female translators if necessary).
- Outward expressions of grief are considered as showing respect for the dead.
- Middle Eastern families often offer gifts to caregivers. Small gifts (candy) that can be shared should be accepted graciously, but for other gifts, the families should be advised graciously that accepting gifts is against hospital policy.
- Middle Easterners often require less personal space and may stand very close.

ASIAN PATIENTS

There are considerable differences among different Asian populations, so cultural generalizations may not apply to all, but nurses caring for Asian patients should be aware of common cultural attitudes and behaviors:

- Nurses and doctors are viewed with respect, so traditional Asian families may expect the nurse to remain authoritative and to give directions and may not question, so the nurse should ensure that they understand by having them review material or give demonstrations and should provide explanations clearly, anticipating questions that the family might have but may not articulate.
- Disagreeing is considered impolite. "Yes" may only mean that the person is heard, not that they agree with the person. When asked if they understand, they may indicate that they do even when they clearly do not so as not to offend the nurse.
- Asians may avoid eye contact as an indication of respect. This is especially true of children in relation to adults and of younger adults in relation to elders.

Caring for Asian patients requires understanding of cultural differences:

- Patients/families may not show outward expressions of feelings/grief, sometimes appearing passive. They also avoid public displays of affection. This does not mean that they don't feel, just that they don't show their feelings.
- Families often hide illness and disabilities from others and may feel ashamed about illness.

- Terminal illness is often hidden from the patient, so families may not want patients to know they are dying or seriously ill.
- Families may use cupping, pinching, or applying pressure to injured areas, and this can leave bruises that may appear as abuse, so when bruises are found, the family should be questioned about alternative therapy before assumptions are made.
- Patients may be treated with traditional herbs.
- Families may need translators because of poor or no English skills.
- In traditional Asian families, males are authoritative and make the decisions.

RELIGIOUS OBJECTIONS TO TREATMENT

JEHOVAH'S WITNESSES

Jehovah's Witnesses have traditionally shunned transfusions and blood products as part of their religious beliefs. In 2004, the *Watchtower,* a Jehovah's Witness publication, presented a guide for members. When medical care indicates the need for blood transfusion or blood products and the patient and/or family members are practicing Jehovah's Witnesses, this may present a conflict. It's important to approach the patient/family with full information and reasons for the transfusion or blood components without being judgmental, allowing them to express their feelings. In fact, studies show that while adults often refuse transfusions for themselves, they frequently allow their children to receive blood products, so one should never assume that an individual would refuse blood products based on the religion alone. Jehovah's Witnesses can receive fractionated blood cells, thus allowing hemoglobin-based blood substitutes. The following guidelines are provided to church members:

Basic **blood standards for Jehovah's Witnesses**:

- **Not acceptable**: Whole blood: red cells, white cells, platelets, plasma.
- **Acceptable**: Fractions from red cells, white cells, platelets, and plasma.

CHRISTIAN SCIENTISTS

Christian Science, a religion developed by Mary Baker Eddy in 1879, promotes the belief that sickness is most effectively treated through prayer alone. While Christian Scientists do not avoid all medical interventions, their beliefs are conservative regarding medical treatment. Most notably, Christian Scientists, for the most part, do not believe in vaccinations and may only agree to such if required by law, as they do acknowledge the importance of community health. They have widely appreciated the use of exemptions from mandatory vaccines, but as these exemptions have become more limited, religious leaders have given their members the right to decide upon vaccinations.

IMPACT OF CULTURE AND RELIGION ON DIETARY PREFERENCES

When performing a dietary assessment, the nurse should remember that culture and religion might dictate which foods and spices are used. The manner in which food is prepared, cooked, and served may also be specified. The utensils used at the meal as well as the persons who may eat together may be important. Mealtimes and required fasts should be determined. Holidays may be accompanied by particular foods. Alcohol (including extracts made with alcohol) and caffeine may be prohibited. The culture may also consider obesity a sign of affluence and success. The nurse should evaluate the foods that are eaten in light of the patient's medical condition. The patient may not wish to eat the usual hospital fare and may need to have a special diet prepared or food brought from home. The nurse can guide the patient and family to foods that are acceptable and within the patient's requirements for health.

GRIEF

Grief is an emotional response to a **loss** that begins at the time a loss is anticipated and continues on an individual timetable. While there are identifiable stages or tasks, it is not an orderly and predictable process. It involves overcoming anger, disbelief, guilt, and a myriad of related emotions. The grieving individual may move back and forth between stages or experience several emotions at any given time. Each person's grief response is unique to their own coping patterns, stress levels, age, gender, belief system, and previous experiences with loss.

KUBLER-ROSS'S FIVE STAGES OF GRIEF

Kubler-Ross taught the medical community that the dying patient and family welcomes open, honest discussion of the dying process and felt that there were certain **stages** that patients and family go through. The stages may not occur in order, but may vary or some may be skipped. Stages include:

- **Denial**: The person denies the diagnosis and tries to pretend it isn't true. During this time, the person may seek a second opinion or alternative therapies. They may use denial until they are better able to emotionally cope with the reality of the disease or changes that need to be made. Patients may also wish to save family and friends from pain and worry. Both patients and family may use denial as a coping mechanism when they feel overwhelmed by the reality of the disease and threatened losses.
- **Anger**: The person is angry about the situation and may focus that rage on anyone.
- **Bargaining**: The person attempts to make deals with a higher power to secure a better outcome to their situation.
- **Depression**: The person anticipates the loss and the changes it will bring with a sense of sadness and grief.
- **Acceptance**: The person accepts the impending death and is ready to face it as it approaches. The patient may begin to withdraw from interests and family.

> **Review Video: Patient Treatment and Grief**
> Visit mometrix.com/academy and enter code: 648794

ANTICIPATORY GRIEF

Anticipatory grief is the mental, social, and somatic reactions of an individual as they prepare themselves for a **perceived future loss**. The individual experiences a process of intellectual, emotional, and behavioral responses in order to modify their self-concept, based on their perception of what the potential loss will mean in their life. This process often takes place ahead of the actual loss, from the time the loss is first perceived until it is resolved as a reality for the individual. This process can also blend with past loss experiences. It is associated with the individual's perception of how life will be affected by the particular diagnosis as well as the impending death. Acknowledging this anticipatory grief allows family members to begin looking toward a changed future. Suppressing this anticipatory process may inhibit relationships with the ill individual and contribute to a more difficult grieving process at a later time. However, appropriate anticipatory grieving does not take the place of grief during the actual time of death.

DISENFRANCHISED GRIEF

Disenfranchised grief occurs when the loss being experienced cannot be openly acknowledged, publicly mourned, or socially supported. Society and culture are partly responsible for an individual's response to a loss. There is a **social context** to grief; if a person incurring the loss will be putting himself or herself at risk if grief is expressed, disenfranchised grief occurs. The risk for disenfranchised grief is greatest among those whose relationship with the individual they lost was not known or regarded as significant. This is also the situation found among bereaved persons who are not recognized by society as capable of grief, such as young children, or needing to mourn, such as an ex-spouse or secret lover.

GRIEF VS. DEPRESSION

Normal grief is preoccupied with self-limiting to the loss itself. Emotional responses will vary and may include open expressions of anger. The individual may experience difficulty sleeping or vivid dreams, a lack of energy, and weight loss. Crying is evident and provides some relief of extreme emotions. The individual remains socially responsive and seeks reassurance from others.

Depression is marked by extensive periods of sadness and preoccupation often extending beyond 2 months. It is not limited to the single event. There is an absence of pleasure or anger and isolation from previous social support systems. The individual can experience extreme lethargy, weight loss, insomnia, or hypersomnia, and has no recollection of dreaming. Crying is absent or persistent and provides no relief of emotions. Professional intervention is required to relieve depression.

Loss

Loss is the blanket term used to denote the absence of a valued object, position, ability, attribute, or individual. The aspect of **loss** as it is associated with the death of an animal or person is a relatively new definition. Loss is an individualized and subjective experience depending on the **perceived attachment** between the individual and the missing aspect. This can range from little or no value of attachment to significant value. Loss also can be represented by the **withdrawal of a valued relationship** one had or would have had in the future. Depending on the unique and individual responses to the perception of loss and its significance, reactions to the loss will vary. Robinson and McKenna summarize the aspects of loss in three main attributes:

- Something has been removed.
- The item removed had value to that person.
- The response is individualized.

Mourning

Mourning is a public grief response for the death of a loved one. The various aspects of the mourning process are partially determined by **personal and cultural belief systems**. Kagawa-Singer defines mourning as "the social customs and cultural practices that follow a death." Durkheim expands this to include the following: "mourning is not a natural movement of private feelings wounded by a cruel loss; it is a duty imposed by the group." Mourning involves participation in religious and culturally appropriate customs and rituals designed to publicly acknowledge the loss. These rituals signify they are adjusting to the change in their relationships created by the loss, as well as mark the beginning of the reorganization and forward movement of their lives.

Bereavement

Bereavement is the emotional and mental state associated with having suffered a **personal loss**. It is the reactions of grief and sadness initiated by the loss of a loved one. Bereavement is a normal process of feeling deprived of something of value. The word bereave comes from the root "reave" meaning to plunder, spoil, or rob. It is recognized that the lost individual had value and a defining role in the surviving individual's life. Bereavement encompasses all the acts and emotions surrounding the feeling of loss for the individual. During this grieving period, there is an increased mortality risk. A **positive bereavement experience** means being able to recognize the significance of the loss while still recognizing the resilience and value of life.

Risk Factors Complicating Bereavement

The caregiver should assess for multiple **life crises** that take energy away from the grieving process. An important factor is the grieving individual's history with past grieving experiences. Assess for other recent, unresolved, or difficult losses that may need to be addressed before the individual can move toward resolution of the current loss. Age, mental health, substance abuse, extreme anger, anxiety, or dependence on the individual facing the end of life can add additional stressors and handicap natural coping mechanisms. Income strains, community support, outside and personal responsibilities, the absence of cultural and religious beliefs, the difficulty of the disease process, and age of the loved one lost can also present additional risk factors.

Interventions for Patients and Family Experiencing Loss and Grief

Loss is painful and frightening. Loss can occur through death or loss of health, self-esteem, or relationships. Loss can also occur from threats, such as fire, flood, theft, or severe weather. The severity of the loss, preparation for it, and the maturity, stability, and coping mechanisms of the person all affect the grieving process. Multiple losses and substance abuse can complicate grief and recovery. Previous life experience and cultural and religious beliefs can help in resolution of grief. Many emotions are triggered, and if the loss is not acknowledged, the person may become depressed or develop health problems. **Interventions** for those experiencing grief and loss include:

- Teach patients to recognize symptoms, such as SOB, empty feelings in the chest or abdomen, deep sighing, lethargy, and weakness as signs of grief.
- Assist the patient and family to heal themselves by accepting the loss, recognizing the pain from it, making changes to adapt to and assimilate the loss, and moving toward new relationships and activity.
- Refer to groups or counseling for more intense support if needed.

SUPPORTING FAMILIES AND PATIENTS AS THEY RECEIVE BAD NEWS

It is often best if the patient can **receive bad news** while being **supported** by family, friends, physicians, nurses, support staff, social workers, and clergy if they so desire. However, the patient may not want family members or others to be present, and this too should be respected.

- Provide privacy and ensure that there will be no interruptions.
- Provide seating for all participants.
- Do not provide too much information at once, as the opening statement may be all that the patient can comprehend at one time.
- Allow time for reactions before providing more information.
- Wait for the patient to signal the need for more information and then provide an honest answer in layman's terms. Information may not be absorbed and may need to be repeated as the patient and family are ready for it later after the initial conference.
- Use techniques of therapeutic communication. People may need others to sit and listen and provide comforting empathy many times before having a conversation about problem solving.

SPIRITUALITY

Spirituality provides a connection of the self to a higher power and a way of finding meaning in life experiences. It provides guidance for behavior and can help to clarify one's purpose in life. It can offer hope to those who are ill or facing loss and grief and can give comfort, support, and guidance. **Spirituality** is not always connected to a religion and is highly individualized. A person may lose faith and confidence in his/her spiritual beliefs during trying times:

- Ask patients about their spiritual beliefs.
- Listen attentively and do not offer opinions about their beliefs or share your own unless invited.
- Show respect for their views and offer to obtain spiritual support by calling a spiritual leader or setting up a spiritual ritual that has meaning for them.

This support can help them to regain their beliefs and endure illness by helping them to rise above their suffering and find meaning in this experience.

PALLIATIVE AND HOSPICE CARE

Palliative care attempts to make the rest of the patient's life as comfortable as possible by treating distressing symptoms to keep them controlled. It does not attempt to cure but only to control discomfort caused by the disease. Palliative care does not require terminal illness/prognosis and can be implemented for any patient with chronic disease and suffering.

Hospice care uses palliative care as it supports the patient and family through the dying process. Hospice teams support the daily needs of the patient and family and provide needed equipment, medical expertise, and medications to control symptoms. They offer spiritual, psychological, and social support to the patient and family as needed and desired. Assistance with end-of-life planning is given to help the patient and family accomplish goals important to them. Bereavement support is also given. The team consists of the attending physician, hospice physician advisor, nurses, social worker, clergy, hospice aides, and volunteers. Hospice care is given in the home when the patient has family who are willing to assume care with the assistance of the hospice team. Hospice care also occurs in hospice facilities, hospitals, and extended care facilities. To qualify for Hospice care, the patient must be deemed terminal and given a 6-month or less life expectancy by two separate physicians. Should the patient survive 6 months in hospice, they can be extended for two 90-day periods, and then an unlimited number of 60-day periods per physician order.

Nursing Ethics

ETHICAL PRINCIPLES

Autonomy is the ethical principle that the individual has the right to make decisions about his or her own care. In the case of children or patients with dementia who cannot make autonomous decisions, parents or family members may serve as the legal decision maker. The nurse must keep the patient and/or family fully informed so that they can exercise their autonomy in informed decision-making.

Justice is the ethical principle that relates to the distribution of the limited resources of healthcare benefits to the members of society. These resources must be distributed fairly. This issue may arise if there is only one bed left and two sick patients. Justice comes into play in deciding which patient should stay and which should be transported or otherwise cared for. The decision should be made according to what is best or most just for the patients and not colored by personal bias.

Beneficence is an ethical principle that involves performing actions that are for the purpose of benefitting another person. In the care of a patient, any procedure or treatment should be done with the ultimate goal of benefitting the patient, and any actions that are not beneficial should be reconsidered. As conditions change, procedures need to be continually reevaluated to determine if they are still of benefit.

Nonmaleficence is an ethical principle that means healthcare workers should provide care in a manner that does not cause direct intentional harm to the patient:

- The actual act must be good or morally neutral.
- The intent must be only for a good effect.
- A bad effect cannot serve as the means to get to a good effect.
- A good effect must have more benefit than a bad effect has harm.

NURSING CODE OF ETHICS

There is more interest in the **ethics** involved in healthcare due to technological advances that have made the prolongation of life, organ transplants, prenatal manipulation, and saving of premature infants possible, sometimes with poor outcomes. Couple these with healthcare's limited resources, and **ethical dilemmas** abound. Ethics is the study of **morality** as the value that controls actions. The American Nurses Association Code of Ethics contains nine statements defining **principles** the nurse can use when faced with moral and ethical problems. Nurses must be knowledgeable about the many ethical issues in healthcare and about the field of ethics in general. The nurse must help a patient to reveal their values and morals to the health care team so that the patient, family, and team can resolve moral issues pertaining to the patient's care. As part of the healthcare team, the nurse has a right to express personal values and moral concerns about medical issues.

BIOETHICS

Bioethics is a branch of ethics that involves making sure that the medical treatment given is the most morally correct choice given the different options that might be available and the differences inherent in the varied levels of treatment. In the health care unit, if the patients, family members, and the staff are in agreement when it comes to values and decision-making, then no ethical dilemma exists; however, when there is a difference in value beliefs between the patients/family members and the staff, there is a bioethical dilemma that must be resolved. Sometimes, discussion and explanation can resolve differences, but at times the institution's ethics committee must be brought in to resolve the conflict. The primary goal of bioethics is to determine the most morally correct action using the set of circumstances given.

ETHICAL DECISION-MAKING MODEL

There are many ethical decision-making models. Some general guidelines to apply in using ethical decision-making models could be the following:

- Gather information about the identified problem
- State reasonable alternatives and solutions to the problem
- Utilize ethical resources (for example, clergy or ethics committees) to help determine the ethically important elements of each solution or alternative
- Suggest and attempt possible solutions
- Choose a solution to the problem

It is important to always consider the **ethical principles** of autonomy, beneficence, nonmaleficence, justice, and fidelity when attempting to facilitate ethical decision-making with family members, caregivers, and the healthcare team.

ETHICAL ASSESSMENT

While the terms *ethics* and *morals* are sometimes used interchangeably, ethics is a study of morals and encompasses concepts of right and wrong. When making **ethical assessments,** one must consider not only what people should do but also what they actually do, as these two things are sometimes at odds. Ethical issues can be difficult to assess because of personal bias, which is one of the reasons that sharing concerns with other internal sources and reaching consensus is so valuable. Issues of concern might include options for care, refusal of care, rights to privacy, adequate relief of suffering, and the right to self-determination. Internal sources might include the ethics committee, whose role is to make decisions regarding ethical issues. Risk management can provide guidance related to personal and institutional liability. External agencies might include government agencies, such as the public health department.

ETHICAL ANALYSIS OF A SITUATION

Assessment of the situation is done to reveal the ethical, legal, and professional **conflicts** that are present. Those who are involved are identified, including the patient, family, and healthcare personnel. The decision maker is determined if it is not the patient. Information about the situation is collected to determine medical facts about the disease and condition of the patient, options for treatment, and nursing diagnoses. Any pertinent legal information is included. The patient and family's cultural, religious, and moral values are determined. Possible courses of action are listed and compared in terms of outcomes for the patient using the utilitarian or deontological theory of ethics. Professional codes of ethics are also applied. A decision is made and evaluated as to whether it is the most morally correct action. Ethical arguments for and against the decision are given and responded to by the decision maker.

PROFESSIONAL BOUNDARIES

GIFTS

Over time, patients may develop a bond with nurses they trust and may feel grateful to the nurse for the care provided and want to express thanks, but the nurse must make sure to maintain professional boundaries. Patients often offer **gifts** to nurses to show their appreciation, but some adults, especially those who are weak and ill or have cognitive impairment, may be taken advantage of easily. Patients may offer valuables and may sometimes be easily manipulated into giving large sums of money. Small tokens of appreciation that can be shared with other staff, such as a box of chocolates, are usually acceptable (depending upon the policy of the institution), but almost any other gifts (jewelry, money, clothes) should be declined: "I'm sorry, that's so kind of you, but nurses are not allowed to accept gifts from patients." Declining may relieve the patient of the feeling of obligation.

SEXUAL RELATIONS

When the boundary between the role of the professional nurse and the vulnerability of the patient is breached, a boundary violation occurs. Because the nurse is in the position of authority, the responsibility to maintain the boundary rests with the nurse; however, the line separating them is a continuum and sometimes not easily defined. It is inappropriate for nurses to engage in **sexual relations** with patients, and if the sexual behavior is coerced or the patient is cognitively impaired, it is **illegal**. However, more common violations with adults, particularly elderly patients, include exposing a patient unnecessarily, using sexually demeaning gestures or language (including off-color jokes), harassment, or inappropriate touching. Touching should be used with care, such as touching a hand or shoulder. Hugging may be misconstrued.

ATTENTION

Nursing is a giving profession, but the nurse must temper giving with recognition of professional boundaries. Patients have many needs. As acts of kindness, nurses (especially those involved in home care) often give certain patients extra attention and may offer to do **favors**, such as cooking or shopping. They may become overly invested in the patients' lives. While this may benefit a patient in the short term, it can establish a relationship of increasing **dependency** and **obligation** that does not resolve the long-term needs of the patient. Making referrals to the appropriate agencies or collaborating with family to find ways to provide services is more effective. Becoming overly invested may be evident by the nurse showing favoritism or spending too much time with the patient while neglecting other duties. On the other end of the spectrum are nurses who are disinterested and fail to provide adequate attention to the patient's detriment. Lack of adequate attention may lead to outright neglect.

COERCION

Power issues are inherent in matters associated with professional boundaries. Physical abuse is both unprofessional and illegal, but behavior can easily border on abusive without the patient being physically injured. Nurses can easily **intimidate** older adults and sick patients into having procedures or treatments they do not want. Regardless of age, patients have the right to choose and the right to refuse treatment. Difficulties arise with cognitive impairment, and in that case, another responsible adult (often the patient's child or spouse) is designated to make decisions, but every effort should be made to gain patient cooperation. Forcing the patient to do something against his or her will borders on abuse and can sometimes degenerate into actual abuse if physical coercion is involved.

PERSONAL INFORMATION

When pre-existing personal or business relationships exist, other nurses should be assigned care of the patient whenever possible, but this may be difficult in small communities. However, the nurse should strive to maintain a professional role separate from the personal role and respect professional boundaries. The nurse must respect and maintain the confidentiality of the patient and family members, but the nurse must also be very careful about **disclosing personal information** about him or herself because this establishes a social relationship that interferes with the professional role of the nurse and the boundary between the patient and the nurse. The nurse and patient should never share secrets. When the nurse divulges personal information, he or she may become vulnerable to the patient, a reversal of roles.

PATIENT RIGHTS AND RESPONSIBILITIES

Empowering patients and families to act as their own advocates requires that they have a clear understanding of their **rights and responsibilities.** These should be given (in print form) and/or presented (audio/video) to patients and families on admission or as soon as possible:

- **Rights** include competent, non-discriminatory medical care that respects privacy and allows participation in decisions about care and the right to refuse care. They should have clear understandable explanations of treatments, options, and conditions, including outcomes. They should be apprised of transfers, changes in care plan, and advance directives. They should have access to medical records and billing information.

- **Responsibilities** include providing honest and thorough information about health issues and medical history. They should ask for clarification if they don't understand information that is provided to them, and they should follow the plan of care that is outlined or explain why that is not possible. They should treat staff and other patients with respect.

> **Review Video: Patient Advocacy**
> Visit mometrix.com/academy and enter code: 202160

INFORMED CONSENT

The patient or their legal guardian must provide informed consent for all treatment the patient receives. This includes a thorough explanation of all procedures and treatment and associated risks. Patients/guardians should be apprised of all options and allowed to have input on the decision-making process. They should be apprised of all reasonable risks and any complications that might be life threatening or increase morbidity. The American Medical Association has established **guidelines for obtaining informed consent:**

- Explanation of the diagnosis
- Nature and reason for the treatment or procedure
- Risks and benefits of the treatment or procedure
- Alternative options (regardless of cost or insurance coverage)
- Risks and benefits of alternative options, including no treatment

Obtaining informed consent is a requirement in all states; however, a patient may waive their right to informed consent. If this is the case, the nurse should document the patient's waiving of this right and proceed with the procedure. Informed consent is not necessary for procedures performed to save life or limb in which the patient or guardian is unable to consent.

CONFIDENTIALITY

Confidentiality is the obligation that is present in a professional-patient relationship. Nurses are under an obligation to protect the information they possess concerning the patient and family. Care should be taken to safeguard that information and provide the privacy that the family deserves. This is accomplished through the use of required passwords when family call for information about the patient and through the limitation of who is allowed to visit. There may be times when confidentiality must be broken to save the life of a patient, but those circumstances are rare. The nurse must make all efforts to safeguard patient records and identification. Computerized record keeping should be done in such a way that the screen is not visible to others, and paper records must be secured.

Nursing Research

ELEMENTS OF RESEARCH

The following are elements of research:

- **Variable**: An entity that can be different within a population
- **Independent variable**: The variable that the researchers change to evaluate its effect
- **Dependent variable**: The variable that may be changed by alterations in the independent variable
- **Hypothesis**: The proposed explanation to describe an expected outcome in a study
- **Sample**: The selected population to be studied
- **Experimental group**: The population within the sample that undergoes the treatment or intervention
- **Control group**: The population within the sample that is not exposed to the treatment of intervention being evaluated

The nurse must be taught and must understand the process of critical analysis and know how to conduct a survey of the literature. **Basic research concepts** include:

- **Survey of valid sources**: Information from a juried journal and an anonymous website or personal website are very different sources, and evaluating what constitutes a valid source of data is critical.
- **Evaluation of internal and external validity**: Internal validity shows a cause-and-effect relationship between two variables, with the cause occurring before the effect and no intervening variable. External validity occurs when results hold true in different environments and circumstances with different populations.
- **Sample selection and sample size**: Selection and size can have a huge impact on the results, but a sample that is too small may lack both internal and external validity. Selection may be so narrowly focused that the results can't be generalized to other groups.

Evidence-Based Practice

CLASSES OF EVIDENCE-BASED PRACTICE

Evidence-based practice is treatment based on the best possible evidence, including a study of current research. Literature is searched to find evidence of the most effective treatments for specific diseases or injuries, and those treatments are then utilized to create clinical pathways that outline specific multi-departmental treatment protocols, including medications, treatments, and timelines. Evidence-based guidelines are often produced by specialty organizations that undertake the task of searching and analyzing literature to produce policies, procedures, and guidelines that become the standard of care for the disease. These guidelines are then used when a patient fits the disease criteria for that guideline.

Evidence-based nursing aims to improve the quality of nursing care by examining the reasons for all nursing practices and determining those that have the most positive outcomes. Evidence-based nursing focuses on the individual nurse utilizing evidence-based observations to influence decision-making.

EVIDENCE-BASED PRACTICE GUIDELINES

The creation of evidence-based practice guidelines includes the following components:

- **Focus on the topic/methodology:** This includes outlining possible interventions and treatments for review, choosing patient populations and settings, and determining significant outcomes. Search boundaries (such as types of journals, types of studies, dates of studies) should be determined.
- **Evidence review:** This includes review of literature, critical analysis of studies, and summarizing of results, including pooled meta-analysis.
- **Expert judgment:** Recommendations based on personal experience from a number of experts may be utilized, especially if there is inadequate evidence based on review, but this subjective evidence should be explicitly acknowledged.
- **Policy considerations:** This includes cost-effectiveness, access to care, insurance coverage, availability of qualified staff, and legal implications.
- **Policy:** A written policy must be completed with recommendations. Common practice is to utilize letter guidelines, with "A" being the most highly recommended, usually based on the quality of supporting evidence.
- **Review:** The completed policy should be submitted to peers for review and comments before instituting the policy.

CRITICAL PATHWAYS

Clinical/critical pathway development is done by those involved in direct patient care. The pathway should require no additional staffing and cover the entire scope of an illness. Steps include:

1. Selection of patient group and diagnosis, procedures, or conditions, based on analysis of data and observations of wide variance in approach to treatment and prioritizing organization and patient needs
2. Creation of interdisciplinary team of those involved in the process of care, including physicians to develop pathway
3. Analysis of data including literature review and study of best practices to identify opportunities for quality improvement
4. Identification of all categories of care, such as nutrition, medications, and nursing
5. Discussion and reaching consensus
6. Identifying the levels of care and number of days to be covered by the pathway
7. Pilot testing and redesigning steps as indicated
8. Educating staff about standards
9. Monitoring and tracking variances in order to improve pathways

LEVELS OF EVIDENCE IN EVIDENCE-BASED PRACTICE

Levels of evidence are categorized according to the scientific evidence available to support the recommendations, as well as existing state and federal laws. While recommendations are voluntary, they are often used as a basis for state and federal regulations.

- **Category IA** is well supported by evidence from experimental, clinical, or epidemiologic studies and is strongly recommended for implementation.
- **Category IB** has supporting evidence from some studies, has a good theoretical basis, and is strongly recommended for implementation.
- **Category IC** is required by state or federal regulations or is an industry standard.
- **Category II** is supported by suggestive clinical or epidemiologic studies, has a theoretical basis, and is suggested for implementation.
- **Category III** is supported by descriptive studies, such as comparisons, correlations, and case studies, and may be useful.
- **Category IV** is obtained from expert opinion or authorities only.
- **Unresolved** means there is no recommendation because of a lack of consensus or evidence.

OUTCOME EVALUATION

Outcome evaluation is an important component of evidence-based practice, which involves both internal and external research. All treatments are subjected to review to determine if they produce positive outcomes, and policies and protocols for outcome evaluation should be in place. **Outcome evaluation** includes the following:

- **Monitoring** over the course of treatment involves careful observation and record-keeping that notes progress, with supporting laboratory and radiographic evidence as indicated by condition and treatment.
- **Evaluating** results includes reviewing records as well as current research to determine if outcomes are within acceptable parameters.
- **Sustaining** involves discontinuing treatment but continuing to monitor and evaluate.
- **Improving** means to continue the treatment but with additions or modifications in order to improve outcomes.
- **Replacing** the treatment with a different treatment must be done if outcome evaluation indicates that current treatment is ineffective.

EVIDENCE-BASED NURSING INTERVENTIONS

Evidence-based nursing interventions enable nurses to provide high-quality patient care that is based upon research and knowledge, as opposed to giving care that is based upon tradition or information that is out of date. An evidence-based nursing approach is based on the integration of practical clinical experience with medical and clinical research; it utilizes proven clinical guidelines and assessment practices. Evidence-based nursing interventions allow nurses to make patient care decisions based on cutting-edge research that has been scientifically validated. Studies show that evidence-based nursing practice yields improved patient outcomes, enables nurses to practice up-to-date methods, improves nurse confidence and decision-making skills, and enhances Joint Commission standards.

RESOURCES

There are numerous information resources for evidence-based nursing interventions. These resources include evidence-based textbooks; databases such as CINAHL Plus, COCHRANE library, Mosby's Nursing Index, NursingConsult, and Nursing@Ovid; evidence-based nursing metasites such as the Academic Center for EBN, Joanna Briggs Institute, McGill University, ONS-EBN section, and EBN-University of Minnesota; online evidence-based nursing journals such as Clinical Nurse Specialist, Clinical Nursing Research, Evidence-Based Nursing, Journal of Nursing Care Quality, Journal of Advanced Nursing, Journal of Nursing Scholarship, Nurse

Researcher, Nursing Research, Western Journal of Nursing Research, and Worldviews on Evidence-Based Nursing; and various online tutorials.

OBTAINING RESULTS OF RESEARCH TO USE IN EVIDENCE-BASED PRACTICE

When searching for **current evidence** in print and online literature, the nurse should look for **systematic reviews, analyses, and reports**. PUBMED lists all literature and can be searched for all published articles on a particular subject. These articles can be analyzed to determine treatments that have the best evidence of efficacy. Subject and methodological terms and clinical filters can be used to find necessary information, including a specific medical subject heading (MH), subheading (SH), publication type (PT), and text word (TW). The nurse should also search the National Guideline Clearinghouse, Cochrane Databases, Agency for Healthcare Research and Quality, and US Preventive Services Task Force Recommendations for evidence and guidelines. When trials of a treatment provide evidence of effectiveness, the evidence is weighed for strength and confidence. Those that provide the strongest evidence of efficacy become recommendations and guidelines for use in the field. Research is also done on a smaller scale by specialists who publish in peer-reviewed journals their research results related to the use of a particular intervention.

Medical-Surgical Nurse Practice Test #1

Want to take this practice test in an online interactive format?
Check out the bonus page, which includes interactive practice questions and much more: **mometrix.com/bonus948/medsurgnurse**

1. When making purchasing decisions about new medical equipment, the healthcare administration is concerned about cutting costs. Which type of study would provide the most information about the financial impact?

  a. A cost-benefit analysis
  b. An efficacy study
  c. A product evaluation
  d. A cost-effectiveness analysis

2. An older adult patient is very reluctant to assume any self-care, repeatedly stating that she is "too old and too dumb" to learn new things. According to Erikson's theory of development, this suggests that the patient has failed to accomplish which of the following developmental tasks?

  a. Identify versus role confusion
  b. Initiative versus guilt
  c. Ego integrity versus despair
  d. Intimacy versus isolation

3. A 30-year-old patient has been diagnosed with advanced ovarian cancer. The patient says, "This is all my fault." Which of Kübler-Ross's five stages of grief is the patient probably experiencing?

  a. Denial
  b. Anger
  c. Depression
  d. Acceptance

4. A 68-year-old man with mild COPD refuses to exercise because he tires easily. He spends most of every day sitting in a chair watching television. What is the most appropriate nursing diagnosis?

  a. Ineffective health maintenance
  b. Impaired physical mobility
  c. Risk for disuse syndrome
  d. Activity intolerance

5. The hospital has invested in robotic surgery equipment and needs to assess its costs and health outcomes compared to traditional surgery. Which type of study is indicated?

  a. A cost-benefit analysis
  b. An efficacy study
  c. A cost-utility analysis
  d. A cost-effectiveness analysis

6. A Hispanic patient is admitted to a hospital unit where a nurse is to obtain the patient's admission history, but the patient speaks very little English. What should the nurse do?

    a. Ask the patient's 12-year-old son, who is fluent in English, to interpret

    b. Use sign language and pictures to supplement questions

    c. Arrange for an interpreter

    d. Ask the patient's wife, who speaks fair English, to answer the questions for the patient

7. A famous patient underwent surgery, and when a staff member who cared for the patient but was not authorized to provide information was asked about the patient's condition by a reporter, the staff member acknowledged that the person was a patient and was doing well after a hip replacement. What type of Health Insurance Portability and Accountability Act of 1996 (HIPAA) violation does this represent?

    a. Privacy violation, impermissible disclosure

    b. Right to access health records

    c. Security violation

    d. No violation

8. The nurse is teaching a 45-year-old woman with a colostomy to perform a colostomy irrigation. The nurse has prepared written directions and a video, but the patient ignores them. Instead, the patient picks up the equipment and looks at each part, trying to figure it out. The patient's learning style is probably:

    a. auditory.

    b. visual.

    c. kinesthetic.

    d. mixed.

9. A patient was admitted at the change of shift with a severe headache and confusion, but the order for a cranial computed tomography scan was not forwarded to the imaging department. The nurse went home and failed to report on the patient, and the patient was left alone for more than 2 hours because no staff was assigned to the patient. When staff members recognized the mistake, the patient had already died. When carrying out a root cause analysis of the event, the best definition of the problem would be:

    a. negligence.

    b. disregard for the patient's welfare.

    c. communication failure.

    d. breach of duty.

10. Which of the following should define the quality (purpose and role) of a healthcare institution?

    a. Mission statement

    b. Vision statement

    c. Goals and objectives

    d. Hierarchy

11. An Alzheimer patient walked away from the hospital and was found hiding in the parking lot. The most appropriate nursing diagnosis to account for his behavior is:

    a. acute confusion.

    b. risk prone health behavior.

    c. impaired memory.

    d. wandering.

12. Clinical pathways should be based on:

 a. a survey of current practices in the area.
 b. committee recommendations.
 c. evidence-based research.
 d. staff preferences.

13. An 80-year-old patient is dying of cancer and has been in and out of consciousness. The family should be encouraged to:

 a. go home, as the patient does not know they are present.
 b. talk to the patient, as hearing is usually the last sense to fail.
 c. offer the patient frequent sips of water to avoid dehydration.
 d. raise the head of the patient's bed if respirations become rattling to help the patient clear secretions.

14. A patient with gastroenteritis has been diagnosed with severe dehydration (>15% fluid loss). Typical symptoms include:

 a. dry mouth and increased thirst.
 b. dizziness, lethargy, reduced skin turgor, and orthostatic hypotension.
 c. resting hypotension, confusion, tachycardia, and oliguria.
 d. marked hypotension and anuria in addition to other symptoms.

15. A 30-year-old woman is hospitalized with severe depression and is incontinent of urine, although the urinary system is normal. The most appropriate nursing diagnosis is:

 a. functional urinary incontinence.
 b. stress urinary incontinence.
 c. overflow urinary incontinence.
 d. urge urinary incontinence.

16. A cost-savings study showed that a free medical clinic ordered 17 different types of dressing supplies because of varying staff preferences. Because of this large number, the clinic was not able to buy in sufficient bulk to receive a large-quantity discount. The best solution to this problem is to:

 a. continue to order the same types of supplies to keep the staff happy.
 b. create an ad hoc team to survey staff preferences and agree on a reduced number of dressing supplies.
 c. reduce the number of dressing supplies ordered according to administrative preference.
 d. complete a 6-month survey of the use of dressing supplies.

17. A 76-year-old female with lung cancer was placed on hospice care by her physician 6 months earlier (two 90-day periods), but she is still alive. Her family asks the nurse if the patient will be removed from hospice care. The best response is:

 a. "She will be removed from hospice care until her condition worsens because she has exceeded the 6-month period."
 b. "She has exhausted all of her hospice care benefits and will be removed from hospice care."
 c. "She can continue with hospice care as long as the physician authorizes the care every 60 days."
 d. "She can continue with hospice care if the physician continues to authorize care every 90 days."

18. The best question to elicit information about a patient's pain is:

 a. "Are you having pain?"
 b. "Will you describe your pain for me?"
 c. "What kind of pain are you having?"
 d. "What is your pain on a scale of 1 to 10?"

19. As part of quality improvement for a hospital system, the processes for patient admission and discharge have been revised. Before utilization, which type of analysis can be done to try to ensure positive outcomes?

   a. Find, organize, clarify, uncover, start
   b. Plan-do-check-act
   c. Focus, analyze, develop, execute
   d. Failure mode and effects analysis

20. How do team members usually deal with issues of power?

   a. By observing and emulating the leader
   b. By arguing
   c. By following strict rules of discourse
   d. By rotating leadership roles

21. Which assessment tool for dementia involves remembering and repeating the names of 3 common objects and drawing the face of a clock with all 12 numbers and hands indicating the time specified by the examiner?

   a. Mini-mental state exam (MMSE)
   b. Mini-cog
   c. Digit Repetition Test
   d. Confusion Assessment Method

22. A 66-year-old male on Medicare is being discharged home. He has an open, draining abdominal wound that he is unable to care for independently because of poor vision. His 14-year-old grandson lives with him. The best solution is:

   a. transferring the patient to an extended care facility.
   b. keeping the patient in the hospital until the wound has healed.
   c. teaching the man's 14-year-old grandson to provide wound care.
   d. making a referral to a home health agency to provide in-home care.

23. When preparing materials to teach a 28-year-old male auto mechanic about wound care, the first thing the nurse should do is:

   a. prepare an audiotape.
   b. prepare visual materials, such a pictures and diagrams.
   c. assess the patient's learning style.
   d. prepare manipulatives, as mechanics are kinesthetic learners.

24. The Occupational Safety and Health Administration (OSHA) regulates:

   a. patient right to privacy.
   b. disposal methods for sharps, such as needles.
   c. reimbursement for services.
   d. patient surveys.

25. A patient with end-stage bone cancer has elected hospice and palliative care. The patient is experiencing severe bone pain from a tumor, and the physician orders radiotherapy to reduce the tumor's size and to reduce pain. Is this treatment acceptable under hospice care criteria?

   a. No, the patient has elected to forego curative treatment, so Medicare will not pay for the radiotherapy
   b. No, the patient needs to be removed from hospice care first
   c. Yes, hospice recommends only palliative care but curative treatment is acceptable
   d. Yes, if the purpose of the treatment is to relieve pain, it is essentially palliative

26. A patient has developed a pressure ulcer over the left ischial tuberosity. The ulcerated area is exposed with loss of epidermis and dermis, and underlying fatty tissue is visible but no muscle, tendons, ligaments, cartilage, or bones. Some slough is present, and there is undermining of 2 cm extending from 1 to 3 o'clock. Using the National Pressure Injury Advisory Panel (NPIAP) Staging System, the wound would be classified as:

    a. stage II.
    b. stage III.
    c. stage IV.
    d. unstageable.

27. The nurse is forming an interdisciplinary team to review processes as part of the mission to improve quality. When choosing team members, which of the following should have priority?

    a. Personality
    B. Skills and knowledge
    c. Eagerness to participate
    d. Personal friendly relationship

28. A patient is very confused and disoriented and insists that the sound of an ambulance is actually someone screaming. What is the best nurse response?

    a. "That sound was an ambulance siren."
    b. "No one is screaming."
    c. "How about if I turn on the TV for you?"
    d. "She has stopped screaming now, so everything's ok."

29. A 60-year-old male is being treated for a myocardial infarction. While he is progressing well physically, he becomes upset when asked to make independent decisions and he rings the call bell constantly asking for reassurance that he will get well. This psychological response to stress is an example of:

    a. dependence.
    b. passivity.
    c. depression.
    d. confusion.

30. If using Lean Six Sigma as a method for performance improvement, the focus is likely going to be on:

    a. improving staff training.
    b. engaging in the community.
    c. flattening the hierarchical structure.
    d. reducing error and waste.

31. The American Geriatrics Society's "Guideline for the Prevention of Falls in Older Persons" recommends (among other things):

    a. remediation of visual deficits where possible (e.g., glasses).
    b. home health aide care.
    c. stretching exercises.
    d. dietary modifications.

32. Which of the following is one of the 23 leading health indicators (determinants of health) outlined in Healthy People 2030?

    a. Mental health
    b. Chronic disease
    c. Annual influenza vaccination
    d. Family support

33. When conducting interviews as part of the development of evidence-based practice guidelines, the initial results show that different interviewers achieved markedly different results. What intervention is indicated?

    a. No intervention is indicated.
    b. Replace the interviewers.
    c. Improve training for the interviewers.
    d. Question the interviewers' biases.

34. A 32-year-old single mother of a 4-year-old child is being discharged after a hysterectomy for cervical cancer. She states she is very depressed because she has lost her job, cannot feed her family, and will soon be homeless. Which referral is most appropriate?

    a. Food bank
    b. Homeless shelter
    c. Social worker
    d. Mental health clinic

35. A patient is being treated for renal disease and exhibits the following: ventricular arrhythmia with increasing ECG changes, weakness with ascending paralysis and hyperreflexia, diarrhea, and increasing confusion. The patient most likely has:

    a. hyperkalemia.
    b. hypokalemia.
    c. hypocalcemia.
    d. hypercalcemia.

36. When teaching a patient to carry out clean intermittent catheterization, the patient is reluctant to handle the equipment but takes notes and asks the nurse to draw diagrams. According to the theory of learning preferences, this suggests that the patient is what type of learner?

    a. Visual
    b. Auditory
    c. Kinesthetic
    d. Tactile

37. The Instrumental Activities of Daily Living (IADL) tool includes an assessment of:

    a. bathing.
    b. toileting.
    c. ascending or descending stairs.
    d. financial responsibility.

38. According to the World Health Organization pain ladder (sometimes called the "analgesic ladder"), a patient with cancer and mild pain should begin treatment with:

    a. acetaminophen or aspirin, followed by NSAIDs.
    b. NSAIDs
    c. acetaminophen or aspirin with codeine or a similar adjuvant.
    d. complementary therapies, such as acupuncture.

39. Which nurses should be covered by malpractice insurance?

a. Advance practice nurses only
b. Nurse practitioners only
c. All licensed nursing personnel
d. All licensed and unlicensed nursing personnel

40. The best time to initiate conflict resolution is:

a. when those in conflict have had time to reflect upon their differences.
b. when conflict first emerges.
c. when conflict interferes with function.
d. when those involved ask for conflict resolution.

41. A 30-year-old male complains of frequent nosebleeds, abdominal pain, and nausea. He has burns on his fingers and a slight cough but no needle marks, and his pupils are constricted. He sniffs repeatedly because of nasal irritation. He has a slight fever and tachycardia, and he is malnourished. What substance has he likely been abusing?

a. Cocaine
b. Heroin
c. Marijuana
d. Methadone

42. The psychological theory that characterizes a hierarchy of needs culminating in self-actualization was developed by:

a. Jung.
b. Havighurst.
c. Maslow.
d. Freud.

43. A patient is admitted with COVID-19 infection and exhibits hypoxemia and requires increasing amounts of conventional oxygen therapy (not per a high-flow device, noninvasive ventilation, invasive mechanical ventilation, or extracorporeal membrane oxygenation). Which of the following treatments is recommended by the Centers for Disease Control (CDC)?

a. Dexamethasone plus remdesivir
b. Remdesivir only
c. Dexamethasone only
d. Hydroxychloroquine plus dexamethasone

44. Which type of pain is best treated with opioids?

a. Chronic back pain of more than 3 months duration
b. Acute pain in response to illness or injury
c. Psychogenic pain
d. Phantom pain after amputation

45. The nurse is interviewing a 40-year-old Chinese woman. The woman seems relaxed and answers all the questions fully, but she keeps her eyes downcast and does not make eye contact. This probably indicates:

a. respect.
b. fear.
c. depression.
d. dishonesty.

46. If a physician insists that a nurse carry out a procedure that is outside of the nurse's scope of practice and the nurse feels confident and able to actually do the procedure, the nurse should:

    a. ask a supervisor if it is appropriate to do the procedure.
    b. do the procedure.
    c. ask the physician to supervise while doing the procedure.
    d. refuse to do the procedure.

47. The nurse enters a patient's room just after he talks to the doctor and finds the patient shaking and distraught. What is the best nurse response?

    a. "What's wrong?"
    b. "You are shaking and seem worried."
    c. "Do you want me to call your family?"
    d. "You don't need to worry. Everything will be all right."

48. A nursing team leader delegates a task to an unlicensed assistant. Who is responsible for patient outcomes?

    a. The unlicensed person who completes the task
    b. Both the team leader and the unlicensed person who completes the task
    c. The team leader who delegates the task
    d. The administrative staff

49. A 40-year-old male patient goes into septic shock after surgical repair of a ruptured bowel. Lab results show increased prothrombin time, partial thromboplastin time, thrombin time, D-dimer, and fibrin split products (FSP), while fibrinogen and antithrombin III are decreased. Platelet count is 85,000. This profile is indicative of:

    a. pulmonary emboli.
    b. disseminated intravascular coagulation (DIC).
    c. multi-organ dysfunction syndrome.
    d. deep vein thrombosis (DVT).

50. The patient for whom the use of transcutaneous electrical nerve stimulation (TENS) to relieve pain is most appropriate is:

    a. a man with chest pain and a pacemaker.
    b. a woman with pain in the anterior neck.
    c. a man with moderate dementia related to Alzheimer's disease.
    d. a woman with chronic low back pain.

51. According to Bloom's revised taxonomy, knowledge of categories, classifications, principles, theories, and models is which type of knowledge?

    a. Factual
    b. Conceptual
    c. Procedural
    d. Metacognitive

52. A 50-year-old Middle Eastern woman from Saudi Arabia has a radical mastectomy. On postoperative day-1 a male nurse prepares to change her dressings. She becomes very upset and refuses care. Which is the best response?

   a. Explain that he is the only nurse available to do this treatment and that the hospital does not consider gender in assignments
   b. Chart that the patient refused care and skip the dressing change
   c. Reassure the patient that he understands her concerns and will make arrangements for a female nurse to change the dressing
   d. Explain that she has no right to refuse care since she signed the surgery permit

53. A 75-year-old male patient had a stroke 2 months previously. He has residual left-sided paresis, a left visual field defect, and impaired motor skills. His language skills are intact, but he behaves impulsively, has difficulty following directions, and has short-term memory loss. His stroke most likely occurred in the:

   a. right hemisphere.
   b. left hemisphere.
   c. brain stem.
   d. cerebellum.

54. The nurse is caring for an asthmatic patient receiving nebulizer therapy. Which of the following can the nurse delegate to nursing assistive personnel?

   a. Reporting any observable changes in patient condition/equipment
   b. Changing the oxygen's flow rate for the nebulizer
   c. Carrying out a respiratory assessment
   d. Monitoring the nebulizer equipment

55. A 26-year-old woman with 2nd degree burns on her hands has received repeated doses of morphine intravenously. She now has a respiratory rate of 8/minute, hypotension, and pinpoint pupils. What treatment is appropriate?

   a. Naloxone (Narcan®)
   b. Flumazenil
   c. N-acetylcysteine (NAC)
   d. Charcoal

56. A patient is admitted to the unit after vomiting excessively for 4 days at home. The patient's serum pH is elevated, PCO_2 is relatively normal, and urine pH is >6. The patient is dizzy, confused, and is exhibiting tremors, seizures, tingling, tachycardia, arrhythmias, and hypoventilation. The patient is most likely exhibiting symptoms of:

   a. respiratory alkalosis.
   b. metabolic alkalosis.
   c. respiratory acidosis.
   d. metabolic acidosis.

57. Failing to provide reasonable care based upon appropriate standards and expertise is an example of:

   a. malpractice.
   b. poor judgment.
   c. negligent conduct.
   d. inadequate supervision.

58. A 35-year-old female patient attempted suicide by stabbing herself in the chest but caused only minor injury. She had made two previous attempts at suicide using pills and has no family or close friends. Her affect remains flat, but she states that the antidepressant is helping her and she no longer feels depressed. Which best characterizes her risk for suicide?

    a. Low risk because she was probably just trying to get attention
    b. High risk because she used a knife and had previous suicide attempts
    c. Low risk because she is responding well to the antidepressant
    d. No risk because she is no longer depressed

59. While suctioning a tracheostomy, the nurse should:

    a. suction intermittently during both insertion and withdrawal.
    b. suction continuously during both insertion and withdrawal.
    c. suction continuously during insertion only.
    d. suction intermittently during withdrawal only.

60. The Disaster-Preparedness Committee is responsible for:

    a. instituting infection control procedures.
    b. establishing guidelines for the use of patient restraints.
    c. posting exit routes from each area of the hospital.
    d. ensuring compliance with air ventilation guidelines.

61. During an interview with a patient, what type of patient response provides the most useful information about the patient?

    a. Verbal responses
    b. Nonverbal responses
    c. Silence
    d. Both verbal and nonverbal responses

62. Providing professional guidance and being someone to whom other staff can bring questions or concerns may be described as:

    a. mentoring.
    b. role modeling.
    c. supervising.
    d. coaching.

63. The best determinant of the effectiveness of patient education is:

    a. patient satisfaction.
    b. a patient's ability to demonstrate a procedure.
    c. a patient's ability to explain a procedure and demonstrate understanding.
    d. a patient's behavior modification and compliance rates.

64. After a spinal tap, the patient complains of severe headache, visual disturbances, and nausea. An autologous blood patch may be injected epidurally near the puncture site in order to:

    a. prevent infection.
    b. relieve local pain at the puncture site.
    c. plug the puncture hole in the dura.
    d. reduce edema at the puncture site.

65. Which right is included in the Patients' Bill of Rights?

    a. affordable healthcare.

    b. pain control.

    c. right to sue.

    d. access to latest medical technology.

66. The nurse is conducting an in-home functional assessment to determine safety issues. The patient had a mild stroke and is alert and able to ambulate with a walker but has some residual weakness of the left side. Which of the following findings should be the priority concern?

    a. A long hallway is lit with only one small 30-watt lightbulb.

    b. The older gas stove in the kitchen must be lit with a match or lighter.

    c. The house has hardwood floors with numerous throw rugs and clutter.

    d. The bathroom is 15 feet from the patient's bed.

67. A patient with liver disease and a history of depression commits suicide after repeatedly ringing the call bell and telling a nurse that he wanted to die. Which of the following is an act of negligent omission?

    a. Giving the patient the wrong dosage of the antidepressant

    b. Failing to notify the crisis management team or appropriate authorities of the patient's suicidal statements

    c. Documenting that the patient was attention seeking

    d. Moving the call bell out of the patient's reach

68. A 26-year-old gay male has suffered a concussion, ruptured eardrum, facial cuts, and large bruises on his back and both arms. The patient and his partner, who stays with the patient, both state that the patient fell down the stairs but they provide inconsistent explanations. These types of injury most suggest that:

    a. the patient is probably telling the truth.

    b. the patient may have been drinking or taking drugs, causing him to fall.

    c. the patient probably had a different type of accident than the one reported.

    d. the patient may be a victim of domestic abuse.

69. A burn patient is upset and argues loudly with the nurse, refusing wound care and stating that the treatment is too painful. Which response is an example of therapeutic communication?

    a. "You should stop arguing with the nurses."

    b. "Everyone gets upset at times."

    c. "Let's talk about this and see if we can figure out a way to make the treatment more comfortable for you."

    d. "You should be happy that the burns are healing so well."

70. Which of the following complies with the American Medical Association guidelines for informed consent?

    a. A patient with a meningioma is provided a list of treatment options: Wait and observe, radiosurgery, or craniotomy

    b. A patient with possible breast cancer is told that her only option for diagnosis is a fine needle aspiration

    c. A preoperative patient is advised that she has nothing to worry about because gall bladder surgery poses almost no risks

    d. A patient with 4th stage pancreatic cancer is advised that he must have chemotherapy, or he will die

71. The primary reason for completing continuing education courses is:

    a. to meet state requirements for licensure.

    b. to remain current in the field of nursing.

    c. to meet institution requirements for employment.

    d. to meet requirements for salary increase.

72. A woman caring for her elderly father in the home complains that he is frequently incontinent of urine on the way from the living room (where he spends most of the day) to the bathroom near his room. The best solution is:

    a. leave the father in the bedroom during the day, close to the bathroom.

    b. ask the doctor to insert a Foley catheter.

    c. utilize adult diapers.

    d. provide a urinal near his chair in the living room.

73. CDC adult recommendations for the hepatitis B vaccine include:

    a. all those age 65 and older.

    b. those with a history of noninjection drug use.

    c. those with autoimmune disorders.

    d. those with chronic liver disease.

74. An 88-year-old male with moderate Alzheimer's disease has been cared for at home by his frail 84-year-old wife. The man has weight loss related to malnutrition and is not wearing his dentures. His clothes are unkempt and dirty. He clings to his wife, who remains attentive. This man's condition is probably related to:

    a. elder abuse.

    b. active neglect.

    c. passive neglect.

    d. poverty.

75. A 65-year-old woman with renal disease is scheduled for magnetic resonance imaging (MRI) with IV contrast. What screening test should be completed prior to the MRI?

    a. Hematocrit

    b. Creatinine

    c. Sedimentation rate

    d. Prothrombin time

76. A patient has been treated for septicemia and is demonstrating depressed cardiac function, renal failure, respiratory distress syndrome, thrombocytopenia, and disseminated intravascular coagulation (DIC). The most-likely diagnosis is:

    a. systemic inflammatory response syndrome.

    b. sepsis.

    c. septic shock.

    d. multiple organ dysfunction syndrome.

77. Which of the following would NOT be considered a patient restraint that requires a physician's order with a specified duration of use?

    a. Wrist strap restraint

    b. Wrist board to protect an IV

    c. Ketamine to sedate an aggressive patient

    d. Bed half side rails (4 rails)

78. **The nurse should identify learner outcomes as part of plan for an educational offering. A learner outcome for teaching diabetics about insulin reaction is to:**

    a. identify different types of insulin.
    b. list and describe the symptoms of insulin reaction.
    c. identify foods high in carbohydrates.
    d. explain the difference between Type I and Type 2 diabetes.

79. **A legal document that specifically designates someone to make decisions regarding medical and end-of-life care if a patient is mentally incompetent is a(n):**

    a. advance directive.
    b. do-not-resuscitate order.
    c. Durable Power of Attorney for Health Care.
    d. general power of attorney.

80. **A 22-year-old sexually active male complains of difficulty urinating and purulent discharge from the urethra. Epididymitis and prostatitis are found on examination. The most likely cause is:**

    a. gonorrhea.
    b. syphilis.
    c. chlamydia.
    d. trichomoniasis.

81. **A surgical patient develops a wound infection and informs the nurse that she plans to sue the hospital. Which department will deal with this issue?**

    a. The administration
    b. Risk management
    c. Human resources
    d. Infection control

82. **A newly hired nurse is assisting her team leader, who is preparing to insert an IV catheter. The team leader drops the sterile catheter onto the bed linens and then picks up the contaminated catheter and continues to prepare for insertion. What is the best response?**

    a. Wait until the team leader finishes the procedure and ask why she used the contaminated catheter
    b. Report the team leader's behavior to a supervisor after the catheter is inserted
    c. Say nothing to anyone, as the linens were clean
    d. Immediately say: "The catheter was contaminated when it fell. Would you like me to get another setup or stay with the patient while you get it?"

83. **In evaluating nutritional intervention outcomes for a patient with type 1 diabetes mellitus with a fasting blood sugar of 130 mg/dL three months previously, which lab result most indicates dietary compliance:**

    a. fasting blood sugar of 106 mg/dL.
    b. Hemoglobin A1c of 6.6%.
    c. Hemoglobin A1c of 5.5%.
    d. fasting blood sugar of 150 mg/dL.

84. **Jung's theory about development of the personality over the lifespan is referred to as:**

    a. hierarchy of needs.
    b. theory of individualism.
    c. age stratification.
    d. life course.

85. A 33-year-old woman developed multiple genital warts in the anogenital area. The warts recently spread to the inside of the vagina. This is a concern, as genital warts increase the woman's risk of developing:

    a.   infertility.
    b.   gonorrhea.
    c.   syphilis.
    d.   cervical cancer.

86. Which of the following is most likely to lead to medication errors?

    a.   Hand block-printing of all orders
    b.   The use of bar coding and scanners
    c.   The use of medical abbreviations
    d.   Computer generated orders

87. A patient complains of exercise-induced angina, chest pain radiating down the left arm and lasting < 5 minutes. This type of angina is:

    a.   stable.
    b.   unstable.
    c.   coronary artery spasm.
    d.   variant (Prinzmetal's).

88. One advantage of group instruction over one-on-one instruction is:

    a.   it is more cost-effective.
    b.   it requires less planning.
    c.   it allows more time for questions.
    d.   it is more flexible.

89. One of the most common causes of the person-to-person spread of infection in hospitals is:

    a.   crowded conditions.
    b.   poor hand-washing technique.
    c.   inadequate housekeeping.
    d.   antibiotic resistance.

90. Pain Assessment in Advanced Dementia (PAINAD) utilizes:

    a.   a face scale with pictures of smiling or crying faces.
    b.   a "0" (no pain) to "10" (severe pain) scale.
    c.   monitoring of blood pressure changes.
    d.   observations of nonverbal behavior.

91. The Confusion Assessment Method is a tool that covers 9 factors related to mental status. This tool is used to assess for:

    a.   delirium.
    b.   Alzheimer's disease.
    c.   substance abuse.
    d.   brain injury.

92. A wealthy patient who has been on a unit for two weeks gives a nurse an expensive watch out of gratitude. What is the best nurse response?

    a.   "You don't need to pay for nursing care."
    b.   "Thank you so much! I will treasure this!"
    c.   "This is much too expensive for me to accept."
    d.   "I'm sorry. This is so kind of you, but nurses are not allowed to accept gifts from patients."

93. National guidelines recommend that adults engage in exercises of moderate intensity for:

   a. 20 minutes daily to minimum total of 100 minutes weekly.

   b. 30 minutes daily to minimum of 150 minutes weekly.

   c. 60 minutes daily to minimum of 300 minutes weekly.

   d. 10 minutes daily to minimum of 60 minutes weekly.

94. A problem list focuses on:

   a. a prioritized list of patient problems based on assessment, history, and interview.

   b. all identified patient problems based on assessment, history, and interview.

   c. the patient's self-reported problems.

   d. a standardized list of problems related to specific diagnoses.

95. When administering the four-question CAGE substance abuse screening tool, answering "Yes" to how many questions is clinically significant and indicates probable substance abuse?

   a. 1

   b. 2

   c. 3

   d. 4

96. A patient being discharged after treatment for liver disease asks if it is all right to resume taking a number of different vitamins and herbal preparations. The best response is:

   a. "No, it's not safe to take multiple vitamins and herbal medications."

   b. "You should ask your doctor."

   c. "Vitamins and herbal medications are fine to take."

   d. "Some vitamins and herbal preparations interfere with other medications or are cleared from the body through the liver, so you need to discuss each one with the doctor."

97. Which of the following nursing interventions is an example of patient advocacy?

   a. The nurse administers treatments as prescribed by a physician.

   b. The nurse stops by a patient's home to feed the patient's cat.

   c. The nurse assists the patient to compile a list of questions to ask the physician.

   d. The nurse notifies the physician of a change in the patient's condition.

98. Biofeedback has been shown to be an effective treatment for:

   a. diabetic fecal incontinence.

   b. spinal cord injury.

   c. attention deficit hyperactivity disorder.

   d. cardiac arrhythmias.

99. A 30-year-old male with paralysis of his legs and hips uses crutches and braces to ambulate. Which crutch gait is most appropriate?

   a. The swing-to gait

   b. The swing-though gait

   c. A two-point gait

   d. A four-point gait

100. A nurse documents a treatment on the wrong chart. Which is the correct action?

   a. Drawing a line through the entry and writing "Error."

   b. Leaving the initial entry but indicating below that it was documented on the wrong chart.

   c. Whiting out the entry so it's not legible.

   d. Recopying the entire page, omitting the entry.

101. A cooperative 80-year-old patient suffered a stroke and has limited use of her right hand and some forgetfulness. She is very anxious. What type(s) of barriers to self-care would this patient have?

- a. Psychological and cognitive
- b. Physical and cognitive
- c. Physical only
- d. Psychological, physical, and cognitive

102. A 23-year-old Hmong male has acute appendicitis but refuses to sign the consent form until his grandfather arrives. The probable reason is:

- a. The patient has no insurance.
- b. The patient lives with his grandfather and is dependent on him for support.
- c. The patient is afraid to have surgery without family present.
- d. The grandfather is the eldest male in the family and makes the decisions for the family.

103. Which technique utilizes mental visualization to reduce anxiety and promote healing?

- a. Psychotherapy
- b. Guided imagery
- c. Meditation
- d. Relaxation

104. A nurse attempts to start an IV line on an elderly patient, but the patient refuses to cooperate. The nurse tells the patient that she will have the nursing assistant hold him down if he doesn't stop fighting and let her insert the IV. This nurse's response is best characterized as:

- a. non-therapeutic communication.
- b. coercion.
- c. abuse.
- d. poor judgment.

105. The best approach to solving a problem that involves 3 different departments in the hospital is:

- a. forming an interdisciplinary team that works together to find a solution.
- b. to have the administration resolve the problem as a nonbiased party.
- c. for each department to propose a solution to administration.
- d. for all three departments to have a joint meeting to brainstorm possible solutions.

106. A home health nurse visits an older adult and observes that the patient has little food in the house. The patient states he has run out of money and cannot buy groceries, but he does not want his family and friends to know. Which nurse response is appropriate?

- a. Going to the store and buying a small bag of groceries for the patient
- b. Referring the patient to the appropriate social service agencies
- c. Calling the patient's daughter anyway and telling her that the patient needs assistance
- d. Asking the next-door neighbor—who has expressed a willingness to help—to provide meals

107. When positioning a patient after a total hip replacement, it's important to:

- a. avoid flexing the knee of the affected leg beyond 90 degrees.
- b. avoid crossing the affected leg over the other leg.
- c. maintain 90-degree hip flexion while the patient is sitting.
- d. position the patient in side-lying position with the affected leg at 90-degree flexion.

108. Which of the following symptoms is most commonly treated with acupuncture?

a. Pain and nausea
b. Hearing loss
c. Diarrhea and/or constipation
d. Dizziness and/or vertigo

109. A patient with myasthenia gravis has been choking frequently (especially with solids and thin liquids), complaining of regurgitation, experiencing esophageal reflux when supine, and losing weight. The patient has probably developed:

a. aspiration pneumonia.
b. hiatal hernia.
c. gastroesophageal reflux disease.
d. dysphagia.

110. When preparing written materials for patients, what readability level would be appropriate for a homogeneous adult patient group in an affluent area?

a. Grade 6 level
b. Grade 9 level
c. Grade 3 level
d. Grade 12 level

111. Which of Piaget's stages of cognitive development is characterized by the ability to think logically, use abstraction, and test hypotheses?

a. Sensorimotor
b. Preoperational
c. Concrete operational
d. Formal operational

112. A supervisor has a laissez-faire leadership style and exerts little direct control but allows staff members to make decisions with little interference or guidance. What is the likely result of this type of leadership?

a. The staff is highly motivated.
b. The staff is able to accomplish very little.
c. The staff is resistive to changes.
d. The staff is resentful.

113. What assumptions should the nurse make about a patient who, upon initial assessment, fails to make direct eye contact with the nurse?

a. Make no assumptions.
b. The patient is showing respect.
c. The patient is being dishonest.
d. The patient is afraid.

114. A 38-year-old post-operative female is exhibiting signs of pulmonary embolism (tachypnea, tachycardia, cough, fever, rales, anxiety, and hemodynamic instability). Which procedure provides the best diagnostic information?

a. Blood gases
b. Electrocardiogram
c. Chest x-ray
d. Spiral CT

115. A 60-year-old female patient is diagnosed as pre-diabetic and insulin resistant with mild kidney disease. Her hemoglobin A1C is 6.5. She is 5 feet 1 inches tall, weighs 220 pounds, and recently quit work because of back pain. Two sisters are diabetic. The expected blood pressure finding for this patient would be:

    a.   normal blood pressure.
    b.   hypertension.
    c.   hypotension.
    d.   postural hypotension.

116. A nurse is interviewing a patient who is hearing impaired. Which of the following may well be a significant impediment to communication?

    a.   The nurse uses only a normal tone of voice and speaks with short sentences
    b.   The nurse provides assistive devices, such as writing materials
    c.   The nurse is facing the patient at a distance of 5 feet
    d.   The nurse is chewing gum to freshen her breath

117. A 50-year-old man dying from liver disease is Catholic and asks to take final communion even though it is 2 AM. The nurse should:

    a.   contact the patient's priest or a priest on call for the institution and ask him to come right away.
    b.   tell the patient that no priest is available.
    c.   ask the patient if he would be willing to see the Protestant chaplain who is on call.
    d.   tell the patient the priest will be called at 7 AM.

118. A nurse gives the wrong medication to a patient. The nurse should:

    a.   immediately inform the patient.
    b.   document the medication given on the patient's record, indicating that it was a medication error.
    c.   document the medication given only on the incident report.
    d.   document the medication as given on the patient's record, but indicate it was an error on the incident report only.

119. Which of the following most closely characterizes Selye's biological theory of stress and aging?

    a.   The body is a machine that wears out over time
    b.   The body's response to stress is characterized by a generalized adaptation syndrome
    c.   All cells and organisms have a programmed life span
    d.   Over time, mutations occur that interfere with body functioning and cause aging

120. What is a misconception about music therapy?

    a.   Classical music is more effective than pop or rock music
    b.   Previous musical ability is unnecessary
    c.   Music therapy can promote relaxation and relieve pain
    d.   Music therapy increases motivation to exercise

121. A 54-year-old patient is admitted with symptoms of an ischemic stroke verified by CT. He is being considered for thrombolytic therapy with alteplase tissue-type plasminogen activator (t-PA). Which is a contraindication to thrombolytic therapy?

    a.   The patient is 2 hours post-onset of symptoms
    b.   The patient had a mitral valve replacement 1 week previously
    c.   The patient's blood pressure has been 180/90 but is controlled by medication
    d.   The patient had an ischemic stroke 6 months previously

122. The nurse enters a room of a patient who has advanced macular degeneration and has lost most central vision. Which action is appropriate?
- a. Speaking loudly on entering the room to alert the patient to the nurse's presence
- b. Sitting directly in front of the patient while speaking to her
- c. Announcing his presence in a normal tone of voice and explaining relevant actions and movements
- d. Speaking to the patient with simple direct vocabulary

123. A 68-year-old female patient has peripheral vascular disease characterized by arterial insufficiency. Which symptom is typical of peripheral arterial disease?
- a. Brownish discoloration about the ankles and the anterior tibial area
- b. Deep circular painful necrotic ulcers on the toe tips, toe webs, or other pressure areas
- c. Irregular superficial ulcers on the medial or lateral malleolus and sometimes the anterior tibial area
- d. Moderate to severe edema

124. What type of precaution is appropriate under CDC isolation guidelines for a patient with active tuberculosis?
- a. Tier I: Standard precautions
- b. Tier II: Airborne precautions
- c. Tier II: Droplet precautions
- d. Tier II: Contact precautions

125. Which medication order is written correctly?
- a. Maalox 30 cc PO qhs
- b. Lasix 40.0 mg PO daily
- c. MS 4.0 mg IV q 4 hr. prn
- d. Synthroid 0.88 mg PO daily at 0700

126. The best time for a nurse to establish educational goals for teaching patients is:
- a. before creating materials and lesson plans.
- b. while creating materials and lesson plans.
- c. after materials and lesson plans are developed.
- d. after presenting the class and determining patient needs.

127. Two months after an ischemic stroke, a patient still has difficulty understanding and producing language in speaking, reading, and writing. However, the patient can understand gestures, pictures, and diagrams. This type of aphasia is:
- a. global.
- b. transient.
- c. Broca's.
- d. Wernicke's.

128. A 62-year-old male patient has a regular pulse >100 with P waves before the QRS complex, but sometimes preceding the T wave. The QRS pattern is of normal shape and duration. The PR interval is 0.12-0.20 seconds and P: QRS ratio is 1:1. Given this information, the cardiac diagnosis is:
- a. sinus bradycardia.
- b. sinus tachycardia.
- c. sinus arrhythmia.
- d. premature atrial contractions.

129. Dietary management of diabetes mellitus, or medical nutrition therapy (MNT), includes:

    a. calorie-based diet control.
    b. low protein diet control.
    c. standardized diet modifications.
    d. individualized diet modifications.

130. Which of the following theories is characterized by the contention that life is an unending process of changes and transitions?

    a. Life course/Life span
    b. Modernization
    c. Geo-transcendence
    d. Exchange

131. The nurse is interviewing a patient with advanced Parkinson's disease and dysarthria, but without signs of dementia or hearing impairment. Which interview technique is most appropriate?

    a. Using simple sentences and speaking loudly
    b. Asking primarily yes/no questions and observing the patient's facial expressions and gestures
    c. Completing patient's sentences to help the patient communicate more easily
    d. Directing all questions to family members to spare the patient stress

132. When determining outcomes, which of the following types of data provides the lowest form of measurement?

    a. Interval (numerical data that contain no absolute zero, such as the Fahrenheit temperature scale)
    b. Ratio (data similar to numerical but contain absolute zero, such as the Celsius temperature scale)
    c. Nominal (descriptive words, such as "dull" or "sharp")
    d. Ordinal (Likert scale)

133. Interdisciplinary teams that are most effective have:

    a. 4-10 members.
    b. 10-15 members.
    c. 2-4 members.
    d. >15 members.

134. A patient is receiving daily warfarin after treatment for atrial fibrillation. Which of the following may interfere with the drug's effectiveness?

    a. One 8-ounce glass of red wine daily
    b. Green leafy vegetables
    c. A daily multi-vitamin
    d. Milk products

135. When considering the use of an interpreter for a patient who does not speak English, which consideration is most important?

    a. The interpreter has training in medical vocabulary for both languages
    b. The interpreter speaks both languages well
    c. The interpreter knows the patient's history
    d. The interpreter is available onsite

136. A 70-year-old female is assessed for nutritional status. Lab results show that her albumin level is 2.4 g/dL, pre-albumin is 4 mg/dL, and transferrin is 90 mg/dL. These results indicate:

    a. adequate nutrition.
    b. dehydration.
    c. severe malnutrition.
    d. mild to moderate malnutrition.

137. Red blood cell (RBC) casts in the urine indicate:

    a. interstitial nephritis.
    b. myoglobinuria.
    c. renal tubular damage.
    d. glomerular disease.

138. Which of the following biological theories of aging contend that cell mutations and failure of the immune system lead to disease?

    a. Free radical
    b. Programmed/cellular
    c. Autoimmunity
    d. Homeostatic

139. A 75-year-old female patient has been unable to eat after surgery to repair an abdominal aneurysm. She has received total parenteral nutrition (TPN) for four days. What risks are associated with TPN?

    a. Infection and glucose intolerance
    b. Irritation and aspiration
    c. Nausea and vomiting
    d. Skin excoriation

140. At what CD4 count does a patient who is HIV positive convert to a diagnosis of AIDS?

    a. ≤400 cells/mm3
    b. ≤350 cells/mm3
    c. ≤200 cells/mm3
    d. ≤100 cells/mm3

141. Which of the following professional communication skills are used to facilitate communication with intra- and inter-disciplinary teams?

    a. Interpreting the statements of others to facilitate the flow of ideas
    b. Reacting and responding to facts rather than feelings
    c. Providing advice when it appears needed
    d. Asking questions to challenge other people's ideas

142. A 40-year-old male patient complains of daytime somnolence, headache, forgetfulness, increased weight, and impotence. His wife states he has been depressed, has had personality changes, and snores loudly with cycles of holding his breath. Which diagnosis is most likely?

    a. Narcolepsy
    b. Insomnia
    c. Obstructive sleep apnea
    d. Hypothyroidism

143. According to Belbin's team role theory, the action-oriented role of an interdisciplinary team member who is charismatic and dynamic, challenges others to improve performance, and has the ability to find the best solution to problems is that of:

a. implementer.
b. planter.
c. completer-finisher.
d. shaper.

144. A 52-year-old female with a history of bipolar disease has had a hip replacement, and is at post-operative day one. The patient slept only one or two hours during the night and is now speaking rapidly, throwing her belongings at the nurses, and insisting she is going to leave the hospital against medical advice. The nurse should notify:

a. the mental health crisis team.
b. social services.
c. a home health agency.
d. the patient's husband.

145. Which smoking cessation medication must be monitored carefully because of dangerous side effects?

a. Nicotine nasal spray
b. Bupropion (Zyban®)
c. Nicotine inhaler
d. Varenicline (Chantix®)

146. Following a severe auto accident, a 24-year-old patient with a BK amputation is having trouble coping with the change in body image. This is evident by the following sign:

a. the patient refuses to look at the stump or participate in his own care.
b. the patient complains of phantom pain.
c. the patient states he is angry with the other driver.
d. the patient starts crying when talking about rehabilitation.

147. In the nursing process, evaluation should be done:

a. during the implementation phase only.
b. during all phases.
c. during the assessment phase only.
d. during the evaluation stage only.

148. Which is a contraindication to organ donation?

a. Age of 65 years
b. History of alcoholism
c. Active pancreatic cancer
d. Age of 2 years or less

149. If a patient is to receive total parenteral nutrition for 4 to 5 weeks, which vascular access device is recommended?

a. Peripherally inserted central catheter (PICC) line
b. Implanted port
c. Midline peripheral vascular access device (VAD)
d. Short peripheral VAD

150. The nurse is carrying out wound care and notes granulation tissue about the periphery of the wound. What phase of healing does this indicate?

a. Maturation
b. Hemostasis
c. Proliferation
d. Inflammation

Answer Key and Explanations for Test #1

1. A: If, when making purchasing decisions about new medical equipment, the healthcare administration is concerned about cutting costs, the type of study that provides the most information about the financial impact is the cost-benefit analysis. This study looks at all of the costs associated with a purchase and the projected income that will be derived to determine how much profit will be generated by the purchase. The cost-benefit analysis does not necessarily determine whether a purchase is the best option from a patient-care perspective.

2. C: If an older adult patient is very reluctant to assume any self-care, repeatedly stating that she is "too old and too dumb" to learn new things, according to Erik Erikson's theory of development, this suggests that the patient has failed to accomplish the developmental stage of ego integrity versus despair. This is a stage of older adulthood, and failure to work through this stage can lead to despair and a lack of confidence in the ability to manage independently.

3. B: The patient is experiencing the stage of anger. People grieve individually and may not go through all stages, but most go through at least 2 stages. Kübler-Ross's 5 stages of grief include:

- Denial: Refusal to believe, confused, stunned, detached.
- Anger: Directed inward (self-blame) or outward.
- Bargaining: If-then thinking. ("If I go to church, then I will heal.")
- Depression: Sad, withdrawn.
- Acceptance: Resolution.

4. C: The most appropriate nursing diagnosis for a person who is able to exercise but remains sedentary is risk of disuse syndrome because the patient is putting himself at risk for the development of circulatory impairment and muscle atrophy. Failure to exercise may also exacerbate his condition. While his health maintenance may be ineffective, it is directly due to of his lack of activity. He does not have impaired physical mobility or activity intolerance that precludes exercise.

5. D: If a hospital has invested in robotic surgery equipment and needs to assess its costs and health outcomes compared to traditional surgery, the type of study that is indicated is a cost-effectiveness analysis. This type of study can help determine whether robotic surgery or traditional surgery is the least expensive and which one provides the desired outcome or provides the desired outcome for the cost (even if the cost is more expensive). The analysis determines the cost per unit of the proposed outcome.

6. C: The nurse should arrange for an interpreter. Children should never be used as interpreters as they lack sufficient vocabulary and understanding about health matters and may not interpret correctly. The use of a child interpreter may also be awkward or embarrassing, depending upon the topic being addressed. Other adult family members, such as the wife, should not be asked to answer questions for the patient unless the patient is unable to answer questions because of health condition because they may not understand medical terms and may not interpret correctly. Additionally, the patient may have kept information from the family.

7. A: If a patient (famous or otherwise) underwent surgery and a staff member who cared for the patient but was not authorized to provide information was asked about the patient's condition by a reporter and the staff member acknowledged that the person was a patient and was doing well after a hip replacement, this is a violation of the HIPAA Privacy Rule regarding impermissible disclosure. No information, including even acknowledging that the person was a patient, can be provided without the permission of the patient or his or her designated representative.

8. C: Kinesthetic learners learn best by handling, doing, and practicing. Thus, they should be allowed to handle supplies and equipment with minimal directions. They benefit most from demonstrating their understanding by performing the procedure. Visual learners learn best by seeing and reading, and thus benefit most from written directions, videos, diagrams, pictures, and demonstrations. Auditory learners learn best by listening and talking, so procedures should be thoroughly explained during any demonstrations. Auditory learners also benefit from audiotapes and extra time for questions.

9. C: If a patient dies unexpectedly or because of a failure of the system, it is a sentinel event. In this case, when carrying out a root cause analysis of the event, the best definition of the problem would be a communication failure. Root cause analysis is not performed to assign blame but to find the underlying cause for an event. Because the patient was admitted at the change of shift, the patient's needs were overlooked. The order for the computed tomography scan was not communicated to imaging, and information about the patient was not communicated to the oncoming staff, so no nurse was assigned to the patient, leaving the patient to die unattended.

10. A: The mission statement should define the quality (purpose and role) of a healthcare institution. The mission statement generally reflects the current status of an organization and is developed in response to data and program analysis. The mission statement should identify the organization or program, state its function, outline its purpose and strategy, and include a commitment to quality and patient care.

11. D: The most appropriate nursing diagnosis for an Alzheimer patient who walks away from the hospital and hides in the parking lot is wandering. Acute confusion alone does not account for his behavior. While this patient may have risk-prone health behavior because of his dementia, and impaired memory, this particular type of wandering behavior is typical of Alzheimer patients. The reason patients wander is not clear. They may have been looking for a bathroom and gotten lost or perhaps they were looking for someone. Once lost, they often become frightened and compound the problem by hiding.

12. C: Clinical pathways should be based on evidence-based research, which refers to the use of current research and patient values in practice to establish an idealized plan of care. Research may be the result of large studies of best practices, or it may arise from individual research efforts using observations in practice about the effectiveness of a particular treatment. Evidence-based research requires a commitment to ongoing research and outcomes evaluation. Evidence-based research requires a thorough understanding of research methods, including internal and external validity.

13. B: The family should be encouraged to stay and talk to the patient, as hearing is usually the last of the senses to fail. Typical physical changes associated with death include:

- Sensory: Reduced sensations of pain and touch. Decreased vision and hearing.
- Cardiovascular: Tachycardia followed by bradycardia, dysrhythmia, and hypotension.
- Respiratory: Tachypnea, progressing to Cheyne-Stokes respiration.
- Muscular: Muscles relax, the jaw sags, and the ability to swallow and talk is lost.
- Urinary: Output decreases (accompanied by incontinence), and anuria follows.
- Integumentary: Skin becomes cold, clammy, cyanotic, and waxy. Skin in the coccygeal area often tears.

14. D: Severe dehydration is fluid loss >15% and occurs when total body water decreases but sodium does not. It is characterized by marked hypotension and anuria as well as symptoms associated with lesser dehydration. Mild dehydration (5% loss) is characterized by dizziness, lethargy, reduced skin turgor, dry mucous membranes, and orthostatic hypotension. Moderate dehydration (10% loss) is characterized by confusion, resting hypotension, tachycardia, and oliguria/anuria. Dehydration may result from inadequate fluids, excess water loss, NG suctioning, drugs, diarrhea, vomiting, and fever.

15. A: Functional urinary incontinence can occur when physical (impaired mobility) or mental (confusion, depression) disabilities prevent the person from controlling urination. Stress incontinence is characterized by small amounts of involuntary urinary leakage, often during physical activity. Overflow incontinence is also characterized by small leakages of urine, but it results from pressure on an overly-distended bladder. Urge incontinence involves moderate to large amounts of involuntary urinary leakage and is characterized by a sudden urge to urinate coupled with an inability to hold urine.

16. B: The best solution for the free clinic is to create an ad hoc (issue-specific) team to survey staff preferences and agree on a reduced number of dressing supplies so that the clinic qualifies for a discounted price. Reducing costs is critical for the viability of medical clinics and all medical institutions. Having the administrator make this decision invalidates the opinions of the staff and ignores shared governance. A 6-month survey is not necessary as this can be done retrospectively by examining records.

17. C: Initially, the physician must certify that a patient who is eligible under Medicare A is terminal with a life expectancy of 6 months (two 90-day periods). However, if the patient remains alive, the physician can extend coverage by authorizing continued hospice care every 60 days. The goal is to maintain the patient in the home environment with home health aides, homemakers, durable goods, pain management, case management, counseling, and social worker assistance. Routine intermittent home care must comprise 80% of total care, with in-home continuous care and in-patient hospice care available for short augmenting periods only.

18. B: When asking a patient to describe his/her pain, it is best to use an open-ended type of question that elicits specific information. Questions, such as "Are you having pain?" may easily be answered by a simple "yes" or "no" and thus provide little information. "What kind of pain are you having?" may be confusing to patients. The pain scale should be used after the patient has described his/her pain and the nurse has explained in detail, with examples, what the pain scale means.

19. D: If, as part of quality improvement, the processes for admission and discharge have been revised, before utilization, failure mode and effects analysis is done to try to determine if there are any problems that have been overlooked and to ensure positive outcomes. This analysis has 12 steps: definition, team creation, description, brainstorming, identification of the potential cause of potential failures, listing potential adverse outcomes, assignment of severity rating, assignment of frequency/occurrence rating, assignment of detection rating, calculation of the risk priority number, reduction of potential failures, and identification of performance measures.

20. A: Team members usually observe the leader and determine who controls the meeting and how control is exercised, while beginning to form alliances. Arguing is counterproductive, and following strict rules of discourse may not solve power issues and may be too restrictive for small collaborative groups. Group interactions often become less formal as members develop rapport and are more willing to help and support each other to achieve goals. Rotating leadership roles can lead to a lack of focus as styles may vary widely. The leader is responsible for organizing the group, clarifying methods to achieve work, and the means of working together toward a common goal.

21. B: The Mini-cog test assesses dementia by having patients remember and repeat 3 common objects and draw a clock face indicating a particular time. The MMSE assesses dementia through a series of tests, including remembering the names of 3 common objects, counting backward, naming, providing location, copying shapes, and following directions. The Digit Repetition Test assesses attention by asking the patient to repeat a 2-number series, then 3, then 4 and so on. The Confusion Assessment Method is used to assess delirium, not dementia.

22. D: Making a referral to a home health agency to provide in-home care is the best solution, as this ensures that the man will receive skilled nursing care and still be able to stay at home with his grandson, who is too young for the responsibility of wound care. This is a more cost-effective solution than transferring the patient to an extended care facility. Keeping the patient in the hospital is not generally an option, as Medicare will not pay for extended hospitalization for long-term wound treatment.

23. C: The nurse should first assess the patient's learning style. Patients often know how they like to learn, or are able to provide enough information for the nurse to determine their learning styles. Audiotapes are appropriate for auditory learners, and pictures and diagrams for visual learners. While auto mechanics are usually good with their hands, the nurse should not assume that the patient has a particular learning style simply because of his profession or occupation.

24. B: The Occupational Safety and Health Administration (OSHA) regulates workplace safety, including disposal methods for sharps, such as needles. OSHA requires that standard precautions be used at all times and that staff be trained to use precautions. OSHA requires procedures for post-exposure evaluation and treatment, and the availability of the hepatitis B vaccine for healthcare workers. OSHA regulates occupational exposure to infections, and establishes standards to prevent the spread of blood-borne pathogens, as well as regulating the fitting and use of respirators.

25. D: Palliative care provides comfort rather than curative treatment, although curative treatment may also relieve pain or symptoms. Thus, there is no clear line between the two. Palliative care is meant to improve the quality of life and to relieve suffering, but it does not include treatments solely intended to prolong life or hasten death. The goals of palliative care are to provide adequate pain management and relief of symptoms (such as nausea or shortness of breath), to provide support for both the patient and caregivers or family, and to ensure that patients and family receive psychosocial, spiritual, and bereavement support.

26. B: If a patient has developed a pressure ulcer over the left ischial tuberosity; the ulcerated area is exposed with a loss of epidermis and dermis; underlying fatty tissue is visible but no muscle, tendons, ligaments, or bones are visible; and some slough is present with undermining of 2 cm extending from 1 to 3 o'clock, according to the NPIAP Staging System this wound would be classified as stage III. It becomes stage IV when bone, muscle, ligaments, cartilage, or tendons are visible. An unstageable ulcer is one in which the wound is covered by slough or eschar that obscures the wound.

27. B: If the nurse is forming an interdisciplinary team to review processes as part of the mission to improve quality, when choosing team members, the skills and knowledge of the person should be the priority. It can be tempting to include those with whom the nurse has a personal friendly relationship or who are eager to participate, but these people may not be the best suited. The nurse should make a list of the characteristics needed (knowledge of processes, good communication, well-organized, reliable) and look for staff members that have those characteristics.

28. A: When a patient is confused and disoriented, the best response is to say what is true. State, "That sound is an ambulance siren," calmly and without arguing. Saying "No one is screaming" challenges the patient without explanation and may increase confusion. Distracting the patient may be helpful after the explanation, but this should not be the first response. Saying "She has stopped screaming now, so everything's ok" reinforces the patient's faulty perception and does nothing to alleviate confusion. Note: A patient confused and disoriented due to transient illness is very different from one suffering with acute delusions or paranoia from chronic mental illness such as schizophrenia. A confused patient needs clarification and re-orientation, while a paranoid and/or delusional patient may become angry or even violent if their perceptions are negated.

29. A: This patient is exhibiting dependence in response to stress. Typical psychological responses to stress include:

- Dependence: The patient has an inability to make decisions, requires constant reassurance, and calls nurses/families frequently.
- Depression: The patient is withdrawn and sad, fails to take treatments and/or misses appointments, and may be at risk for suicide.
- Anger: The patient is belligerent, uncooperative, and blames others.
- Confusion: The patient is forgetful, disoriented, and bewildered.
- Passivity: The patient defers to others, feeling he/she has no control.

30. D: If using Lean Six Sigma as a method for performance improvement, the focus is likely going to be on reducing error and waste. Process improvement is based on strategic goals rather than on a project-by-project basis, and it focuses on continuous learning and rapid change. Characteristics include long-term goals and strategies for a 1–3 year period, performance improvement as an underlying belief, cost reduction, and use of improvement methodologies (such as plan-do-check-act).

31. A: The American Geriatrics Society's "Guideline for the Prevention of Falls in Older Persons" includes an assessment of falls, gait and balance and makes a number of recommendations for preventing falls, including visual remediation (e.g., glasses, if needed, etc.), exercises for strength and balance, review and possible reduction in medications that cause dizziness or instability, modification of home environment, use of an assistive device, supportive footwear, and control of cardiovascular conditions that might cause dizziness/syncope and thereby precipitate falls.

32. C: Healthy People 2030 outlines leading health indicators (LHIs) to improve health and reduce the risks of disease in order to improve life expectancy and quality of life. Leading health indicators are divided across four categories: (1) All Ages, (2) Infants, (3) Children and Adolescents, and (4) Adults and Older Adults. Within the All Ages category, leading health indicators address various conditions including annual vaccination against seasonal influenza, drug overdose deaths, homicides, and suicides, amongst others. The leading health indicators are core objectives for HP 2030.

33. C: If, when conducting interviews as part of the development of evidence-based practice guidelines, the initial results show that different interviewers achieved markedly different results, the intervention that is indicated is to improve training for the interviewers. To achieve interrater reliability, interviewers must be trained to asked the questions in exactly the same way to each person interviewed and to avoid any coaching or additional questioning.

34. C: Referring the single mother to a social worker is the most appropriate, as social workers have the expertise required to assist a patient to apply for social services, including programs such as Temporary Assistance for Needy Families (TANF) and food stamps. The social worker may be able to help the patient avoid homelessness by assisting her to apply for subsidized or low-cost housing. While the patient may benefit from a referral to a mental health clinic, this will not solve the immediate underlying problem of food and shelter.

35. A: Hyperkalemia often occurs with renal disease and is characterized by ventricular arrhythmia, weakness with ascending paralysis and hyperreflexia, diarrhea, and confusion. Hypokalemia is characterized by weakness, lethargy, nausea and vomiting, paresthesias, dysrhythmias (PVCs, flattened T waves), muscle cramps with hyporeflexia, hypotension, and tetany. Hypocalcemia is characterized by tetany, tingling, seizures, altered mental status, and ventricular tachycardia. Hypercalcemia is characterized by increasing muscle weakness with hypotonicity, constipation, anorexia, nausea and vomiting, and bradycardia.

36. A: If, when teaching a patient to carry out clean intermittent catheterization, the patient is reluctant to handle the equipment but takes notes and asks the nurse to draw diagrams, according to the theory of learning preferences, this suggests that the patient is a visual learner. Visual learners often rely on reading and writing to gain knowledge and enjoy visual representations, such as videos and illustrations. They may be reluctant to carry out procedures until they have a base of knowledge.

37. D: The Instrumental Activities of Daily Living (IADL) tool assesses financial ability (ability to pay bills, budget, and keep track of finances), telephone use, shopping, food preparation, housekeeping, laundry, transportation availability (ability to drive or use public transportation), and medications (ability to manage prescriptions and take medications). The Barthel Index of Activities of Daily Living assesses 10 categories, usually including bathing, toileting, ascending or descending stairs, feeding, mobility, personal grooming, urinary and fecal control, transferring, and ambulatory/wheelchair status.

38. A: A patient with cancer and mild pain (Level 1) should begin treatment with acetaminophen or aspirin followed by NSAIDs. Patients should always start with the medication with the fewest side effects (acetaminophen/aspirin) and then move to stronger medications as necessary. NSAIDs should be used if acetaminophen or aspirin doesn't relieve pain. As patients move up the pain ladder to mild-moderate pain (Level 2) codeine (hydrocodone, tramadol, or oxycodone) with adjuvants will be added, and, finally, with moderate-severe pain (Level 3), opioids (such a fentanyl, morphine, and oxycodone), are used to control pain.

39. C: All licensed nursing personnel should be covered by malpractice insurance. Most institutions carry malpractice insurance for staff, but advance practice nurses are usually insured at a higher rate because they have a wider scope of practice. A nurse may be sued individually or as part of a medical group. A suit is a civil matter, so loss of judgment may not be reported to the state board of nursing. If a charge of negligence is brought to the attention of the board, it may institute investigation and disciplinary action.

40. B: The best time to initiate conflict resolution is when conflict first emerges, but before open conflict and hardening of positions. Resolution steps include:

1. Allowing both parties to present their side without bias.
2. Encouraging cooperation through negotiation and compromise.
3. Maintaining focus and avoiding arguments.
4. Evaluating the need for renegotiation, a formal resolution process, or a 3rd party mediator.
5. Utilizing humor and empathy to diffuse tension.
6. Summarizing and outlining key arguments.
7. Avoiding forced resolution if possible.

41. A: Signs of inhaled cocaine use include nasal irritation and nosebleeds, and signs of smoked cocaine include lip burns and a cough. Constricted pupils, headaches, and abdominal pain are also common. Most abused drugs have similar symptoms. However, heroin users would have needle tracks and would not have nasal irritation. Marijuana users may exhibit tachycardia and cough from lung irritation (similar to tobacco smokers), but usually do not develop nasal irritation or nose bleeds. Methadone abuse can cause constricted pupils and abdominal pain, but does not cause nasal symptoms.

42. C: Maslow stated that human behavior is motivated by various needs, and posited that there is a hierarchy of need beginning with basic needs and progressing to personal needs. Maslow theorized that working toward self-actualization is a lifelong process that may involve progress in multiple directions rather than in one direction. Failure results in depression and diminished feelings of value:

- 1st Level (the base): Physiological needs.
- 2nd Level: Safety and security.
- 3rd Level: Love/Belonging.
- 4th Level: Self-esteem.
- 5th level (the apex): Self-actualization.

43. A: If a patient is admitted with a COVID-19 infection and exhibits hypoxemia and requires increasing amounts of conventional oxygen therapy (not per a high-flow device, noninvasive ventilation, invasive mechanical ventilation, or extracorporeal membrane oxygenation), the treatment is dexamethasone plus remdesivir. Dexamethasone alone may be administered if remdesivir is not available for use for patients with this degree of acuity. If a patient is stable and requires only minimal supplemental oxygen, then only remdesivir is recommended.

44. B: Acute pain in response to illness or injury often responds well to opioids. Chronic back pain responds less well to opioids and more relief may be gained by exercise, corticosteroids, or complementary therapy (massage, acupuncture, TENS). Psychogenic pain is difficult to treat but opioids are not appropriate. Phantom pain after amputation can be severe and is sometimes treated with opioids, but tricyclic antidepressants and anticonvulsants are often more effective and have fewer side effects. Other treatments, such as TENS or acupuncture, may be effective.

45. A: In this case, averting the eyes is probably a sign of respect toward the nurse. In many Asian cultures, it is considered disrespectful to look someone in the eyes, and the eyes are often averted downward to show respect. Although what is generally true for a group is not always true for an individual, the fact that the woman seems relaxed rather than anxious and is forthcoming with her responses suggests that she is not fearful, depressed, or dishonest.

46. D: If a physician insists that a nurse carry out a procedure that is outside of the nurse's scope of practice and the nurse feels confident and able to actually do the procedure, the nurse should refuse to do the procedure, stating, "I can't do this procedure because it is outside of my scope of practice and I could lose my nursing license if I do it." The nurse should also report this event to a supervisor because the physician may need to be educated about the implications of violating the scope of practice.

47. B: "You are shaking and seem worried" acknowledges what is true and evident and leaves an opening for the patient to discuss his feelings if he desires. "What's wrong?" requires a direct response that the patient may not feel like giving. "Do you want me to call your family?" does not deal with the patient's anxiety and is an escape for the nurse. "You don't need to worry. Everything will be all right" is a platitude that has little meaning and may not, in fact, be true. Of additional note, it is usually wise to first confer with the intervening physician, if possible, to become better informed regarding the presenting issue. This can aid in avoiding pitfalls and unnecessary conflicts, and in more meaningfully supporting the patient.

48. C: The nurse who delegates also remains accountable for patient outcomes and for supervision of the person to whom the task was delegated. The scope of nursing includes delegation of tasks to unlicensed assistants, along with ensuring those personnel have adequate training and knowledge. Delegation can be used to manage the workload and to provide adequate and safe care. Delegation should be done in a manner that reduces liability by providing adequate communication.

49. B: This profile of increased clotting times and reduced fibrinogen, antithrombin and platelets is found with disseminated intravascular coagulation (DIC), which is a secondary disorder (i.e., triggered by another). DIC causes both coagulation and hemorrhage through a complex series of events. It includes trauma of a nature that causes tissue factor (transmembrane glycoprotein) to enter the circulation and bind with coagulation factors, triggering the coagulation cascade. This cascade stimulates thrombin to convert fibrinogen to fibrin, causing aggregation and destruction of platelets and forming clots that can be disseminated throughout the intravascular system.

50. D: Transcutaneous electrical nerve stimulation (TENS) is appropriate treatment for a woman with chronic low back pain. TENS is contraindicated for those with pacemakers, as TENS can interfere with pacemaker function. TENS should not be used on the anterior neck and should be used on the head only with careful physician supervision. TENS should not be used by those who have dementia, as they may become confused and fail to use the equipment properly.

51. B: According to Benjamin Bloom's revised taxonomy, knowledge of categories, classifications, principles, theories, and models is conceptual knowledge. Other categories of knowledge include procedural (skill, algorithms, techniques, processes), metacognitive (self-knowledge, strategies), and factual (terminology, details, facts). The educational goals of the revised taxonomy include remembering (recognize, recall), understanding (classify, summarize, infer, compare, interpret, explain), applying (implement), analyzing (organize, differentiate), evaluating (critique, examine), and creating (plan, produce).

52. C: In this case, cultural sensitivity should take precedence over gender equality, and the nurse should reassure the patient and make arrangements for a female nurse to provide the dressing change. This Saudi patient comes from a culture that strictly segregates males and females, and this surgery and follow-up care may threaten her religious and cultural beliefs, her sense of sexuality, and her body image. Further, because nurses care for both males and females, they are not always held in high esteem. Thus, the males in her family may be very upset that the patient allowed a male to change her dressings, adding significantly to her stress.

53. A: These symptoms are typical of a stroke in the right hemisphere. A left hemispheric stroke results in right-sided paresis and visual field defect. Depression and impulsive behavior are commonly sequelae. Patients often have visio-spatial, math, and language difficulties that can include aphasia and difficulty with reading and writing. Patients may have short-term memory loss and difficulty learning new material. Brain stem stroke impairs cardiac and respiratory function and often results in death. Cerebellum strokes result in ataxia, nausea, vomiting, headaches, and dizziness or vertigo.

54. A: If the nurse is caring for an asthmatic patient receiving nebulizer therapy, caring for the patient and assessing the patient's condition cannot be delegated to nursing assistive personnel. However, the nurse can advise the nursing assistive personnel to report any observable changes in patient condition, such as a decrease in oxygen saturation, or any malfunctioning of the equipment. The assistant should also be advised to report any alarms sounding on the monitor.

55. A: Depressed respiratory rate, hypotension, and pinpoint pupils are signs of morphine overdose and should be treated with naloxone (Narcan®) intravenously, as it is an opiate antidote. Flumazenil is an antidote for benzodiazepines. Charcoal may be used for an oral overdose of morphine if little time has passed since ingestion but will not have an effect on morphine that was administered intravenously. N-acetylcysteine is the antidote for overdose of acetaminophen and will have no effect on a morphine overdose.

56. B: These symptoms are typical of metabolic alkalosis: Elevated serum pH, PCO_2 that is relatively normal (if compensated) or increased (if uncompensated), and a urine pH that is >6 (if compensated). The patient is dizzy, confused and is exhibiting tremors, seizures, tingling, tachycardia, arrhythmias. Metabolic alkalosis occurs with decreased strong acid or increased base, with compensatory CO_2 retention by the lungs associated with hypoventilation. Metabolic alkalosis is usually caused by excessive vomiting, gastric suctioning, diuretics, potassium deficit, excessive mineralocorticoids, and/or excessive $NaHCO_3$ intake.

57. C: While laziness, poor judgment, and inadequate supervision may all be factors, failing to provide reasonable care based upon usual and customary standards and expertise is an example of negligent conduct. Reasonable care uses rationale for decision-making in relation to providing care. Gross negligence is willfully providing inadequate care while disregarding the safety and security of another. Contributory negligence involves the injured party contributing to his or her own harm. Comparative negligence assigns a percentage amount of negligence to each individual involved. Malpractice is indicated when the negligent act caused damages to the patient.

58. B: The patient remains at high risk for suicide because of her choice of self-injury (knives and guns increase risk) and the fact that she has had previous suicide attempts. Additionally, the method used is more aggressive and less impulsive, and thus her intent may well have escalated. She also has little or no social support. The fact that the patient states she is no longer depressed is less important than the outward signs of depression, such as a flat affect, as patients are not always truthful when they are suicidal. Finally, the risk of suicide often increases when depression first begins to lift (as it induces greater emotional engagement and potentially a renewed impetus toward suicide). Consequently, this patient is at high risk for suicide and should be hospitalized.

59. D: The suction catheter should be inserted into the tracheostomy without suction, and then intermittent suction used only during withdrawal. The tracheostomy should be secured with ties about the neck. Regular suction of the tracheostomy is needed, especially initially, to remove secretions. The suction catheter should be 50% the size of the tracheostomy tube to allow ventilation during suctioning. Vacuum pressure is 80-100 mm Hg, and the catheter should only be inserted 0.5 cm beyond the tube to avoid tissue damage.

60. C: Posting exit routes from each area of the hospital is the responsibility of the Disaster-Preparedness Committee, which is charged with ensuring the institution can respond quickly and effectively to natural disasters, such as hurricanes or floods, and other disasters, such as terrorist attacks, fires, or pandemics. The Disaster-Preparedness Committee should establish phone trees for rapid contacts upon news of a disaster, and should ensure that fire suppressant equipment is readily available and in working order. This committee is not responsible for infection control issues.

61. D: Both the patient's verbal and nonverbal responses may be of equal importance. Patients may look away or become tense if they are not telling the truth or don't want to answer. Thus, information elicited during an interview should include not only the patient's factual responses but also attitudes and concerns. Nurses should ask open-ended information questions rather than yes/no questions, and should follow-up with clarifying questions. Providing a list of options and rephrasing a patient's statement may encourage the patient to provide more information.

62. A: Mentoring is providing professional guidance, as well as being someone to whom a staff person can bring questions or concerns. Role modeling takes place when one nurse serves as a role for others, such as demonstrating those behaviors and responses that advocate for the patient and show care. Supervising is ensuring that delegated tasks and duties are done correctly. Coaching involves providing staff with tools and ways to respond, or procedures to follow, to help staff become more effective.

63. D: Behavior modification and compliance rates are the best determinants of the effectiveness of patient education. Patients may be satisfied, may understand, and may be able to provide a demonstration, but if they don't utilize what they have learned the education has not been effective for that patient. Behavior modification involves thorough observation and measurement, identifying behavior that needs to be changed and then planning and instituting interventions. Compliance rates should be determined by observation at necessary intervals and on multiple occasions.

64. C: An autologous blood patch (15-20 mL) is injected epidurally near the subarachnoid puncture site to plug the puncture hole in the dura. Post-dural puncture headache (frontal and/or occipital) results from loss of cerebrospinal fluid through the puncture hole, resulting in displacement of the brain posteriorly and stress on supporting structures. Headache onset is usually 12 to 48 hours after the puncture, but may be delayed for weeks or months. Conservative treatment includes bed rest, fluid, and caffeine.

65. B: The right to pain control is part of the Patients' Bill of Rights. Affordable healthcare and access to latest medical technology are not included. The right to sue is not directly included, but patients are entitled to a procedure for registering complaints or grievances. Other provisions include respect for patient, informed consent, advance directives, and end of life care, privacy and confidentiality, protection from abuse and neglect, protection during research, appraisal of outcomes, appeal procedures, an organizational code of ethical behaviors, and procedures for donating and procuring organs/tissues.

66. C: If the nurse is conducting an in-home functional assessment to determine safety issues for a patient who has had a mild stroke and is alert and able to ambulate with a walker but has some residual weakness of the left side, the finding should be the priority concern is the fact that the house has hardwood floors with numerous throw rugs and clutter. Because the patient uses a walker to ambulate, obstructions on the floor markedly increase the risk that the patient will fall.

67. B: Failing to notify the crisis management team or appropriate authorities of the patient's suicidal statements is an act of negligent omission, because reasonable action was not taken to prevent this suicide. Giving the wrong dosage of antidepressant would be an act of negligent commission, as would documentation that the patient was attention-seeking (an incorrect subjective judgment) and moving the call bell out of patient's reach.

68. D: Gay and lesbian people are as vulnerable to domestic abuse as heterosexuals (many studies indicate greater abuse rates, up to 18 times higher), but this is often overlooked by healthcare providers. Partners who commit abuse often stay with the patient to ensure that the victim does not report the abuse, and abused males are particularly unlikely to report. The inconsistencies in this report are also cause for alarm. This patient has injuries consistent with domestic abuse:

- Facial and head injuries, including ruptured eardrum, suggests blows to the head.
- Bilateral injuries of both arms suggest defensive wounds.
- Bruising on the back suggests the patient was kicked while curled into a defensive posture.

69. C: Collaborating with the patient to find a solution to a problem is an example of effective therapeutic communication. The other responses are non-therapeutic and can serve to block effective communication. "Everyone gets upset at times" devalues the patient's feelings. "You should stop arguing with the nurses" is a negative, confrontational judgment that may anger the patient more and does not deal with the real issue. "You should be happy that the wound is healing" provides unwanted advice and ignores the patient's concerns.

70. A: The patient with meningioma was provided a list of possible treatment options, as required by the guidelines for informed consent. Fine needle aspiration is not the only option for diagnosis of breast cancer and has a high rate of false negatives. While gallbladder surgery is relatively safe, patients should be realistically appraised of the specific risks rather than being given blanket statements. A patient with 4th stage pancreatic cancer has a very low chance of survival even with treatment, and thus should be provided information about the risks and benefits of both having treatment and foregoing treatment.

71. B: The primary reason for completing continuing education courses is to remain current in the field of nursing. It is every nurse's responsibility to be informed and aware of advances and changes in practice. Many states require continuing education for licensure, and some institutions require continuing education as a condition for continued employment. Taking courses to meet requirements for a salary increase is a personal reason that does not obviate a nurse's professional responsibility for learning.

72. D: The best solution for this man's urge incontinence is to provide a urinal for him to use during the daytime, as he is aware of the need to urinate but is unable to make it to the bathroom in time. Leaving the man in his room would isolate him. Foley catheters are no longer recommended for long-term use to control incontinence because of the danger of infection. Adult diapers would not resolve the problem and would require frequent changing to prevent skin breakdown.

73. D: CDC adult recommendations for the hepatitis B vaccine include those with chronic liver disease and others at risk of hepatitis B infection, including those with human immunodeficiency virus infection and acquired immunodeficiency syndrome (HIV/AIDS), those with sexual exposure risk, injection drug users (current, recent), those with risk of exposure to blood, those who are incarcerated, those who travel to endemic areas, and those who are pregnant and at increased risk for hepatitis B. A two-dose vaccination series (Heplisav-B) or a three-dose vaccination series (Engerix-B, Recombivax HB, Twinrix) is available.

74. C: This type of neglect (malnutrition, no dentures, unkempt and dirty clothing) is probably an example of passive neglect. The patient's wife is also elderly and frail, and caring for an Alzheimer's patient is very difficult as he may be uncooperative. Active neglect is more intentional, and abuse (physical, financial, sexual, emotional) is more serious. The patient does not have injuries consistent with physical abuse and does not appear frightened of his wife (which might suggest physical or emotional abuse). Poverty may be an issue, but is probably not the cause of this neglect.

75. B: Prior to an MRI, a 65-year old woman with renal disease should have a creatinine test. Some institutions also require an eGFR. All current MRI contrast materials contain gadolinium, which has been implicated in the development of a fatal renal disorder in those with end-stage renal disease. For these patients, alternative imaging, such as CT, should be done. If this is not possible, then the patient may need dialysis after completion of the MRI to rapidly remove the gadolinium, which is normally excreted through the kidneys.

76. D: Multiple organ dysfunction syndrome (MODS) is the most common cause of sepsis-related death. It is a progression from an infection that results in bacteremia, septicemia, sepsis, severe sepsis, septic shock, and finally MODS as the infection overwhelms the body's defenses. Cardiac function becomes depressed. Acute respiratory distress syndrome may occur, with renal failure following acute tubular necrosis or cortical necrosis. Thrombocytopenia occurs in 30% of cases and may result in disseminated intravascular coagulation (DIC). Liver and bowel necrosis may also occur.

77. B: Restraints are defined as any physical or chemical means through which a patient is prevented from movement or the ability to access their own body. Hospital/Facility policy is to generally use the least restrictive measures, when possible, to protect the patient and staff. If all other measures have not sufficed and patient and/or staff safety is at risk, physical or chemical restraints may be deemed necessary and must be ordered by the physician. Orders include a duration of use in which the order must be renewed, and a frequency for assessing the patient with regards to the restraint (pressure injuries, constriction, etc.) Physical restraints include wrist or ankle strap restraints that attach each of the patient's extremities to the bed frame, 4 bed side rails in the up and locked position to prevent a patient from getting out of bed, mittens that are tethered to the bed frame, and vests that are tethered to the bed frame, amongst others. Chemical restraints include any drug used to sedate a patient for the purpose of restraint. Ketamine may be ordered as a chemical restraint for an aggressive patient, such as a patient that has overdosed, to keep both the patient and the staff safe. Wrist boards are a common measure to protect the integrity of an IV in the hand or wrist in confused/demented patients and in pediatric patients who may otherwise unawaringly remove an IV. They are also helpful in maintaining the patency of an IV that requires the wrist to remain in a specific position for maximal flow.

78. B: The learner outcome for teaching a patient about insulin reaction should relate directly to that goal: list and describe the symptoms of insulin reaction. While all of the other things (different types of insulin, foods high in carbohydrates, and the difference between Type 2 and Type 2 diabetes) are important, they don't relate to the topic and should not be the learner outcome for this activity. In some cases, one class or session may cover multiple topics with multiple outcomes, but a patient may be overwhelmed by too much information.

79. C: The legal document that designates someone to make decisions regarding medical and end-of-life care if a patient is mentally incompetent is a Durable Power of Attorney for Health Care. This is one type of advance directive, which can also include a living will, a medical power of attorney, and other specific requests of the patient regarding his or her health care. A do-not-resuscitate order is a physician-generated document that is completed when a patient does not want resuscitative treatment in an end-of-life situation. A general power of attorney allows a designated person to make decisions for a person over broader areas, including financial concerns.

80. A: Difficulty urinating, purulent discharge, epididymitis, and prostatitis are classic symptoms of gonorrhea in the male. Females are often asymptomatic but may have abdominal pain, cystitis, or mucopurulent cervicitis, which can lead to pelvic inflammatory disease and chronic pain if left untreated. Women and homosexual males may also present with rectal infections. Untreated gonorrhea may become a systemic infection with petechial or pustular skin lesions, arthralgias, fever, malaise, and septic arthritis. Treatment is with antibiotics, such as Cefixime 400 mg orally in one dose.

81. B: Risk management department often include medicolegal staff that address lawsuits against a health care organization. Risk management is also an organized and formal method of decreasing liability, financial loss, and risk of harm to patients, staff or others by completing an assessment of risk and introducing risk mitigation strategies. Duties of the risk management staff include:

- Risk identification
- Risk analysis
- Risk prevention
- Assessment/evaluation

82. D: As an advocate for the patient, the nurse must prevent possible injury to a patient: "The catheter was contaminated when it fell," states the problem. "Would you like me to get another setup or stay with the patient?" suggests a solution without assigning blame. A contaminated catheter could cause a serious infection. Reporting the team leader's behavior to the supervisor, while appropriate, does not protect the patient. Saying nothing may (but is not guaranteed to) protect either nurse from possible secondary repercussions (i.e., subsequent infection) but it is also negligent and unprofessional conduct.

83. C: Hemoglobin A1$_c$ of 5.5% most indicates dietary compliance. Hemoglobin AIC comprises hemoglobin A with a glucose molecule because hemoglobin holds onto excess blood glucose, so it shows the average blood glucose levels over a 3-month period and is used primarily to monitor long-term diabetic therapy: Normal value: <6% and elevation >7%. Fasting blood sugar (FBS) results can vary widely and show only a current serum level. Thus, a person who stays on a diet for only a few days and fasts before the test may show a near-normal FBS for a short period, even though the patient is frequently non-compliant. Normal FBS: 70-99 mg/dL.

84. B: Jung proposed the theory of individualism. He theorized that one's personality continued to develop over the lifespan. Personality comprises ego, personal unconsciousness, and collective unconsciousness. Personality can be introverted or extroverted, but a balance is necessary for emotional health. Jung theorized that during middle age, people begin to question their values, beliefs, and attainments. As they continue to age, they turn more inward. Successful aging is when people value themselves more than the concern they have for external things, losses, and physical limitations.

85. D: Genital warts, caused by the human papillomavirus (HPV), increase a woman's chance of developing cervical cancer because the virus induces changes in the cervical mucosa. There are about 40 different HPVs that are sexually transmitted. Over 99% of cervical cancer is caused by HPV and 70% is caused by HPVs 16 and 18. The HPV vaccine, Gardasil®, protects against HPVs 6, 11, 16, and 18, but does not convey protection if a female is already infected, so the initial dose is recommended between ages of 11-12 years.

86. C: The use of medical abbreviations is one of the leading causes of medication errors. While institutions usually have an approved list of abbreviations, sometimes these lists are overly extensive. In many cases abbreviations and symptoms should be avoided altogether, or at least restricted to a limited list. Illegible handwriting also leads to errors, so orders should be block-printed or computer generated. Institutions should establish protocols for medication administration, such as double identification of each patient, and should provide lists of similarly-named medications.

87. A: These are classic symptoms of stable angina. Unstable angina (pre-infarction), a medical emergency, is a progression of coronary artery disease. Pain may increase and last >5 minutes. Coronary artery spasm can cause angina pain and ischemia and is sometimes related to cocaine use. Variant (Prinzmetal's) angina is also related to coronary artery spasm but symptoms are more predictable. It is usually cyclical, occurring at rest and at the same time each day, and is characterized by elevation of ST segments. It may be associated with substance abuse.

88. A: Group instruction is more cost effective than one-on-one instruction because a number of patients/family can be served at one time. Group presentations are usually more rigidly scripted and scheduled for a particular time period, so family and patients have less control. Questions may be more limited, but group instruction also allows patients/families with similar concerns to interact. Group instruction is particularly useful for general types of instruction, such as managing diet or other lifestyle issues.

89. B: Inadequate or poor hand-washing technique is one of the most common causes of the person-to-person spread of infection in hospitals. Hands should be washed before and after every patient contact or when removing gloves. Hand-washing should be done under running water with plain soap, scrubbing the hands, nails, and wrists thoroughly, and turning the faucet off by using the elbow, upper arm, or paper towel. Alcohol-based rubs used for hand disinfection (at least 15 seconds) are effective against *Staphylococcus aureus* but are not effective against *Clostridium difficile*.

90. D: Pain Assessment in Advanced Dementia (PAINAD) scale utilizes careful observation of nonverbal behavior to evaluate pain, noting changes in:

- Respirations: Rapid, labored, with short periods of hyperventilation or Cheyne-stokes
- Vocalization: Negative or absent speech, moaning, and crying out as pain increases
- Facial expression: Sad, frightened, frowning, grimacing
- Body language: Tense, fidgeting, pacing, clenching fists, and lying in a fetal position as pain increases
- Consolability: Less easily distractible or consolable as pain increases

91. A: The Confusion Assessment Method is used to assess the development of delirium and is intended for use by those without psychiatric training. The assessment tool covers 9 factors:

- Onset: Acute changes in mental status
- Attention: Inattentive, stable, or fluctuating
- Thinking: Disorganized, rambling, switching topics, illogical
- Level of consciousness: Altered (ranging from alert to coma)
- Orientation: Time, place, person
- Memory: Impaired
- Perceptual disturbances: Hallucinations, illusions
- Psychomotor abnormalities: Agitations or retardation
- Sleep-wake cycle: Awake at night, sleepy in the daytime

92. D: Small tokens of appreciation, such as candy or flowers that can be shared among staff are usually acceptable as gifts from patients (depending on facility policy), but almost any other gifts (clothes, jewelry, watches, etc.) should be politely declined with an explanation: "I'm sorry. This is so kind of you, but nurses are not allowed to accept gifts from patients." Patients often offer gifts, and some patients, especially those who are older or cognitively impaired, may be easily manipulated into giving away valuables or money.

93. B: National guidelines recommend that adults exercise 30 minutes daily to a minimum of 150 minutes weekly with moderate intensity exercises (walking, bicycling, gardening) or 20 minutes of vigorous intensity exercises (running, aerobics, heavy physical work) to a minimum of 60 minutes a week. In addition, adults should engage in strengthening exercises (pushups, sit-ups, weight-lifting) at least twice weekly. Exercise sessions should be at least 10 minutes long to achieve health benefits.

94. A: A problem list focuses on a prioritized list of patient problems based on assessment data, history, and interview. Trying to deal with all patient problems without prioritizing them to determine which are the most critical can result in ineffective care. Patients are not always aware of their own needs regarding health care or intervention, and standardized lists of problems may be used as a guide but will not always match the individual's circumstances.

95. B: When administering the four-question CAGE substance abuse screening tool, answering "Yes" to at least two questions is clinically significant and indicates probable substance abuse. The CAGE tool was developed to assess alcohol abuse but is often modified to assess for drug abuse as well. Questions include (1) Have you ever felt you need to reduce drinking/drug use? (2) Have people annoyed you/criticized your drinking/drug use? (3) Have you felt bad/guilty about your drinking/drug use? (4) Have you ever had a drink or used drugs first thing in the morning to steady nerves/get rid of a hangover?

96. D: The best response regarding the use of herbal or alternative therapies is one that provides a reason. Many vitamins and herbal preparations are safe to use, but some interfere with medications or contain the same or similarly acting ingredients. Others, such as vitamin A, can more easily result in overdose. Some are cleared through the liver or kidneys, so a patient with liver or kidney failure may be at increased risk of harm. The ultimate decision remains with their doctor.

97. C: A nursing intervention that is an example of patient advocacy is the nurse assisting the patient to compile a list of questions to ask the physician. Patient advocacy involves assisting patients to communicate with physicians and other healthcare providers and assisting patients to receive the medical attention they need, such as by making appointments. Administration of treatments and notifying the physician of a change in condition are part of the routine duties of the nurse. Feeding a patient's cat (although kind) is a boundary violation.

98. A: Although biofeedback has been used as treatment for many different types of disorders, evidence to support its effectiveness is limited for most disorders. However, biofeedback has shown positive results with diabetic fecal incontinence, fibromyalgia, headaches (associated with tension/stress), and Raynaud's phenomenon. Biofeedback may also be effective for urinary incontinence that is relieved by strengthening the pelvic floor muscles because biofeedback helps to increase the patient's squeeze pressure.

99. A: The swing-to gait, in which the crutches are advanced together and the body swings to meet the crutches, is most appropriate for a patient with paralysis of the lower extremities. A swing-through gait swings the body past the crutches and requires better balance and coordination. A two-point gait (with the right crutch and left foot advancing together and vice versa) requires partial weight bearing on each foot. A three-point gait alternates between weight bearing on two crutches and an unaffected limb. A four-point gait requires weight bearing on both legs and moves each foot and crutch independently (i.e., left crutch and right foot, followed by right crutch and left foot, and so on).

100. A: Once an entry is made, it must be left in place and remain legible. The correct procedure is to draw a single line through the incorrect entry and write "Error" after the entry. It is never appropriate to whiteout an entry or otherwise render it illegible. Hand entries should always be made with blue or black permanent ink, and no erasable pen or pencil should be used for any documentation on a patient's permanent record. Recopying a page to omit an error is not acceptable.

101. D: The barriers to self-care that this patient faces after the stroke are psychological, physical, and cognitive:

- Psychological: She is very anxious, and this may interfere with her ability to manage her own care.
- Physical: The stroke has left her with motor impairment that may prevent her from carrying out necessary daily activities or procedures.
- Cognitive: This patient is forgetful, so she may require repeated instructions, prompts, and reminders to adequately manage her own care.

102. D: The Hmong culture is patriarchal and the eldest male makes the decisions. More traditional families may shun Western medicine and rely on healers, but Christian Hmong and others who are less traditional may rely on Western medicine or some combination. Hmong believe that illness occurs when the spirit, soul, and body are out of balance. They believe people have multiple souls and sickness occurs when one or more soul is lost or taken by other spirits. These souls must be reclaimed by a healer for healing to occur.

103. B: Guided imagery uses mental visualization (mental imagery) to reduce anxiety and promote healing. It may incorporate relaxation techniques as well. Patients often use audiotapes but additional techniques include:

- Getting into a comfortable position and concentrating on breathing slowly.
- Closing the eyes and concentrating on an image while engaging as many image-related senses as possible (i.e., color, sound, smell, feel, etc.).
- Bringing the mind back to the image if it wanders and ending with a positive image.

104. B: Threatening to force a patient to undergo a treatment is a form of coercion. Nurses can easily intimidate patients into having procedures or treatments they don't want. Regardless of age, patients have the right to choose and refuse treatment. Forcing a patient to do something against his or her will borders on abuse and can sometimes degenerate into actual abuse if physical coercion is involved. If patients are cognitively impaired, other family members may be designated to make decisions, but every effort should be made to gain cooperation.

105. A: The best approach to solving a problem that involves 3 different departments is to form an interdisciplinary team of representative participants to work together and find a solution. This allows all parties to have a voice and to work toward compromise, while avoiding the confusion caused by too many competing interests. If administration makes a decision independently, or picks one of the proposed solutions over another, all or many staff members may feel their voices weren't heard. Trying to gather all members of 3 departments together for brainstorming is usually impractical, and an unnecessary use of employee time and resources.

106. B: Making referrals to the appropriate social services agencies is the appropriate response. Older patients often have many needs, but buying groceries is a sign of overinvestment in a patient's life, will not solve the problem in the long run; it can also establish a relationship of dependency. Calling the daughter or discussing the matter with a neighbor would be a violation of the patient's right to privacy and should be done only with patient's permission.

107. B: The patient has been told to avoid crossing the affected leg over the other leg since this position could dislocate the implant. Although there is no reason to flex the knee on the affected leg more than 90 degrees, doing so would not adversely impact the hip joint. An abduction pillow should be used between the legs while the patient is in bed or turned on the side. Ninety-degree flexion of the affected hip should be avoided in both the sitting and lying position. The patient should be cautioned to avoid bending over to pull on shoes or socks. The toilet seat should be raised, and chairs should have cushions or platforms to raise the seats.

108. A: While acupuncture is sometimes used for a variety of disorders, in the United States it is most commonly used for the treatment of pain. NIH studies indicate acupuncture is effective for treating nausea and vomiting related to surgery or chemotherapy. Acupuncturists insert small gauge needles into "acupoints," usually leaving them in place for 20-40 minutes. Electrical stimulation or moxibustion (burning moxa herb on the end of the needle) to heat the needles may be used to increase circulation.

109. D: Dysphagia may develop as the result of stroke, neuromuscular disease (Parkinson's disease, myasthenia gravis, MS, ALS), drugs (phenothiazines), achalasia, and esophageal strictures, diverticulum, or cancer. Dysphagia is a common cause of aspiration pneumonia. A diagnosis is made through presenting symptoms, barium swallow testing, and endoscopy. Management includes treating the underlying cause, sitting upright to eat, avoiding eating prior to lying down, chewing foods carefully, sipping water, thickening thin liquids, limiting bite sizes (in part by using smaller utensils), doing strengthening exercises, and taking medications to relax the esophagus.

110. A: The best readability level is grade 6. The average American reads effectively at the 6th to 8th grade level (regardless of education achieved), and research shows that even people with much higher reading skills learn medical and health information most effectively when the material is presented at the 6th to 8th grade readability level. A grade 3 level would be too simplified for most native speakers of English, but might be appropriate for immigrant populations with limited English.

111. D: Piaget's stages of cognitive development relate to changes in cognitive abilities related to age and development, and the "formal operational" stage is characterized by logical thinking and the use of abstraction:

- Sensorimotor (0-2): Infants learn about cause and effect and the permanence of objects.
- Preoperational (2-7): Thinking is concrete and tangible at the preconceptual stage, and later becomes intuitive. These children are egocentric.

- Concrete operational (7-11): Children develop the concept of conservation and reasoning becomes inductive.
- Formal operational (11-15): Adolescents develop the ability to use abstract thought and to develop and test hypotheses.

112. B: If a supervisor has a laissez-faire leadership style and exerts little direct control but allows staff members to make decisions with little interference or guidance, the likely result is that little is accomplished. This type of leadership is generally only effective if staff members are highly skilled and motivated and use their own initiative to plan and work together, but more often the staff members are rudderless and avoid innovation or efforts at performance improvement.

113. A: The nurse should make no assumptions about a patient who, on the initial assessment, fails to make direct eye contact with the nurse. Although body language can provide clues about a patient's emotional state (fear, respect, dishonesty, social anxiety), these observations can be easily misconstrued and are difficult to interpret without a deeper understanding of the patient. Making an assumption may lead to a bias that colors the evaluation of the patient.

114. D: Spiral (helical) CT provides a definitive diagnosis for pulmonary embolism. Blood gases provide supporting information (hypoxemia, hypocarbia, and respiratory alkalosis). A chest x-ray may be used to rule out other disorders, but is not adequate for a definitive diagnosis as an x-ray may indicate a false negative. Electrocardiogram may show typical cardiac abnormalities (tachycardia) but it is not sufficient for diagnosis. Angiography also provides a definitive diagnosis, but is more invasive and is associated with more complications.

115. B: This patient is at risk for hypertension (resulting from a change in cardiac output, peripheral resistance, or both) for a variety of reasons:

- Obesity results in hyperinsulinism that increases peripheral resistance through structural hypertrophy.
- Genetic abnormalities may increase peripheral resistance.
- Stress triggers over activity of the sympathetic nervous system, increasing contractibility and/or renin-angiotensin excess, resulting in increased constriction and resistance.
- Insufficient nephrons result in sodium retention and decreased filtration, causing increased fluid volume and preload.

116. D: Many hearing-impaired patients use some degree of lip-reading, so the nurse should not chew, smoke, or eat while speaking to the patient. The nurse should face the patient at a distance of 2 to 6 feet, use a normal tone of voice and short sentences, and provide assistive devices as necessary, including writing materials and a telecommunications device for the deaf (TDD) phone/relay service. If patients are deaf and know sign language, interpreters should be used for important communication, and the nurse should face the patient during the communication, not the interpreter.

117. A: The nurse should attend to the spiritual needs of the patient by calling a priest even though the hour is not convenient. A Protestant chaplain cannot perform specific rituals that are important to Catholics, and the patient may not survive or be able to receive communion if the call is delayed. Catholic rituals include:

- Sacrament of the Anointing of the Sick: This replaces the last rites (Extreme Unction) and is a bedside blessing.
- Viaticum: This is essentially the "last" Holy Communion and is called the "food for the journey."

118. D: While procedures vary somewhat, generally the nurse should document the medication given on the patient's record as well as the time the physician was notified and any medical orders to prevent or treat adverse effects, but specifically indicate that it was an actual error on the incident report only. Patients are not informed of an error by the nurse involved and, in many cases, are never informed at all. This is an ethical issue that has legal and moral implications. Some healthcare facilities are now utilizing an open policy in which patients are informed, but more often this is not the case.

119. B: Selye's biological theory of stress and aging states that stress is the body's response to demands requiring positive or negative adaptation, characterized by the "generalized adaptation syndrome," which includes 3 stages:

1. Alarm: Fight or flight response.
2. Resistance: The body mobilizes to resist a threat, focusing on those organs most involved in an adaptive response.
3. Exhaustion: As the body is weakened and overwhelmed, organs/systems begin to deteriorate (hypertrophy/atrophy) and can no longer cope with stress, resulting in stress-related illnesses and eventual death.

120. A: There is no evidence that one type of music is more effective than another when used for music therapy. Patients should be encouraged to pick music that pleases them. There is no need for previous musical ability even if patients actively participate, as in drumming to relieve tension. Music therapy is often used passively (listening) to promote relaxation, to motivate patients to exercise, and to relieve pain.

121. B: Contraindications to thrombolytic therapy include hemorrhagic stroke, recent surgery, or bleeding. While, ideally, thrombolytic therapy should be administered within 90 minutes of the onset of symptoms, it may be given within 6 hours. History of any type of stroke within 2 months, AVM, or aneurysm precludes thrombolytic therapy. Severe hypertension (>210/130) that is uncontrolled by medications or that occurs with retinal-vascular disease is also a contraindication. Relative contraindications, such as >75 years of age, pregnancy, pericarditis, and endocarditis, should be evaluated on individual basis.

122. C: The nurse should announce his presence in a normal tone of voice, explaining actions and movements. Visual impairment is unrelated to hearing or intelligence, so speaking loudly or using simple sentences is not necessary. If the central field of vision is impaired, the patient may have better peripheral vision, so the nurse should ask the patient which position is best, and then position himself to the patient's advantage. Braille materials, enlarged text, or manipulatives may also be helpful.

123. B: Peripheral arterial insufficiency is characterized by deep, circular painful necrotic ulcers on the toe tips, toe webs, or other pressure areas, intermittent to constant pain, rubor on dependency and pallor on foot elevation, shiny, pale, skin with loss of hair, thick and ridged nails, weak or absent pulses, and minimal edema. Peripheral venous insufficiency is characterized by irregular superficial ulcers on the lateral malleolus and sometimes on anterior tibial area, aching and cramping pain, pulses present, brownish discoloration about the ankles and anterior tibial area, and moderate to severe edema.

124. B: Tier II, airborne precaution, is appropriate for a patient with active tuberculosis, measles, or varicella. The patient is placed in a private room with negative airflow and a closed door. Staff must use respiratory precautions (masks). Tier II, droplet precautions (private room and masks if within 3 feet of the patient) is used with viral influenza, pertussis, *Neisseria meningitidis*, streptococcal pharyngitis or pneumonia and mumps. Tier II, contact precautions (private room or cohorting and a protective gown for close contact) is used for infections spread by person-to-person contact. Tier I, standard precautions (protection from blood and body fluids), is used for all patients.

125. D: "Synthroid 0.88 mg PO daily at 0700" is correct because the medication is spelled out, the decimal has a leading zero, "PO" is clearly written, and "daily" is used instead of "qd," which can be misinterpreted as "QID" if the nurse uses periods (i.e., "q.d."). Additionally, a 24-hour (military) time designation is used. "Maalox 30 cc" should be "Maalox 30 mL" because "cc" may be misread as "U" for "unit." Instead of "qhs," which can be misread as "qhr," "nightly" should be used. "Lasix 40.0 mg" should be "Lasix 40 mg" because the trailing zero may cause someone to read the order as "400 mg." "MS" could be misread as "magnesium sulfate."

126. A: The nurse should establish educational goals before beginning to develop materials and lesson plans. This is important because all objectives should be directed specifically at the educational goals and expected learner outcomes. Planning should always precede production, or the nurse can waste considerable time preparing materials and lesson plans that are not effective, or that wander off of the topic and confuse the learners. As each educational goal is identified, the nurse should then plan how to specifically achieve that particular goal through the educational process.

127. A: Aphasia is the loss of ability to use and/or understand written or spoken because of damage to speech centers in the brain. Global aphasia is characterized by difficulty understanding and producing language, although patients may still understand gestures, pictures, and diagrams. Transient aphasia is short lasting, often related to transient ischemic episodes. Broca's aphasia (also known as "expressive aphasia") is characterized by difficulty producing verbal (and, usually, written) language, even though the ability to understand others remains intact. Wernicke's aphasia (also known as "receptive aphasia") is characterized by difficulty understanding (i.e., receiving) verbal (and, usually, written) language even while retaining the ability to understand gestures and produce language. Global aphasia is when Broca's and Wernicke's aphasias are combined.

128. B: Sinus tachycardia is characterized by pulse >100. The rapid pulse rate decreases diastolic filling time and reduces cardiac output. The result is hypotension and pulmonary edema. Bradycardia is characterized by pulse <60. Sinus arrhythmia is characterized by cyclic changes in pulse during respirations, and is common in children and young adults. However, it may also occur with vagal stimulation from suctioning, vomiting, or defecating. Premature atrial contractions are essentially extra beats caused by an errant electrical impulse to the atrium before the sinus node impulse, resulting in an irregular pulse.

129. D: Dietary management of diabetes mellitus, medical nutrition therapy (MNT), includes individualized diet modifications. Typically, the type of food consumed is more important than the calories themselves, and a normal protein intake is recommended. Diets may be low fat and low carbohydrate. Saturated fats should be restricted to <7% of total calories and carbohydrates monitored through the use of carbohydrate counting or exchanges. Sugar alcohols and non-nutritive sweeteners (aspartame, Splenda®) may be used. Alcohol intake should be limited to 1 drink daily for females and 2 for males.

130. A: The life course theory of aging is a sociological model that views aging as a lifelong process of social, psychological, and biological changes. The process of change begins in infancy and continues through older adulthood, and is viewed within cultural, economic, social, and historic contexts. Key concepts include:

- The social and historical contexts and environmental location
- Individual, generational, and historical time
- Degrees of heterogeneity or variability
- Social connections
- Personal agency and control, and control cycles
- The past as related to future

131. B: Because the Parkinson's patient with dysarthria has difficulty speaking, the nurse should ask primarily yes/no rather than open-ended information questions (e.g., who, what, when, where, how, why) and should observe the patient's facial expressions and gestures used in "augmentative and alternative communication" (AAC). The patient has no dementia or hearing impairment, so age-appropriate sentences and normal tone of voice should be used. The nurse should not rush the patient, finish sentences, or direct questions at family rather than the patient. Assistive materials (such as computer programs) may be used.

132. C: When determining outcomes, nominal data provide the lowest form of measurement. This may include asking a patient to describe pain by choosing among a number of descriptive words, such as "dull" and "sharp." Even if numbers are assigned to the descriptions, the numbers don't represent an established mathematical difference among the descriptions. The next highest type of data is ordinal followed by interval and ratio-level data (the most reliable in terms of statistics).

133. A: Interdisciplinary teams with 4-10 members are most effective. Very small teams (2-4) may not be sufficiently representative. Large teams are difficult to lead and keep focused. Team members should have complementary skills and should be allowed a reasonable degree of autonomy in producing action plans. They should also have flexibility in working together. Team members are collectively accountable, rather than individually accountable.

134. B: Alcohol intake should be limited to no more than 3 drinks daily. A daily multivitamin should not affect warfarin, but some herbal medications can affect clotting time. Milk products should not affect warfarin, but foods that are high in vitamin K may affect the medication and should be limited and eaten in consistent amounts. These include broccoli, green leafy vegetables (kale, turnip greens, beet greens), cauliflower, and legumes as well as soybean and canola oil.

135. A: The interpreter should have training in medical vocabulary for both languages. Just speaking the languages well does not mean that the translator will adequately interpret specialized vocabulary. It is not necessary for the interpreter to know the patient's history, as the interpreter's job is only to interpret what is said, not add to it or augment it based on prior knowledge. While onsite interpreters are ideal, interpretation can be provided through a speakerphone at a distance.

136. C: The patient is suffering from severe malnutrition, based on these laboratory findings. Value ranges and interpretations include:

- Albumin: Normal 3.5 to 5.5 g/dL. Severe deficiency <2.5 g/dL. Albumin is more sensitive to long-term protein deficiencies than short term.
- Pre-albumin: Normal 16 to 40 mg/dL. Severe deficiency <5 mg/dL. Pre-albumin responds quickly to changes in nutritional status related to protein intake.
- Transferrin: Normal 200 to 400 mg/dL. Severe deficiency <100 mg/dL. Transferrin levels decrease rapidly with protein deficiency but may be affected by many different things, such as liver disease and iron deficiency.

137. D: Urinary casts may be composed of red blood cells, white blood cells, or renal cells. To perform a test for casts, the patient provides a midstream clean-catch urine specimen. RBC casts indicate bleeding into the renal tubule, commonly seen in glomerular diseases such as lupus nephritis, IgA nephropathy, and Wegener's granulomatosis. With renal tubular damage, renal tubular epithelial cell casts are present in the urine. Neither UTIs nor interstitial nephritis is associated with RBC casts.

138. C: The autoimmunity theory states that aging is programmed by cell mutations that occur with aging, creating new proteins. The body mounts an autoimmune defense against these new proteins by producing antibodies, but the antibodies fail to recognize the new cells, allowing them to multiply. Eventually, both B-cell and T-cell function decline, preventing the body from combating invaders such as bacteria, and foreign cells such as malignant cells. Failure of the immune system may lead to diseases related to older age, such as cancer, diabetes, and emphysema.

139. A: Both infection from the IV catheter and glucose intolerance are common side effects of total parenteral nutrition (TPN). A re-feeding syndrome, which can be fatal, can be triggered by an excessive carbohydrate load in malnourished patients. Vitamin and essential fatty acid deficiencies may occur, so nutrition must be monitored carefully. Enteral feeding poses the risk of irritation from NG, ND, or NJ tubes, and skin excoriation from gastrostomy and jejunostomy tubes. The risk for aspiration is high with nasal tubes. Nausea, vomiting, and diarrhea may also occur, especially if the infusion rate is excessive.

140. C: A patient who is HIV positive converts to a diagnosis of AIDS when the CD4 counts falls to ≤200 cells/mm³. CD4 is a protein that is found on immune cells, including T cells, so when the level falls, this is an indication that the immune system is impaired and the person is at risk for opportunistic diseases. The two tests essential for monitoring HIV/AIDS are the CD4 count and the viral load. Generally, as the CD4 count falls, the viral load increases.

141. B: Reacting and responding to facts instead of feelings to avoid confrontations and diffuse anger. Professional communication skills to facilitate team communication also include:

- Avoiding interpreting others statements, interrupting, giving unsolicited advice, or jumping to conclusions—all of which may interfere with the free flow of ideas
- Listening actively and asking questions for clarification rather than challenging other people's ideas
- Clarifying information or opinions to help avoid misunderstandings
- Communicating openly and respecting others' opinions

142. C: These symptoms are typical of obstructive sleep apnea. Diagnosis is per polysomnography and evaluation of O_2 saturation during sleep. ECG may indicate bradydysrhythmia during apnea and tachydysrhythmia during respiration. Erythrocytosis is common. Narcolepsy is characterized by brief sudden episodes of falling asleep, loss of muscle tone, and sleep paralysis. Insomnia has milder symptoms. Patients complain of inadequate sleep or waking up and being unable to go back to sleep. Hypothyroidism can cause similar symptoms to obstructive sleep apnea and should be ruled out with thyroid function tests.

143. D: According to Meredith Belbin's team role theory, the action-oriented role of an interdisciplinary team member who is charismatic and dynamic, challenges others to improve performance, and has the ability to find the best solution to problems is that of shaper. Belbin describes three types of team roles: action focused (shaper, completer-finisher, and implementer), thought focused (plant, monitor-evaluator, and specialist), and people focused (team worker, coordinator, and resource investigator).

144. A: The nurse should call the mental health crisis team. Crisis teams are comprised of mental health professionals. The teams are usually available to non-psychiatric units in order to evaluate the mental status of a patient. In this case, the patient is probably experiencing an exacerbation of her bipolar disease because of the stress related to surgery and could irreparably damage her surgical repair. The crisis team will determine whether the patient is a danger to herself or others, identify any treatment necessary to stabilize the mania the patient appears to be experiencing, and will decide whether she should remain hospitalized for further treatment.

145. D: Varenicline use must be carefully monitored as it can cause mood or behavioral changes, seizures, psychiatric manifestations, and suicidal thoughts. Varenicline is one of the most lethal drugs in terms of injury and death associated with a drug. Other prescription medications include nicotine inhalers, nicotine nasal sprays, and bupropion (Zyban®). Bupropion can cause insomnia and dry mouth. OTC smoking cessation medications include nicotine gum, the nicotine patch, and nicotine lozenges. These can cause local irritation, primarily.

146. A: The patient's refusal to look at the amputation stump or participate in his own care suggests he is having trouble coping with the change in body image. Phantom pain is common after an amputation. Grief at the loss of a limb and some lability in emotions is normal. The other driver is a logical target for anger. Rehabilitation plans may easily become overwhelming for someone who is still coming to terms with new limitations, so crying is probably a normal response.

147. B: While evaluation is a separate phase of the nursing process, it does not take place chronologically. Evaluation is critical, so evaluation and re-evaluation should be done at all phases:

- Assessment: Collecting data, history, and completing a physical exam
- Diagnosis: Analyzing data, determining needs and problems, and applying a nursing diagnosis
- Planning: Setting priorities, setting goals and expected outcomes, and planning interventions and strategies of care

- Implementation: Applying interventions/treatments
- Evaluation: Reassessing and auditing

148. C: Actively spreading cancer, systemic infection, and positive HIV status/AIDS are absolute contraindications for organ donation, but age (young or old) is not in itself a contraindication, as the organs will be examined for suitability. Cancer in and of itself may not be an absolute contraindication; for example, primary brain cancer that has not spread beyond the brainstem is not a contraindication for donation. A history of alcoholism does not necessarily exclude a donor, depending upon the extent of alcohol abuse and any physical damage related to alcohol use.

149. A: If a patient is to receive total parenteral nutrition, the vascular access device that is recommended is a PICC line. Peripheral lines, such as midline peripheral VAD and short peripheral VAD, are typically not used for periods longer than 1 to 2 weeks because of the increased risk of thrombophlebitis. PICC lines are often used for intravenous access when treatments will continue for 4 weeks or longer. Implantable ports are used for longer term intravenous access, such as for months of chemotherapy.

150. C: If the nurse is carrying out wound care and notes granulation tissue about the periphery of the wound, this indicates the proliferation phase of healing. There are four phases to healing:

1. Hemostasis: Begins immediately; platelets are activated and clots form.
2. Inflammation: Days 1 to days 4–6; erythema and edema are present, phagocytosis begins, and macrophages replace white blood cells.
3. Proliferation: Days 5–20; granulation tissue appears and epithelialization occurs.
4. Maturation: Days 21+; remodeling occurs and scarring reduces.

Medical-Surgical Nurse Practice Test #2

To take this additional Medical-Surgical Nurse practice test, visit our bonus page:
mometrix.com/bonus948/medsurgnurse

How to Overcome Test Anxiety

Just the thought of taking a test is enough to make most people a little nervous. A test is an important event that can have a long-term impact on your future, so it's important to take it seriously and it's natural to feel anxious about performing well. But just because anxiety is normal, that doesn't mean that it's helpful in test taking, or that you should simply accept it as part of your life. Anxiety can have a variety of effects. These effects can be mild, like making you feel slightly nervous, or severe, like blocking your ability to focus or remember even a simple detail.

If you experience test anxiety—whether severe or mild—it's important to know how to beat it. To discover this, first you need to understand what causes test anxiety.

Causes of Test Anxiety

While we often think of anxiety as an uncontrollable emotional state, it can actually be caused by simple, practical things. One of the most common causes of test anxiety is that a person does not feel adequately prepared for their test. This feeling can be the result of many different issues such as poor study habits or lack of organization, but the most common culprit is time management. Starting to study too late, failing to organize your study time to cover all of the material, or being distracted while you study will mean that you're not well prepared for the test. This may lead to cramming the night before, which will cause you to be physically and mentally exhausted for the test. Poor time management also contributes to feelings of stress, fear, and hopelessness as you realize you are not well prepared but don't know what to do about it.

Other times, test anxiety is not related to your preparation for the test but comes from unresolved fear. This may be a past failure on a test, or poor performance on tests in general. It may come from comparing yourself to others who seem to be performing better or from the stress of living up to expectations. Anxiety may be driven by fears of the future—how failure on this test would affect your educational and career goals. These fears are often completely irrational, but they can still negatively impact your test performance.

> **Review Video: 3 Reasons You Have Test Anxiety**
> Visit mometrix.com/academy and enter code: 428468

Elements of Test Anxiety

As mentioned earlier, test anxiety is considered to be an emotional state, but it has physical and mental components as well. Sometimes you may not even realize that you are suffering from test anxiety until you notice the physical symptoms. These can include trembling hands, rapid heartbeat, sweating, nausea, and tense muscles. Extreme anxiety may lead to fainting or vomiting. Obviously, any of these symptoms can have a negative impact on testing. It is important to recognize them as soon as they begin to occur so that you can address the problem before it damages your performance.

> **Review Video: 3 Ways to Tell You Have Test Anxiety**
> Visit mometrix.com/academy and enter code: 927847

The mental components of test anxiety include trouble focusing and inability to remember learned information. During a test, your mind is on high alert, which can help you recall information and stay focused for an extended period of time. However, anxiety interferes with your mind's natural processes, causing you to blank out, even on the questions you know well. The strain of testing during anxiety makes it difficult to stay focused, especially on a test that may take several hours. Extreme anxiety can take a huge mental toll, making it difficult not only to recall test information but even to understand the test questions or pull your thoughts together.

> **Review Video: How Test Anxiety Affects Memory**
> Visit mometrix.com/academy and enter code: 609003

Effects of Test Anxiety

Test anxiety is like a disease—if left untreated, it will get progressively worse. Anxiety leads to poor performance, and this reinforces the feelings of fear and failure, which in turn lead to poor performances on subsequent tests. It can grow from a mild nervousness to a crippling condition. If allowed to progress, test anxiety can have a big impact on your schooling, and consequently on your future.

Test anxiety can spread to other parts of your life. Anxiety on tests can become anxiety in any stressful situation, and blanking on a test can turn into panicking in a job situation. But fortunately, you don't have to let anxiety rule your testing and determine your grades. There are a number of relatively simple steps you can take to move past anxiety and function normally on a test and in the rest of life.

> **Review Video: How Test Anxiety Impacts Your Grades**
> Visit mometrix.com/academy and enter code: 939819

Physical Steps for Beating Test Anxiety

While test anxiety is a serious problem, the good news is that it can be overcome. It doesn't have to control your ability to think and remember information. While it may take time, you can begin taking steps today to beat anxiety.

Just as your first hint that you may be struggling with anxiety comes from the physical symptoms, the first step to treating it is also physical. Rest is crucial for having a clear, strong mind. If you are tired, it is much easier to give in to anxiety. But if you establish good sleep habits, your body and mind will be ready to perform optimally, without the strain of exhaustion. Additionally, sleeping well helps you to retain information better, so you're more likely to recall the answers when you see the test questions.

Getting good sleep means more than going to bed on time. It's important to allow your brain time to relax. Take study breaks from time to time so it doesn't get overworked, and don't study right before bed. Take time to rest your mind before trying to rest your body, or you may find it difficult to fall asleep.

> **Review Video: <u>The Importance of Sleep for Your Brain</u>**
> Visit mometrix.com/academy and enter code: 319338

Along with sleep, other aspects of physical health are important in preparing for a test. Good nutrition is vital for good brain function. Sugary foods and drinks may give a burst of energy but this burst is followed by a crash, both physically and emotionally. Instead, fuel your body with protein and vitamin-rich foods.

Also, drink plenty of water. Dehydration can lead to headaches and exhaustion, especially if your brain is already under stress from the rigors of the test. Particularly if your test is a long one, drink water during the breaks. And if possible, take an energy-boosting snack to eat between sections.

> **Review Video: <u>How Diet Can Affect your Mood</u>**
> Visit mometrix.com/academy and enter code: 624317

Along with sleep and diet, a third important part of physical health is exercise. Maintaining a steady workout schedule is helpful, but even taking 5-minute study breaks to walk can help get your blood pumping faster and clear your head. Exercise also releases endorphins, which contribute to a positive feeling and can help combat test anxiety.

When you nurture your physical health, you are also contributing to your mental health. If your body is healthy, your mind is much more likely to be healthy as well. So take time to rest, nourish your body with healthy food and water, and get moving as much as possible. Taking these physical steps will make you stronger and more able to take the mental steps necessary to overcome test anxiety.

Mental Steps for Beating Test Anxiety

Working on the mental side of test anxiety can be more challenging, but as with the physical side, there are clear steps you can take to overcome it. As mentioned earlier, test anxiety often stems from lack of preparation, so the obvious solution is to prepare for the test. Effective studying may be the most important weapon you have for beating test anxiety, but you can and should employ several other mental tools to combat fear.

First, boost your confidence by reminding yourself of past success—tests or projects that you aced. If you're putting as much effort into preparing for this test as you did for those, there's no reason you should expect to fail here. Work hard to prepare; then trust your preparation.

Second, surround yourself with encouraging people. It can be helpful to find a study group, but be sure that the people you're around will encourage a positive attitude. If you spend time with others who are anxious or cynical, this will only contribute to your own anxiety. Look for others who are motivated to study hard from a desire to succeed, not from a fear of failure.

Third, reward yourself. A test is physically and mentally tiring, even without anxiety, and it can be helpful to have something to look forward to. Plan an activity following the test, regardless of the outcome, such as going to a movie or getting ice cream.

When you are taking the test, if you find yourself beginning to feel anxious, remind yourself that you know the material. Visualize successfully completing the test. Then take a few deep, relaxing breaths and return to it. Work through the questions carefully but with confidence, knowing that you are capable of succeeding.

Developing a healthy mental approach to test taking will also aid in other areas of life. Test anxiety affects more than just the actual test—it can be damaging to your mental health and even contribute to depression. It's important to beat test anxiety before it becomes a problem for more than testing.

Review Video: <u>Test Anxiety and Depression</u>
Visit mometrix.com/academy and enter code: 904704

Study Strategy

Being prepared for the test is necessary to combat anxiety, but what does being prepared look like? You may study for hours on end and still not feel prepared. What you need is a strategy for test prep. The next few pages outline our recommended steps to help you plan out and conquer the challenge of preparation.

STEP 1: SCOPE OUT THE TEST

Learn everything you can about the format (multiple choice, essay, etc.) and what will be on the test. Gather any study materials, course outlines, or sample exams that may be available. Not only will this help you to prepare, but knowing what to expect can help to alleviate test anxiety.

STEP 2: MAP OUT THE MATERIAL

Look through the textbook or study guide and make note of how many chapters or sections it has. Then divide these over the time you have. For example, if a book has 15 chapters and you have five days to study, you need to cover three chapters each day. Even better, if you have the time, leave an extra day at the end for overall review after you have gone through the material in depth.

If time is limited, you may need to prioritize the material. Look through it and make note of which sections you think you already have a good grasp on, and which need review. While you are studying, skim quickly through the familiar sections and take more time on the challenging parts. Write out your plan so you don't get lost as you go. Having a written plan also helps you feel more in control of the study, so anxiety is less likely to arise from feeling overwhelmed at the amount to cover.

STEP 3: GATHER YOUR TOOLS

Decide what study method works best for you. Do you prefer to highlight in the book as you study and then go back over the highlighted portions? Or do you type out notes of the important information? Or is it helpful to make flashcards that you can carry with you? Assemble the pens, index cards, highlighters, post-it notes, and any other materials you may need so you won't be distracted by getting up to find things while you study.

If you're having a hard time retaining the information or organizing your notes, experiment with different methods. For example, try color-coding by subject with colored pens, highlighters, or post-it notes. If you learn better by hearing, try recording yourself reading your notes so you can listen while in the car, working out, or simply sitting at your desk. Ask a friend to quiz you from your flashcards, or try teaching someone the material to solidify it in your mind.

STEP 4: CREATE YOUR ENVIRONMENT

It's important to avoid distractions while you study. This includes both the obvious distractions like visitors and the subtle distractions like an uncomfortable chair (or a too-comfortable couch that makes you want to fall asleep). Set up the best study environment possible: good lighting and a comfortable work area. If background music helps you focus, you may want to turn it on, but otherwise keep the room quiet. If you are using a computer to take notes, be sure you don't have any other windows open, especially applications like social media, games, or anything else that could distract you. Silence your phone and turn off notifications. Be sure to keep water close by so you stay hydrated while you study (but avoid unhealthy drinks and snacks).

Also, take into account the best time of day to study. Are you freshest first thing in the morning? Try to set aside some time then to work through the material. Is your mind clearer in the afternoon or evening? Schedule your study session then. Another method is to study at the same time of day that you will take the test, so that your brain gets used to working on the material at that time and will be ready to focus at test time.

STEP 5: STUDY!

Once you have done all the study preparation, it's time to settle into the actual studying. Sit down, take a few moments to settle your mind so you can focus, and begin to follow your study plan. Don't give in to distractions or let yourself procrastinate. This is your time to prepare so you'll be ready to fearlessly approach the test. Make the most of the time and stay focused.

Of course, you don't want to burn out. If you study too long you may find that you're not retaining the information very well. Take regular study breaks. For example, taking five minutes out of every hour to walk briskly, breathing deeply and swinging your arms, can help your mind stay fresh.

As you get to the end of each chapter or section, it's a good idea to do a quick review. Remind yourself of what you learned and work on any difficult parts. When you feel that you've mastered the material, move on to the next part. At the end of your study session, briefly skim through your notes again.

But while review is helpful, cramming last minute is NOT. If at all possible, work ahead so that you won't need to fit all your study into the last day. Cramming overloads your brain with more information than it can process and retain, and your tired mind may struggle to recall even previously learned information when it is overwhelmed with last-minute study. Also, the urgent nature of cramming and the stress placed on your brain contribute to anxiety. You'll be more likely to go to the test feeling unprepared and having trouble thinking clearly.

So don't cram, and don't stay up late before the test, even just to review your notes at a leisurely pace. Your brain needs rest more than it needs to go over the information again. In fact, plan to finish your studies by noon or early afternoon the day before the test. Give your brain the rest of the day to relax or focus on other things, and get a good night's sleep. Then you will be fresh for the test and better able to recall what you've studied.

STEP 6: TAKE A PRACTICE TEST

Many courses offer sample tests, either online or in the study materials. This is an excellent resource to check whether you have mastered the material, as well as to prepare for the test format and environment.

Check the test format ahead of time: the number of questions, the type (multiple choice, free response, etc.), and the time limit. Then create a plan for working through them. For example, if you have 30 minutes to take a 60-question test, your limit is 30 seconds per question. Spend less time on the questions you know well so that you can take more time on the difficult ones.

If you have time to take several practice tests, take the first one open book, with no time limit. Work through the questions at your own pace and make sure you fully understand them. Gradually work up to taking a test under test conditions: sit at a desk with all study materials put away and set a timer. Pace yourself to make sure you finish the test with time to spare and go back to check your answers if you have time.

After each test, check your answers. On the questions you missed, be sure you understand why you missed them. Did you misread the question (tests can use tricky wording)? Did you forget the information? Or was it something you hadn't learned? Go back and study any shaky areas that the practice tests reveal.

Taking these tests not only helps with your grade, but also aids in combating test anxiety. If you're already used to the test conditions, you're less likely to worry about it, and working through tests until you're scoring well gives you a confidence boost. Go through the practice tests until you feel comfortable, and then you can go into the test knowing that you're ready for it.

Test Tips

On test day, you should be confident, knowing that you've prepared well and are ready to answer the questions. But aside from preparation, there are several test day strategies you can employ to maximize your performance.

First, as stated before, get a good night's sleep the night before the test (and for several nights before that, if possible). Go into the test with a fresh, alert mind rather than staying up late to study.

Try not to change too much about your normal routine on the day of the test. It's important to eat a nutritious breakfast, but if you normally don't eat breakfast at all, consider eating just a protein bar. If you're a coffee drinker, go ahead and have your normal coffee. Just make sure you time it so that the caffeine doesn't wear off right in the middle of your test. Avoid sugary beverages, and drink enough water to stay hydrated but not so much that you need a restroom break 10 minutes into the test. If your test isn't first thing in the morning, consider going for a walk or doing a light workout before the test to get your blood flowing.

Allow yourself enough time to get ready, and leave for the test with plenty of time to spare so you won't have the anxiety of scrambling to arrive in time. Another reason to be early is to select a good seat. It's helpful to sit away from doors and windows, which can be distracting. Find a good seat, get out your supplies, and settle your mind before the test begins.

When the test begins, start by going over the instructions carefully, even if you already know what to expect. Make sure you avoid any careless mistakes by following the directions.

Then begin working through the questions, pacing yourself as you've practiced. If you're not sure on an answer, don't spend too much time on it, and don't let it shake your confidence. Either skip it and come back later, or eliminate as many wrong answers as possible and guess among the remaining ones. Don't dwell on these questions as you continue—put them out of your mind and focus on what lies ahead.

Be sure to read all of the answer choices, even if you're sure the first one is the right answer. Sometimes you'll find a better one if you keep reading. But don't second-guess yourself if you do immediately know the answer. Your gut instinct is usually right. Don't let test anxiety rob you of the information you know.

If you have time at the end of the test (and if the test format allows), go back and review your answers. Be cautious about changing any, since your first instinct tends to be correct, but make sure you didn't misread any of the questions or accidentally mark the wrong answer choice. Look over any you skipped and make an educated guess.

At the end, leave the test feeling confident. You've done your best, so don't waste time worrying about your performance or wishing you could change anything. Instead, celebrate the successful completion of this test. And finally, use this test to learn how to deal with anxiety even better next time.

> **Review Video: 5 Tips to Beat Test Anxiety**
> Visit mometrix.com/academy and enter code: 570656

Important Qualification

Not all anxiety is created equal. If your test anxiety is causing major issues in your life beyond the classroom or testing center, or if you are experiencing troubling physical symptoms related to your anxiety, it may be a sign of a serious physiological or psychological condition. If this sounds like your situation, we strongly encourage you to seek professional help.

Thank You

We at Mometrix would like to extend our heartfelt thanks to you, our friend and patron, for allowing us to play a part in your journey. It is a privilege to serve people from all walks of life who are unified in their commitment to building the best future they can for themselves.

The preparation you devote to these important testing milestones may be the most valuable educational opportunity you have for making a real difference in your life. We encourage you to put your heart into it—that feeling of succeeding, overcoming, and yes, conquering will be well worth the hours you've invested.

We want to hear your story, your struggles and your successes, and if you see any opportunities for us to improve our materials so we can help others even more effectively in the future, please share that with us as well. **The team at Mometrix would be absolutely thrilled to hear from you!** So please, send us an email (support@mometrix.com) and let's stay in touch.

> **If you'd like some additional help, check out these other resources we offer for your exam: http://MometrixFlashcards.com/MedicalSurgical**

Additional Bonus Material

Due to our efforts to try to keep this book to a manageable length, we've created a link that will give you access to all of your additional bonus material:

mometrix.com/bonus948/medsurgnurse